The People's Health

Recent Titles in
Contributions in Medical Studies

Cancer Factories: America's Tragic Quest for Uranium Self-Sufficiency
Howard Ball

The AIDS Pandemic: Social Perspectives
Howard Ball

Childbed Fever: A Scientific Biography of Ignaz Semmelweis
K. Codell Carter and Barbara R. Carter

James Cook and the Conquest of Scurvy
Francis E. Cuppage

Romance, Poetry, and Surgical Sleep: Literature Influences Medicine
E. M. Papper

Sex, Disease, and Society
Milton Lewis, Scott Bamber, and M. Waugh, editors

Histories of Sexually Transmitted Diseases and HIV/AIDS in Sub-Saharan Africa
Philip W. Setel, Milton Lewis, and Maryinez Lyons, editors

The History of Modern Epilepsy: The Beginning, 1865–1914
Walter J. Friedlander

The Legend of Nietzsche's Syphilis
Richard Schain

Drama and Discovery: The Story of Histoplasmosis
Thomas M. Daniel and Gerald L. Baum

Dis-ease in the Colonial State: Medicine, Society, and Social Change Among the AbaNyole of Western Kenya
Osaak A. Olumwullah

The People's Health

Public Health in Australia, 1950 to the Present

Milton J. Lewis

Contributions in Medical Studies, Number 49, Volume 2

PRAEGER

Westport, Connecticut
London

Library of Congress Cataloging-in-Publication Data

Lewis, Milton James.
The people's health : public health in Australia, 1950 to the present / Milton J. Lewis.
p. cm.—(Contributions in medical studies, ISSN 0886–8220 ; no. 49, volume 2)
Includes bibliographical references and index.
ISBN 0–313–32045–4 (alk. paper)
1. Public health—Australia—History. 2. Medical care—Australia—History.
3. Medicine—Australia—History. I. Title. II. Series.
RA553.L495 2003
362.1′0994—dc21 2001054099

British Library Cataloguing in Publication Data is available.

Library of Congress Catalog Card Number: 2001054099
ISBN: 0–313–31090–4 (Vol. 1)
0–313–32045–4 (Vol. 2)
0–313–32595–2 (Set)
ISSN: 0886–8220

First published in 2003

Praeger Publishers, 88 Post Road West, Westport, CT 06881
An imprint of Greenwood Publishing Group, Inc.
www.praeger.com

Printed in the United States of America

The paper used in this book complies with the Permanent Paper Standard issued by the National Information Standards Organization (Z39.48–1984).

10 9 8 7 6 5 4 3 2 1

Contents

Tables

Acknowledgments

A research grant from the National Health and Medical Research Council enabled me to research and write this history of public health in Australia from 1950 to 2000. For this I am most grateful. Many people have provided invaluable assistance during the course of the project: members of the Commonwealth Department of Health and Aged Care, Canberra; the staff of the Burkitt-Ford, the Medical, and the Fisher Library at the University of Sydney, of the Library of the Commonwealth Department of Health and Aged Care, of the National Library of Australia, and of the Noel Butlin Archives Centre at the Australian National University; and the many individuals from politics, health bureaucracies, academia, and other backgrounds from around the country with whom I discussed the development of public health in Australia. Finally, I want to thank Charles Kerr, emeritus professor of preventive and social medicine, University of Sydney, for reading critically the early draft of this study.

Introduction

What George Rosen saw as the biosocial nature of human beings requires that some area of social activity be devoted to the protection of the public's health. All societies have to arrange ways of dealing with such collective health matters as an adequate supply of quality water and food, cleaning of the physical environment, and control of communicable disease. What ways are pursued will depend, on the one hand, on how the causes of health and disease are understood, and on the other, on the social, economic, political, and cultural (including religious and ideological beliefs) context. In the most general terms, then, the history of public health is the record of the various ways in which the community has acted to deal with inescapable health problems that arise from the biosocial being of humans. These ways have changed with changing knowledge and changes in the social context in which that knowledge has been located.[1]

Modern public health evolved in Western Europe between about the sixteenth and the twentieth centuries, and it came to maturity in the last 150 to two hundred years. Unprecedented economic growth, industrialization and urbanization in a capitalist economic mode created the need for it, as well as the financial and material resources with which to construct it. The history of European settlement in Australia, from its inception in 1788, fits almost exactly into this period of maturation of modern public health in Europe; there was little or no time lag between the development of public health knowledge, practices and institutions in Australia and the development in the heartland of modern public health.

HEALTH IN THE PREMODERN ERA

Personal and environmental health were pursued in the classical world for both spiritual-cum-religious and material reasons. Conscious pursuit of personal health was the preserve of the well-to-do elite. Collective sanitary practises were pursued by the members of the governing classes for reasons of personal comfort and social prestige, and as part of the demonstration of their status as representatives of a civilized lifestyle. Salaried physicians had been employed by Greek communities to serve all citizens as early as the fourth century B.C., and Roman cities in the imperial era also employed public physicians. The Greek conception of philanthropy did not specifically focus on the poor; it embraced all members of the *polis,* all citizens. Early imperial Rome likewise did not make special collective provision for the sick poor. This classical "egalitarianism" contrasts with the tradition of obligatory good works for the poor arising from the religious beliefs of ancient Egypt and Israel. Developing out of this same religion-based concern for care of the disadvantaged came the Judeo-Christian focus on good works, and the Christian obligation to relieve the suffering of the indigent sick. True, the humanitarianism of Stoic philosophy helped engender a new sense of aristocratic obligation to the poor in the Roman imperial era. This translated sometimes into material gifts to support needy citizens. But Stoicism and other contemporary philosophical systems taught indifference to physical suffering, and special concern did not extend to the sick poor. Moreover, the fact of slavery's association with manual labor generally degraded the laboring free poor in the eyes of the leisured elite. Thus, the *valetudinaria,* the hostels or "hospitals" for treatment of sick slaves or sick soldiers, did not serve the needs of the free poor. The work of slaves and soldiers was vital to the economic and defence needs of the empire; both groups lacked the kinship networks that traditionally cared for sick and disabled Romans.[2]

By the 340s the Christian Church in Antioch was operating *xenodocheia,* or *xenones*, hostels to house the poor. Monasteries also cared for the poor and sick. One of the earliest figures to offer specifically medical care in these hospices was Aeteus, a Syrian physician. There was, however, no clear distinction between a *xenon,* a hostel, and a *nosokomeion,* a house for the sick. By the fifth and sixth centuries, towns in the Eastern Empire commonly had at least one hospital. The first *xenon* in the Latin West was founded in Rome by Fabiola in about 397. She had been inspired by Eastern examples. The first in Gaul was established after A.D. 500. The end of the empire in the West saw the infirmaries of monasteries carry on the care of the sick, and monastic medicine flourished from the fifth century to the tenth century. Larger hospitals in the 800s declined for lack of public revenue, consequent on the decline of Charlemagne's Holy Roman Empire. In the East some hospitals grew quite large. By A.D. 600, hospitals of six hundred beds existed in Antioch and Constantinople. From the ninth century, large specialized hospitals were established in the great cities of the Islamic world, like Baghdad and Cairo. With Christianity integral to the process of state formation in Western Europe after the fall of Rome, collective institutional provision for the sick poor became an established feature of Western society.[3]

Some ancient civilizations performed substantial public health engineering feats concerning drainage or conveyance of clean water to cities. But these works were undertaken for reasons of ritual cleanliness and for aesthetic rather than hygienic reasons. The ruins of Kohun (2100–1700 B.C.) and Tel-el-Amarna (1400 B.C.) in Egypt reveal that masonry gutters drained water from streets. The Cretan-Mycenean culture used conduits to supply water to cities. The palace at Knossos (2000 B.C.) had baths and flushing toilets. Half a world away, the Indus Valley cities of Harappa, Mohenjo-daro and Lothal (3000–1500 B.C.) possessed public water tanks, probably for communal bathing to purify ritually the inhabitants. Paved streets were drained by covered sewers. India's first great empire, the Mauryan State, was established in the fourth century B.C. Megasthenes, a Seleucid ambassador to the court of Chandragupta Maurya, noted public health practices carried out by committees of physicians, including concern with the statistics of births and deaths and with antenatal care.[4]

The bureaucratic feudalism of ancient China lent itself to preventive practices, and prevention was as highly valued in Chinese medicine as in statecraft and administration. *The Yellow Emperor's Treatise on Internal Medicine* (produced mainly in the early Han period, the second to first centuries B.C.) states, "The sage does not cure the sick only when they are such but he prevents the illness arising. In the same way he does not put right upheavals in the body politic, he prevents them from ever taking place."[5] The imperial court of the Chou dynasty (the middle of the first millennium B.C.) employed an "imperial dietitian" as well as an "imperial physician." The Confucian Analects (about 500 B.C.) forbade the consumption of damaged food. The practice of eating food cooked at high temperature (preventing the spread of food-borne infection) began about this time, and water to be consumed was always boiled. In the imperial capital, vermin exterminators were employed, rotting corpses of humans and animals were routinely removed from public areas, and streets were regularly swept. In the Chin and Han periods, some cities obtained water from a distance through bamboo, sometimes earthenware, conduits. The growth of Buddhist abbeys with bathing facilities from the second century reinforced existing bathing customs arising from Taoist purification ceremonies. In the Sung era, public bathhouses multiplied, and from the eleventh century commercial bathhouses became more common.

From ancient times, bamboo implements and water were employed to clean the body after defecation. Following the invention of paper about A.D. 100, improved lavatory hygiene spread more widely. Systematic removal of night soil each morning from cities dates from early times. As in Rome and other strongly hierarchical societies, those at the bottom of Chinese society were more exposed to environmental hazards. Helminth and other fecally transmitted infections were occupational dangers for peasants, who used human waste as crop fertilizer.[6]

Greek cities added water drawn from external sources—Athens obtained water from surrounding hills as early as the sixth century B.C.—to that obtained from wells and rainwater cisterns. But the Romans's public health engineering was unsurpassed in the ancient world. For Romans, clean water was part of everyday life and was not particularly connected with public or private health. Frontinus, water commissioner from A.D. 97, reported in *The Aquaducts of Rome* that the censor, Crassus, built the first aqueduct in 312 B.C. Nine aqueducts operated by Frontinus's time. Millions of gallons a day supplied public fountains and baths, but a private supply required imperial approval. Other cities throughout the empire were supplied by aqueducts. By the early imperial era, a board administered the water supply, and *aediles* supervised public baths, street cleaning and maintenance and the food markets, although how diligently is unclear.

The Roman sewerage system dated from republican times. In the time of Constantine, public latrines numbered as many as 150. But social inequality made for maldistribution of the benefits of public health engineering. The poor in the upper levels of Rome's slums still emptied chamber pots into the streets. Severe crowding and homelessness characterized slum life. Drainage in individual homes was often unconnected to public drains and sewers, as the ruins of Pompeii attest. Latrines did not have running water. Cesspits could contain dead bodies of the poor, carcasses of animals, sewage and garbage. It is worth remembering that for Romans, Greeks and other ethnic groups of the imperial world, average life expectancy was only twenty-five years.[7]

In Greco-Roman medicine, hygiene sought to preserve the health of the individual, by modification of lifestyle and of environmental factors. Classical hygiene did not seek to promote the health of the whole community. The ideal (male) citizen of the Greek *polis* was someone of cultivated mind possessing a physically fit and aesthetically pleasing body. Athletics brought fitness, and special instruction developed in bathing, massage, gymnastics, exercise and diet. The personal hygienic regimen recommended by Greco-Roman physicians was possible only for members of a leisured class, people whose lifestyles were supported by the labor of slaves.

The Hippocratic and Galenic texts on hygiene remained the source of ideas about individual health until at least the sixteenth century. They still influenced Western medicine in the nineteenth century, when the meaning of hygiene narrowed to equate with cleanliness but its focus widened from the individual to the group or population. The longevity of classical hygiene arose from various factors: because classical knowledge persisted due to the authority of the written text, the absorption of classical learning into medieval Christian culture, and the revival of interest in classical texts in the Renaissance; because the way of life of pre-industrial societies up to about the eighteenth century was not radically different from that of the ancient Greeks; and because before the development of scientific chemistry and bacteriology, the individual continued to have to rely on his or her own senses to assess the healthiness of air, food, and water.[8]

The Middle Ages and the Renaissance saw the promotion of the ideas of classical hygiene through the medium of new texts, the most famous of which was the thirteenth-century *Regimen Sanitatis Salernitanum,* attributed to the medical school of Salerno in Italy. The *Regimen,* like the illustrated handbooks on health, discussed Galen's "six non-naturals," or the categories of hygiene (air; food and drink; sleep and working; movement and rest; retention and evacuation; and the emotions) as well as therapeutics. Intended for the upper and "middle" classes, books on hygienic regimen were popular. In 1486–1604, they represented 115 of 392 editions published on medicine in English. Only when the state required the norms of hygiene to be observed by the whole population—a requirement expressed in nineteenth-century public health legislation (although it is foreshadowed in plague-control measures and intermittent use of quarantine from the fourteenth century)—was the transition to the focus on the group completed. The transition demanded not only the advent of new technologies (like cast-iron pipes) and state legislative and administrative action but a large-scale cultural transformation in hygienic habits. From the eighteenth century, the habit of personal cleanliness became more and more widely accepted. As a matter of routine, people washed their bodies and clothes, and in various other ways followed hygienic practices.[9]

FORERUNNERS OF MODERN PUBLIC HEALTH

In the aftermath of the fall of Rome, cities and trade gave way to a largely rural way of life. However, by the fourteenth century, cities of a hundred to 150,000 people were flourishing in Europe. Influenced by their reading of Roman legal texts, the governing elites of Italian cities reestablished the Greco-Roman office of public physician in the twelfth and thirteenth centuries. They also reestablished Roman public facilities like fountains, baths, and sewers, and the practice of regulating refuse disposal and food markets. Indeed, it was not until the creation of boards of public health in the fourteenth century that Italian cities moved beyond the classical world in public sanitation, although in medieval Europe both the church and the state organized care for lepers in residential hospitals.

Plague ravaged Europe in the fourteenth century. The republican city-states, Florence and Venice, introduced the innovation of lay health committees during epidemic crises. These oversaw the cleansing of the environment, kept public order, and implemented emergency legislation. A number of Italian city-states had established permanent health boards by the beginning of the sixteenth century; the boards now also attended to the regular sanitary supervision of their cities. Physicians acted usually only as advisers, and lay members of the governing classes continued to dominate the boards. The boards developed into significant arms of government in Italy and other parts of the Mediterranean region. They regularly gathered information about the health status of foreign states, in the light of which health magistracies could take strong action like imposing quarantine and destroying incoming goods (thought to convey contagion) in an effort to halt the ingress of epidemic disease. Quarantine was another city-state invention. In 1377 Ragusa, a Venetian colony, first imposed a suspension of trade and travel (then only thirty days, but later forty) to prevent incursion of plague. Originally, this was a passive procedure—"a cordon sanitaire"—but it subsequently came to involve action to isolate active cases of infection. Infected cases were collected in a *lazaretto,* or pesthouse. In the beginning a way of caring for the sick poor, from the mid-fifteenth century it was part of the system of isolating the infected from the healthy citizen.

The sanitary approach inherited from Rome reflected one explanation of disease—that polluted air (or exhalations) adversely changed the healthy "humoral" balance in humans and animals. Another explanation—that disease was spread by contact with diseased persons or with infected intermediate inanimate objects (contagion)—was, except in relation to lepers, not widely accepted among educated people in the classical or medieval periods. It became better established in the early modern period, as the growth of quarantine and isolation practices after the 1450s indicates. The human and material costs of plague in the late sixteenth and seventeenth century Mediterranean were huge. The damage wrought, together with the transfer of the center of trade and economic activity north of the Alps and the rise of strong monarchical states in northern Europe, meant that the future of public health development lay in France, Britain and Germany.[10] From Britain, modern public health spread later to British settlements, like the American and Australian colonies.

The northern European countries that pioneered modern public health did not simply reproduce the permanent public health magistracies of the Italian city-state type, although they did from time to time use such Italian epidemic-control measures as quarantine and temporary health boards. Seventeenth- and eighteenth-century ideological movements influenced in fundamental ways the evolving conception of public health. Mercantilism taught that to maximize national power and wealth the state had to "grow" a healthy and numerous population. The health of the people as a whole became a key objective of the state. Enlightenment rationalists would apply rational organization and collective responsibility to the prevention of disease, as they would apply them to other areas of human affairs. Good health for all became a matter of establishing rational social and political institutions and providing rational education for the individual.

Industrialization and urbanization under unregulated industrial-capitalist conditions in the early nineteenth century and the continuing threat of serious epidemic disease heightened the urgency of finding new mechanisms to protect the health of the laboring population, the living and working conditions of whom were degraded. Too many workers were falling, because of ill health, into unproductive penury and dependence on their parishes. Sanitation in Britain promised not only to advance the health of all the people but in doing so to relieve the financial burden on the propertied classes of supporting those in the lower classes reduced to poverty by sickness. Later in the nineteenth century, "neomercantilist" ideas of a numerous and healthy population as a vital resource in the growing economic and military "struggle for survival" among Western nation-states and empires came to influence public health strongly. At the same time, the rise to political power of the labor movement, and the more collectivist orientation of fin-de-siècle liberalism in a context of increasing democratization of the state, began to give rise to the conception of health as a right of citizenship rather than as a state resource, although the latter view remained alive at least up to the mid-twentieth century.

The severe international economic depression of the 1930s, the inhumanity of the totalitarian Fascist regimes, the destructiveness of World War II, and the postwar economic and political problems of many former colonies and Third World countries all promoted consciousness of human rights, including the right to health. The Universal Declaration of Human Rights (1948) included a right to a standard of living adequate for health. Notions of social justice and equity in postwar decades replaced, or at least overlaid, instrumentalist, healthy-population-as-productive-resource justifications for public health. Good health for all people (and peoples) as a matter of social justice was most fully recognized in formal terms at the international level in the 1970s, when the World Health Organization of the United Nations adopted its strategy of "Health for All by the Year 2000." In the 1980s, official acceptance of the WHO strategy by Australia reinforced, at least in principle, an emerging national commitment to better health for the whole population as an issue of social justice.

ORGANIZATION OF THIS VOLUME

A number of themes are addressed in this history of public health in Australia from the beginning of European settlement in 1788 to about 1950.

One important theme is the interaction between the internal history of ideas and practices in public health and medicine, and the changing social, political, economic and cultural context. A second theme concerns the institutional, professional and ideological relations between public health and clinical medicine—between disease prevention and health promotion addressed to the population as a whole, on the one hand, and treatment, rehabilitation and palliation directed to the individual, on the other.

Public health may refer to the professional knowledge and practices, social institutions, and public policy devoted to the advancement of the collective health. It may also refer to the actual state of health of the people—that is, the health status of the population as a whole. The health status of the Australian people has improved markedly over the last 150 years, the period in which modern public health was transplanted to, and matured in, that country. The reasons for this long-term improvement constitute the third theme.

A fourth theme involves the setting of the Australian history in international perspective. To this end much comparative material, especially from the British and American experiences, is presented. No other countries have had greater cultural influence on Australia than these two. Their influence has been substantial as well in the specific culture of public health and medicine. Britain, as the "mother country" and center of the empire and Commonwealth, was the key external reference point and examplar for Australia from 1788 to at least World War II. The United States increasingly assumed that position in the next fifty years. However, even in the early twentieth century, America had direct influence on the development of public health in Australia. A prime example is the critical role that the Rockefeller Foundation played in the establishment of the Federal Health Department in 1920. Moreover, because of the shared cultural, political, social and economic heritage of the three English-speaking countries, there are interesting, and perhaps instructive, similarities and differences between the history of public health here in Australia, in Britain and in the United States.

This volume ends chronologically at about 1950. A second volume will cover the period from 1950 to 2000. There is a certain unity to public health in the period from the nineteenth to the mid-twentieth century. First, the pattern of diseases with which public health dealt remained the same over most of this period. Infections bulked large as causes of mortality and morbidity. Only late in the period did chronic, "degenerative" disorders like cardiovascular disease and cancer begin to replace communicable illnesses as the main causes of death and disability. Even then, it took some years for public health experts and policy to "retool" in order to deal with the new epidemiological situation. Second, an instrumental approach to public health, as mentioned earlier, largely prevailed in those years. In the mid-nineteenth century spending on sanitary measures was thought worthwhile to reduce the cost of supporting the lower-class casualties of the diseases allegedly spread by filth in the environment. Later, it was considered worthwhile to spend on public health to produce a healthy and numerous population as a vital economic and military resource in a world of increasing international competition.

In the period after about 1950 as well, public health has a certain unity. The epidemiology fundamentally changed. The "diseases of affluence" have dominated the health agenda. By their nature they have called for different responses from public health. Health education and health promotion, persuading and working with people—not legislated mandatory action, the threat of legal sanction, or attempted control of behavior—are seen to be the way forward. The diseases themselves have required a more democratic, cooperative approach from professionals and the state alike, an approach that engaged, not forced, community compliance. At the same time, the extensive spread of democratic and "egalitarian" values fueled a quest for social justice and equity in health, a quest that had been initiated by the labor movement and social reformers in the earlier period. The difference in this post-1950 period is that the desire for social justice becomes a more central force of public health development.

Chapter 1 looks at the emergence of modern public health as a socially organized effort to protect the health of the whole population. This emergence took place in Western Europe between the sixteenth and the nineteenth centuries. As suggested earlier, its development depended on progress in understanding the nature and causes of disease, and on a conducive political, economic and social environment. Prominent in this environment were the rise of the strong, modern state; urbanization and industrialization in a capitalist mode; mercantilist ideas of population as a state resource; and Enlightenment-based faith in the educability of a rational humankind. These general forces were mediated by national cultures and political systems so that public health development followed particular national paths.

Chapter 2 discusses the transportation of European infections to Australia and their devastating impact on the Aboriginal tribes of Terra Australis. The Australian Aboriginal experience is compared with that of other indigenous peoples in the Americas and Oceania. The growth of public health measures in early colonial Australia is outlined against the backdrop of contemporary European public health, especially with respect to quarantine and smallpox vaccination.

Rapid urbanization and the growth of an industrial base in Australia in the second half of the nineteenth century resulted in serious deterioration in the quality of the urban environment and in public health problems similar to those of much older European cities. Chapter 3 discusses the transfer of the "sanitary idea" from Britain to the Australian colonies. The creation of classical public health administrations here, as in Britain and the United States, was spurred by the threat of epidemic. The role of public health measures in the decline of mortality in the United Kingdom, the United States and Australia is assessed. The advent of the first wave of public health professionals—the beginning of professionalization of public health—is recounted.

Chapter 4 focuses on an important turning point in public health development around the beginning of the twentieth century. In Australia, as in other parts of the Western world, public health began to expand into provision of personal services for social groups like mothers and babies. The organized medical profession ensured that the growth of such public services did not threaten the viability of private practice. "National efficiency" (as part of a "neomercantilist" climate) was a buzzword across the Western world at this time. This was a significant motive for the growth of state support for infant, maternal, and school health services. These new departures in public health in the United Kingdom and the United States, as well as in Australia, are outlined.

J.H.L. Cumpston, the first Commonwealth Director General of Health and the outstanding figure in Australian public health in the first half of the twentieth century, set out in the interwar years to construct a truly national public health system. This and other aspects of the interwar history of public health are discussed in chapter 5. Cumpston and his professional allies believed, reasonably enough, that more health gain was to be had at this time from prevention than from treatment. As in the United States, the federal division of powers between the center and states made it very difficult for the national health authorities to act effectively without the full cooperation of the states. In 1930, just before the economic depression severely restricted funds, the Commonwealth, at Cumpston's urging, established a national school of public health at the University of Sydney to train public health professionals and to carry out research. In the following decade, the first mass immunization projects began with campaigns against diphtheria. Mass campaigns to control tuberculosis and poliomyelitis were to be pursued successfully two decades later.

The Labor Party began in the early twentieth century to feel its way toward the idea of equal access to health care as a right of citizenship. The period of 1941–49, which is covered in chapter 6, was marked by fierce debate about the merits of the federal Labor government's plans for a tax-funded national health scheme. But it was Cumpston and other public health doctors who formulated the first detailed plan for a national health scheme integrating preventive and curative services. The plan called for a national salaried service, a concept opposed by the organized medical profession. After constitutional challenges and a bitter, protracted struggle between the Labor government and the medical community, the government finally enacted legislation establishing a national health service. This service supported fee-for-service practice. Still, the profession feared the government, even as part paymaster, and it rejected the scheme. Labor left office in late 1949.

By about 1950, in Australia, as in Britain and the United States, curative medicine's star was rising. It took credit for the "defeat" of infectious diseases—when, in fact, well before it became effective, public health had been contributing significantly to the long-term decline in mortality from infection. Chapter 7, the last chapter, discusses this and other matters relating to the state of the health system in the middle years of the twentieth century.

Even in Britain, where the collective provision of health services was taken farther than in Australia or the United States, the new National Health Service was overwhelmingly focused on clinical services for the individual. However, changing disease and demographic patterns in the 1950s were bringing to the fore in affluent Western countries chronic "degenerative" conditions for which no cures existed. Government and health professionals became interested again in the behavioral and social causes of disease. The rocketing costs of technologically driven curative medicine reinforced interest in less costly preventive, public health measures. These and other issues relating to the period between 1950 and 2000 will be discussed at length in the second volume of this history of public health, *The People's Health: Public Health in Australia, 1950 to the Present.*

LIMITS TO THE SCOPE OF THIS HISTORY

The history of occupational health and safety in Australia, while closely connected with the history of public health, is not systematically discussed in this history of public health. So extensive and important a subject should be treated at length in a monograph of its own. Similarly, the history of psychiatric services, while touched upon, is by no means exhaustively discussed. Those interested in the latter might want to consult Milton Lewis, *Managing Madness: Psychiatry and Society in Australia, 1788–1980* (1988).

NOTES

1. G. Rosen, *From Medical Police to Social Medicine: Essays on the History of Health Care* (New York: Science History Publications, 1974), 176.

2. G.B. Risse, *Mending Bodies, Saving Souls: A History of Hospitals* (New York: Oxford University Press, 1999), 44–56; A.G. Carmichael, "History of Public Health and Sanitation in the West before 1700," in *The Cambridge World History of Human Disease*, ed. K.F. Kiple (Cambridge: Cambridge University Press, 1993), 195.

3. G.B. Risse, *Mending Bodies, Saving Souls: A History of Hospitals* (New York: Oxford University Press, 1999), 81–95; D. Porter, *Health, Civilization and the State: A History of Public Health from Ancient to Modern Times* (London: Routledge, 1999), 22–23.

4. G. Rosen, *A History of Public Health* (Baltimore: Johns Hopkins University Press, 1993), 1–3; S.C. Seal, "A Short History of Public Health in India," *Indian Journal of History of Medicine* 16 (1971), 26–28; R. Porter, *The Greatest Benefit to Mankind: A Medical History of Humanity from Antiquity to the Present* (London: HarperCollins, 1997), 84–85, 136–38.

5. Quoted in J. Needham and Lu Gwei-Djen, "Hygiene and Preventive Medicine in Ancient China," *Journal of History of Medicine and Allied Sciences* 17 (1962), 433.

6. J. Needham and Lu Gwei-Djen, "Hygiene and Preventive Medicine in Ancient China," *Journal of History of Medicine and Allied Sciences* 17 (1962), 435–38, 449–57, 463–67; I. Polunin, "Disease, Morbidity, and Mortality in China, India, and the Arab World," in *Asian Medical Systems: A Comparative Study,* ed. C. Leslie (Berkeley: University of California Press, 1976), 126–27.

7. Rosen, *A History of Public Health,* 14–25; A.G. Carmichael, "History of Public Health and Sanitation in the West before 1700," 193–94.

8. A. Wear, "The History of Personal Hygiene," in *Companion Encyclopedia of the History of Medicine,* Vol. 2, eds. W.F. Bynum and R. Porter (London: Routledge, 1993), 1283–90; Rosen, *A History of Public Health,* 6–13; Porter, *The Greatest Benefit to Mankind,* 84–85, 136–38.

9. Wear, "The History of Personal Hygiene," 1297, 1304–5.

10. A.G. Carmichael, "History of Public Health and Sanitation in the West before 1700," 196–99.

Chapter 1

Toward a Social Conception of Health

INTRODUCTION

The People's Health: Public Health in Australia, 1788–1950, the companion volume to this study, discusses the history of public health in Australia from 1788 to about 1950. This volume covers the period 1950 to 2000. As in the earlier volume, much comparative material drawn from the United Kingdom and the United States is introduced in the present work, because no other countries have had greater influence on the development of public health and medicine in Australia. One notable difference between the earlier and later periods is in the background ideology that shapes public health, and this difference reflects changes in larger social and political values. From the late nineteenth to the mid-twentieth century, as noted in *The People's Health*, volume 1, an ideology of "national efficiency" and "race fitness" significantly influenced public health, while the doctor as authoritative expert dominated the practice of the discipline. Public health was, as it were, "done to" a passive citizenry, with the ultimate aim of producing a fit people, able to advance the economic power and defensive capacity of the nation. But the more egalitarian, democratic and participatory values of the last four decades or so have shifted the ideological emphasis toward social justice and a public health that, ideally at least, is practiced in active partnership with citizens, and in which persuasion and participation figure more prominently than legal coercion. Public health is now "done" in cooperation with an informed and involved citizenry. However, it should be noted that as discussed in volume 1, the Labor Party in pursuit of social justice had been haltingly elaborating since the 1900s the idea of health as a right of democratic citizenship, even if for a long time it saw the right in terms of access to clinical services. The idea of the citizen's democratic right to health goes back still farther, being articulated by the National Constituent Assembly and the National Convention in Revolutionary France in the 1790s. Moreover, at the international level, the Universal Declaration of Human Rights of 1948 recognized the right to a living standard adequate for maintenance of health, and in the 1970s the World Health Organization (WHO) policy of "Health for All by the Year 2000" identified good health as an issue of social justice.

One notable continuity between the periods of the first and second volumes is the problematic relationship between curative medicine and public health. In terms of policy significance, resources and prestige, public health, despite some gains, continued after 1950 to take second place to clinical medicine.

By about 1950, curative and restorative medicine in Australia, and in the other two countries as well, enjoyed the high regard of both governments and citizens. It was given the credit for the historical defeat of infectious diseases, an attribution made the more plausible by the wondrous effectiveness of the new antibiotics against bacterial infections. In contrast, public health was almost invisible. Even in the United Kingdom, where state provision of health services had, under the National Health Service, proceeded considerably farther than in Australia or the United States, public health doctors had lost their prewar importance and had failed to establish a significant new role in a health system dominated by hospital medicine in particular, and curative medicine generally. In Australia, following the failure of federal labor governments to establish a tax-funded national health service similar to Britain's, the conservative Menzies Liberal-Country Party government created in the 1950s a federal funding scheme underwriting the existing system of fee-for-service, private medicine, in the practice of which preventive work had but a minor place.[1] As in the United States and Britain in the immediate postwar decades, hospital-based medicine, often engaged in dramatic struggles to save the lives of identifiable, individual patients, was far more visible than public health, which worked with populations and employed interventions not directly concerned with the fate of the individual.

THE NATURE OF EPIDEMIOLOGY

However, by the 1950s demographic and epidemiologic patterns were changing notably. The populations of Australia, Britain and America were aging, and chronic, "degenerative" diseases were replacing infectious diseases as the main causes of death and disability in the affluent societies of the West. Indeed, by the 1970s, Australia faced the threat of epidemics of coronary heart disease and lung cancer. At first, both health professionals and governments responded to these new threats to the people's health by pointing to the need for individual preventive action, especially through education-mediated lifestyle modification. Only slowly was it generally recognized that social and economic factors constrain the capacity of the individual to take responsibility for his or her health. A social conception of health was then, and still is, incompletely established. Even within the public health establishment, epidemiology, the premier tool of understanding of health and disease, was beset by an individualistic bias that did not permit a large enough place for social factors and that therefore did not encourage interventions promoting change at the societal and environmental levels. Indeed, it might be argued that historically, two professional views of public health have been in competition. One of them sees public health as a subdivision of medicine; it focuses on the actions of individuals and on individual-level, proximate risk factors for disease (reporting statistically significant associations between the disease and some variable). The other considers medicine to be a subdivision of public health. It sees public health as a multidisciplinary field of inquiry and a sociopolitical activity concerned with interventions at various levels of social organization: "The key word is 'health,' not 'medicine'; the universe of concern is the health of the public, not the discipline of medicine."[2]

Adherents of the first view pursue the "causes" of disease laterally and, while identifying an ever larger number of risk factors, essentially continue on the same plane of explanation. Adherents of the second pursue a hierarchical approach to causation, a schema involving levels of explanation: "What gets cancer—the genes, the cell, the organism, or perhaps even the population? . . . [T]hese are levels of explanation that may be more or less coherent within themselves but provide even more information when they exist in a framework provided by all of the explanatory modes."[3] This hierarchical approach, as McKinlay and Marceau point out, offers great benefits. First, it allows different levels of analysis to be integrated—from the topmost level of social determinants down through geographical and environmental influences and, farther down, through lifestyle and behavioral influences to the influence of biophysiological and family history on the individual. Second, it entails different actions or interventions at each level. Thus, a multilevel approach to diabetes would entail at the level of biophysiology, clinical action to correct imbalances of metabolism; at the individual behavior level, action to persuade at-risk people to change dietary and physical activity patterns; at the environmental, community level, workplace interventions like screening; and at the social-structural level, public policy initiatives. The burgeoning concern of researchers with the social determinants of health and disease leads inevitably to the hierarchical approach to explanation and to intervention.

As public health confronts the emerging health issues of the early part of the twenty-first century, it requires research methods and interventions appropriate to the issues of the time—to growing health status inequalities within and between nations, and environmental threats of global proportions like climate change and rupture of ecosystems that, in concert with modern air travel, spread deadly new infections, for example, globally and at unprecedented speed.[4]

During the second half of the twentieth century, epidemiologists developed a conceptual and methodological framework to study multiple risk factors for chronic, noncommunicable diseases because these conditions were replacing the major infectious diseases as the significant causes of death in the economically advanced countries, where most epidemiologists worked. Assuming that populations were simply aggregates of individuals, epidemiologists largely failed to come to grips with the social patterning of disease. They mostly gave up the quest to understand the determinants and distribution of disease within populations. One recent critic has asserted that epidemiology in the main has "ceased to function as part of a multidisciplinary approach to understanding the causation of disease in populations and has become a set of generic methods for measuring associations of exposure and disease in individuals."[5] Other critics have pointed out that it has no theory of what shapes population patterns of disease.

SOCIAL MODELS OF CAUSATION OF DISEASE

The history of public health in the nineteenth and twentieth centuries reveals the waxing and waning of broader social and environmental models of disease causation. In the earlier nineteenth century, Louis René Villermé in France and Rudolf Virchow in Germany pointed to the fact that disease was associated with social or environmental factors like urban poverty and dangerous working conditions. Friedrich Engels pointed out that death rates of Manchester families occupying the worst housing were double those of people occupying the best. From the mid-nineteenth century, the exponents of Edwin Chadwick's "sanitary idea," stressing the importance of the physical environment, identified miasmas, or emanations from decaying organic matter, as the proximate cause of disease. They offered a narrow, sanitary-engineering solution—the disposal of urban wastes and the provision of clean water. The great advance of bacteriology in the last decades of the nineteenth century promoted another powerful idea—specific aetiology, the concept that particular diseases were caused by particular infectious agents. The idea of "specific cause" was reinforced in the early twentieth century by the identification of specific vitamin deficiencies and particular occupational exposures as the causes of nutritional disorders and cancers, respectively. In the 1920s and 1930s, the interactive model of host, environment and agent lifted disease causality to a broader level, while the work of Major Greenwood in Britain and that of Joseph Goldberger and Edgar Sydenstricker in the United States pointed up the importance of the social and economic environment. But from the 1950s on, concern with multiple, proximate risk factors for chronic diseases cut across any revival of interest in social causes. The result has been that epidemiology has not forwarded our understanding of distribution of disease within populations. Recently, some epidemiologists have urged recognition of the role of the history, culture and social structure of a population in determining the distribution of disease risk. As Tony McMichael has noted, at the beginning of the twenty-first century epidemiology is extending its spatial-temporal frame of reference and moving away from its established preoccupation with proximate, individual-level risk factors.[6]

Interest in how social structures affect the people's health has grown in recent years. While the pathways connecting social status and health status are complex and as yet not well understood, it seems that psychosocial factors like social support and sense of control of one's life play a significant mediating role. Various governments of states belonging to the Organization for Economic Cooperation and Development (OECD) have supported both research on, and policy initiatives to reduce, inequalities in health status. The "Healthy People 2010" program, sponsored by the U.S. government, was intended both to end health disparities by 2010 and to increase life expectancy and quality of life. The British government's white paper "Saving Lives: Our Healthier Nation" (1999) likewise was intended to reduce significantly health status inequalities while also increasing life expectancy and the number of disability-free years. For almost a decade and a half, the Netherlands government has supported both research and interventions concerning socioeconomic determinants of health. In 1998 Australia's Commonwealth Department of Health and Aged Care gave the National Centre for Epidemiology and Population Health (NCEPH) at the Australian National University the task of studying the feasibility of a research and development collaboration concerning health inequalities. The Commonwealth Department of Health then asked NCEPH to set up the Health Inequalities Research Collaboration (HIRC) as an "institute without walls." The HIRC established three research networks—one on the impact of early life on health in later life, one on what makes a healthy community, and one on the effect of primary health care as a source of health advantage or disadvantage. All three were to look at both socioeconomic and urban-rural gradients in health status.[7]

WHO Europe, impressed with the growing evidence of the importance of the social determinants of health, in the late 1990s commissioned Michael Marmot's International Centre for Health and Society to put together the core evidence in a form convenient for policy makers and citizens to read. The result was *Social Determinants of Health: The Solid Facts.* This publication shows how the effect of material deprivation may be reinforced by psychosocial factors like anxiety and lack of social integration to make the health of those on the lower rungs of the social ladder worse than that of people on higher rungs. Michael Marmot and Richard Wilkinson, who coauthored *The Solid Facts,* confidently advance the following propositions:

1. Differences in health between social groups result from social factors, not differences in health care.
2. Disease rates of people change with their social and cultural environments.
3. Relative material deprivation alone does not produce poor health.
4. The health gradient may change quickly, as was the case in Eastern Europe after the fall of communist regimes.
5. The health gradient does not result from selection; in the main, social status determines health, not vice-versa.

A comprehensive model of the social determinants of health would connect social structure to health along material, psychosocial, behavioral and biophysiological pathways. Genetic, cultural and early-life factors permeate the series of pathways.[8]

Sociologists of health have long stressed the impact of social structure on health. Thus, Conrad and Kern, in a 1981 text on the sociology of health and illness, stated as an explicit assumption of their approach that health problems and health inequalities are related to the "particular historically located social arrangements and the cultural values of any society."[9] The difficulty with a social-structural explanation of health is that it leaves no room for human agency—for individual intention and action. The social, political, economic and cultural conditions are taken as given. But in truth the interaction of individual subjects with such structures modifies these givens: "Society forms people[,] who then transform and reproduce society."[10]

Sociological theories tend to divide between those based on an individualistic, behavioral approach and those that hold to a social-structural, systems approach. According to van der Maesen and Nijhuis, modern public health must connect the two domains; they propose the notion of "social quality" as a mediating concept. Social quality is "the extent to which citizens are able to participate in the social and economic life of their communities under conditions which enhance their wellbeing and individual potential."[11] Social quality involves an accepted minimum level of economic security, a basic level of social inclusion, residence in a community that exhibits social cohesion, and empowerment allowing development of competencies. The concept thus connects "public" (the collective level) and "health" (the individual level) in "public health."

Social quality relates to the health-conferring conditions arising from the interaction between citizens and social systems like cultural, educational, economic and health care institutions and behaviors. Where in medicine quality relates to the efficacy and ethical circumstances of individual medical interventions, in public health the key is the social quality of living conditions and social systems. "Healthy" populations are those that enjoy a high degree of social quality. Contemporary public health thus has three social tasks—to promote social conditions producing health; to prevent social conditions threatening health; and to neutralize social conditions causing ill health. Contemporary public health is inescapably caught up in the problems of social and economic relationships, and social inequalities in particular, at the national and international levels.[12]

THE ROLE OF THE STATE

Whether public health will be successful with the social-policy-level interventions that are necessary to promote social quality depends on the state's itself being willing to act—the state being defined as "that set of institutions that are recognizably 'public' in that they are responsible for the collective organization of social existence and are funded at the public's expense."[13] While more effective interventions and more sophisticated research methods are important to the success of public health, the real key is the will of the state to act.

It does not augur well for strong state action that in Australia and the United States "new right," or neoconservative, administrations control the national governments. Even the Blair Labor government in Britain is constrained by the free-market ideology and policy agenda that have swept Western countries over the last two to three decades. Hostile to state intervention in economic and social life, neoconservatism looks overwhelmingly to the market, not government, to be the mechanism for allocating national resources. It sees the state as a parasite upon individual freedom and upon economic growth. It even rejects the claim that the state may usefully act to stabilize capitalism by reducing class tension. Rather, it views the state as pursuing its own interests in expanding its power and prestige, which it believes are separate from those of society.

If the role of the state will be a critical force shaping public health in the first decades of the new millennium, so also will two closely connected phenomena—privatization and globalization. Privatization, or the turning over of functions of the state to private individuals and institutions, is commonly associated with the late-twentieth-century advance of neoconservatism, but even "left-wing" governments have moved important services from the public to the private arena. At the same time, the emergence of a global economy has restricted the power and reach of nation-states, reducing greatly the capacity of government to direct the national economy toward high levels of employment and steady economic growth. The actions of various supranational entities—multinational companies, international financial markets, transnational communication systems and supranational bodies like the World Bank—greatly impinge on the freedom of action of the nation-state. They function beyond the control of even significant nation-states.[14] Politics, in the sense of the distribution and effects of power in society, is thus deeply connected to the future of public health, as it was to the origins of modern public health in Britain a century and a half ago. Indeed, two contemporary commentators on the historical lessons offered by Edwin Chadwick's famous Public Health Act of 1848 suggest that above all else it showed that "communities and nations can transform themselves for better health . . . but that they do not do so automatically and necessarily."[15] The state thus had, and continues to have, a pivotal role in protecting and promoting the people's health, but the extent to which the state is willing and able to pursue an effective role is in doubt.

THE POPULATION PERSPECTIVE AND THE SOCIAL CONCEPTION OF HEALTH

A distinguished British epidemiologist, Geoffrey Rose, drew attention some years ago to the fact that risk of disease is in most cases distributed along a continuum, such that when the distribution is shifted even in a small favorable way, the health of the population improves to a larger extent. Risk of disease in an individual must be viewed against the disease risk of the population to which he or she belongs. Most cases of disease are located in the bulk of the population who are positioned outside the distribution curve's "tail" of high risk. A Finn is more likely than a Japanese to suffer premature death from heart disease, not simply because the Finn has a high cholesterol level but also because the distribution of cholesterol levels in the Finnish population is to the right of the distribution in the Japanese population. Rose's point was anticipated in the 1890s in the conclusion of the French sociologist Emile Durkheim that the suicide rate is a social phenomenon. There may be many reasons for an individual's suicide, but the social rate of suicide remains predictable. The rate of suicide is not a simple summation of individual suicidal tendencies; it reflects such characteristics of the population as social values, the morality of suicide, and the pattern of social relations. In the same way, at the individual level, low income correlates with poor life expectancy. However, at the population level, income and health relate differently. Differences in average life expectancy between countries do not correlate well with average income. Moreover, life expectancy correlates inversely with income inequality. The relation does not simply result from the poor health of the materially deprived; it reflects health across the range of incomes.

Some researchers believe that the poor health of given populations arises from low levels of what Harvard sociologist Robert Putnam has called "social capital"—where the difference between the well-to-do and the disadvantaged is great, levels of mistrust and hostility are higher and the extent of cooperative relations expressed in community organizations is minimal. Those wedded to an individualistic explanation would relate onset of disease to chronic stress and insecurity in individuals. Those pursuing society-level explanations would point to alienation, violence, and risk behaviors for disease (and a history of such) as the sources of the population's poor health.

A good historical example of how social, political and cultural features of a population impact on health is the experience of indigenous peoples in Australia, North America and New Zealand. The low life expectancies of Aboriginal, Amerindian and Maori populations were in part determined by the oppressive and alienating character of settler society and the unequal relations between indigenes and whites. Constitutional features of populations, like herd immunity, income inequality and social morale, appear to influence health "at a supra-individual level, in addition to any manifestation of risk . . . at the individual level."[16]

The neoconservative view of society (strong, as noted above, in Australia, the United States and Britain) as a mass of individuals whose primary reason for being is economic competition in the marketplace may need to be supplemented by a Durkheimian emphasis on the social. Methodological individualism (the progenitors of which are utilitarianism, liberal political theory and neoclassical economics) sees complexity as something that must be broken down into the parts of the whole; society is "really" only an aggregation of individuals. In contrast, in Durkheim's collectivist epistemology social wholes are seen as social facts, and an irreducible social reality is the point of departure for a social explanation. Social subsystems subserve the whole and society is a set of collectivities linked by rights and duties. A social conception of health will need to include a Durkheimian appreciation of the reality of the social.[17]

THE ORGANIZATION OF THE BOOK

The basic theme of this history of public health in Australia in the last fifty years of the twentieth century is the development of a social conception of health—evolving appreciation of the key role of social factors in the determination of health status and commitment to promotion of social justice, especially reduction of social inequalities in health. Chapter 2 discusses the emergence in the 1950s and 1960s of professional and government concern with chronic degenerative diseases and other health problems of affluence; the solution offered at that stage was largely individual behavior change. Chapter 3 discusses the rise and fall of the idea of a national network of community health centers and its legacy of adherence by some health professionals to a social view of health. Chapter 4 traces the rise, at the international level and then in Australia, in the 1970s and 1980s of the "new public health" with emphasis on health promotion, community participation and intersectoral collaboration in policy development and execution. In chapter 5 the significance of concern with social justice as a driving force in public health in the 1980s and 1990s is explored. In the final chapter, chapter 6, an answer is attempted to the question, whither public health at the beginning of the new millennium? I suggest that public health can take a broad path, concerning itself with social causes of disease, health status inequalities, human rights and global environmental issues, or it can follow a narrow path, focussing on individual risks of disease, disease prevention and cost containment.

Efforts to push public health along the broad road will be made difficult by the dominance of a market-oriented ideology in public policy discourse. They will be made even more difficult by the constraints placed by economic globalization on the freedom of action of nation-states. The history of public health shows that the people's health advanced significantly in nineteenth-century Britain when state intervention—in the form of publicly funded waste-disposal and clean-water systems—was used to distribute to the poorer urban classes some of the greater social amenities created by the unprecedented productivity of industrial capitalism. At the beginning of the twenty-first century, this process of civilizing capitalism has to be addressed at the international level—social and environmental agreements must be established to supplement agreements liberalizing trade and investment—if health inequalities created by free-market capitalism are to be reduced. Collective intervention in the name of social justice must rectify the inequities that the market inevitably produces.

NOTES

1. Underlying the Australian federal government's expanded role in health matters was a strong growth in the power of the commonwealth in relation to that of the states during the 1940s. The constitution had been constructed to protect the powers of the states while also ensuring achievement of the primary aims of federation: creation of a national market, establishment of a national defense system, and realization of a national restrictive immigration ("White Australia") policy. The only health responsibility given the commonwealth was full but concurrent power over quarantine. Not until a 1946 referendum conferred responsibility for medical and social services did the commonwealth extend its constitutional power in the field of health. At least as important was its acquisition of control over the purse strings. In World War II, under the defense power, the commonwealth had almost complete control over the economic and social life of the nation. The uniform taxation legislation of 1942 gave it clear financial superiority as the states vacated the income tax area in return for grants from the commonwealth. Upholding the legislation, the High Court of Australia indicated that it flowed from the commonwealth's power of taxing, not the defense power. Thus, the arrangement could continue beyond any wartime arrangements. In 1957 the legislation survived another constitutional challenge in the High Court. See M.J. Lewis, "Editor's Introduction," in J.H.L. Cumpston, *Health and Disease in Australia: A History,* ed. M.J. Lewis (Canberra: AGPS Press, 1989), 7, 22, and 31.

2. Quoted in J.B. McKinlay and L.D. Marceau, "Public Health Matters: To Boldly Go . . . ," *American Journal of Public Health* 90(1) (2000): 27.

3. Quoted in ibid., 27–28.

4. Ibid., 27–31.

5. Quoted in A.J. McMichael, "Prisoners of the Proximate: Loosening the Constraints on Epidemiology in an Age of Change," *American Journal of Epidemiology* 149(10) (1999): 888.

6. Ibid., 888–96; G. Rosen, *A History of Public Health* (Baltimore: Johns Hopkins University Press, 1993), 390.

7. J.M. Dixon, R.M. Douglas, and R.M. Eckersley, "Making a Difference to Socioeconomic Determinants of Health in Australia: A Research and Development Strategy," *Medical Journal of Australia* 172 (2000): 541–42.

8. J. Dixon, "Resource Reviews: Social Determinants of Health," *Health Promotion International* 15(1) (2000): 87–88.

9. P. Conrad and R. Kern, "General Introduction," in *The Sociology of Health and Illness. Critical Perspectives,* ed. P. Conrad and R. Kern (New York: St. Martin's Press, 1981), 6.

10. L.J.G. van der Maesen and H.G.J. Nijhuis, "Continuing the Debate on the Philosophy of Modern Public Health: Social Quality as a Point of Reference," *Journal of Epidemiology and Community Health* 54 (2000): 135.

11. Quoted in ibid., 136.

12. Ibid., 134–39.

13. Quoted in J.B. McKinlay and L.D. Marceau, "Upstream Healthy Public Policy: Lessons from the Battle of Tobacco," *International Journal of Health Services* 30(1) (2000): 61.

14. Ibid., 61–66.

15. C. Hamlin and S. Sheard, "Revolutions in Public Health: 1848 and 1998," *BMJ* 317 (7158) (1998): 591.

16. McMichael, "Prisoners of the Proximate," 893.

17. van der Maesen and Nijhuis, 137–38.

Chapter 2

The Health Problems of Affluence

THE ADVANCE OF CURATIVE MEDICINE

In the popular imagination, the great wartime advances of penicillin and DDT represented the triumph of scientific medicine. Biomedicine was credited not only with wartime achievements of heroic proportions and the prospect of further achievements in peacetime but with the historical victory over infectious diseases. Public health failed to assert its rightful claim to major credit in controlling infectious diseases in the Western world. The arrival of effective chemotherapy—the antibiotic treatment of bacterial infections—revolutionized clinical medicine. It conferred an unprecedented effectiveness on biomedical therapy. In Australia, the sulfonamides (sulfapyridine in 1938 and sulfadiazine in 1940) and then penicillin (first produced in the second half of 1943 at the Commonwealth Serum Laboratories) were soon followed by streptomycin, chlortetracycline, chloramphenicol, and erythromycin. Streptomycin (1948), para-aminosalicyclic acid (1950) and isoniazid (1952) radically transformed the treatment of tuberculosis and helped shut down sanatoria in Australia, as well as in other Western countries. As the case of tuberculosis itself shows, the focus on the social causes of disease tended to recede. Concern with an individualistic aetiology of disease was reinforced.[1]

In Australia in the 1950s and 1960s, health policy was marked by the dominance of curative and restorative medicine after the Menzies Liberal-Country Party government established a national medical service, an arrangement that was aptly described by a British medical visitor, Sir Theodore Fox, as "private practice publicly supported."[2] Fox went on to say that "the English system is geared more to the patient's satisfaction than the doctor's. Australia, and to a less extent New Zealand, illustrate advantages in systems which favour the profession."[3] The possibility of a new, integrated relationship between curative medicine and public health, which the national hygienists had planned (see *The People's Health*, volume 1) and which survived in a attenuated form in the Chifley Labor government's ultimate version of the national health service, disappeared altogether in the scheme introduced by the Menzies government's health minister, Dr. Earle Page. Individual responsibility for health care and an individualistic conception of disease informed Page's approach: "Any such scheme should contain elements of self reliance and a sense of personal responsibility. Also it should stress the obligation of the individual to make a least a part of his contribution directly to the . . . cost of the scheme."[4] On another occasion he declared, "No disease runs an exactly similar course in every person. Its course is determined by the constitution and heredity, previous diseases and condition of other organs. It is obvious, therefore, that human disease cannot be overcome by mass treatment."[5]

Page, who was a member of the Australian Branch of the British Medical Association (BMA) and a founding fellow of the Royal Australasian College of Surgeons, saw his scheme as a bulwark against socialized medicine. It involved voluntary participation, functioned within the existing system of medical and hospital services, and sought to cover a large percentage of the people. Private, nonprofit bodies, like benefit funds, would provide health insurance. Individuals receiving federal pensions would be eligible for free services; all others had to hold medical insurance from a private fund and contribute to the cost of other services.

The scheme had four aspects: pharmaceutical benefits, hospital benefits, medical benefits and pensioner medical services. The pharmaceutical benefits, introduced in August 1950, and the pensioner medical service, February 1951, proved comparatively straightforward to implement. The hospital and medical benefits were more difficult to introduce, because, in the case of hospital benefits, arrangements already were in place under the Labor government's Hospital Benefits Act, 1945–48; in the case of medical benefits, the BMA continued to push its own barrow, while private funds competent to participate were not plentiful. Only the most costly, life-saving drugs were provided free. Subsequently, non-pensioners were required to pay small charges for hitherto free drugs, but the range of subsidized drugs was increased; pensioners were eligible for a full range at no cost. The pharmacists were won over by requiring that life-saving drugs on the list be dispensed by registered pharmacists (salaried doctors in smaller hospitals no longer qualified) and accepting prices set by the Pharmacy Guild. Doctors could prescribe any brand within the list—a provision that, in effect, encouraged manufacturers to increase prices while using nonprice competition, such as promotion to doctors, to win larger shares of the market for their products. With such inbuilt features, cost-increase pressures were powerful from the outset. The first estimates had allowed for 2.5 million pounds in the first year, but in 1951–52 actual costs were above five million pounds. The hope that the BMA would restrain the prescribing behavior of doctors was not fulfilled. From 1960, a full range of drugs was provided, but patients were required to pay five shillings toward the cost of a prescription. The aim was to contain costs by eradicating the inducement for doctors to prescribe the costly drugs on the existing free list. Moreover, since it now purchased on a larger scale, the federal government could use its market power to obtain drugs at lower prices. The pensioner medical service provided free general practitioner services for pensioners, and for dependants, on a fee-for-service basis. From 1955 eligibility was narrowed to pensioners able to pass a means test but was widened again in 1966 to allow all access to the service. The restricted access had been urged by the BMA because doctors believed that the government, not the profession, should bear the cost involved in providing pensioner consultations at a fee somewhat lower than normal. Cost-increase problems beset this service as they did the pharmaceutical benefits scheme. The BMA was able to get agreement to link fee increases to basic wage increases. Moreover, the Health Department became concerned about allegedly widespread overservicing, although few cases were investigated at this time.

Health Minister Page was not keen to antagonize the BMA while the medical benefits scheme had yet to be finalized, so state committees of pharmacists and doctors were allowed to exercise self-regulation. But soon other ways of containing costs were tried. As noted above, access to the pensioner scheme was confined in 1955 to those receiving the full pension, with the result that a few years later more than 25 percent of pensioners did not qualify for the free service. This residual welfare component of the conservative Menzies government's national health service was the only area in which doctors would accept direct payment of fees by the government.

In 1952, the hospital benefits scheme was launched. The states agreed that the commonwealth would contribute—benefits first had been introduced by the Chifley Labor government in 1948—at a per diem rate of eight shillings per patient, with twelve shillings for pensioners and dependants. With the aim of promoting voluntary private insurance, the commonwealth paid a further four shillings for insured individuals (and their dependants) who qualified for fund benefits of six shillings or more. By the mid-1950s, free public ward accommodation had disappeared in all states except Queensland, which refused to abandon its long-standing policy of free hospital care. The scheme worked more or less well for pensioners and those with private insurance, but it did not serve the chronically ill or disabled well at all.

In mid-1953, the centerpiece of the Menzies government's national health service, the medical benefits scheme, was finally introduced. The benefit was paid only to members of registered nonprofit organizations, so there was an inbuilt incentive for private insurance to grow. The fee-for-service principle so important to the BMA was preserved. The majority of friendly societies (not-for-profit, insurance organizations that from the mid-nineteenth century had provided for the provident working and lower middle classes a limited range of medical care delivered by general practitioners under contract arrangements; see *The People's Health*, volume 1) eventually became registered organizations and abandoned contract practice. Organizations could reimburse members (with the fund and government benefit) only up to 90 percent of the cost of medical care, although doctors could levy whatever fees they wished. Page had been impressed by the capacity of the American Blue Cross private funds to persuade the middle classes to take out hospital and medical coverage; in 1951 he visited the United States to observe their work at first hand. But the middle classes in Australia were not nearly as ready to take out private coverage. Here the state had to subsidize insurance arrangements. Initially, Page had envisaged different subsidies for pensioners (the unemployed were ultimately left out), the working and lower middle classes, and the middle classes (incomes greater than 550 pounds a year). The first were to be fully subsidized, while the second were to be subsidized but were also to pay 10 to 20 percent of the cost of the services (which were to be based on established lodge practice). The third were to be subsidized through reimbursement via private insurance organizations and had to pay full fee for service. Page intended by these arrangements to underpin the private medical market yet contain overall costs by retaining contract practice for a substantial part of the population.

The BMA was upset at the major role assigned to friendly societies and lodge practice, fearing that if enforcement of the income limit to membership proved as difficult to achieve as it had in the past, contract practice would colonize totally medical services. The BMA then set out to end altogether the threat of contract practice itself. With New South Wales in the vanguard, the state branches indicated that they would cease to provide contract practice facilities by the close of 1950. In Victoria, where the friendly societies had historically been most powerful, their capitulation was delayed till late 1951. The BMA still feared that the friendly societies, which became registered organizations, might form a group hostile to the doctors' interests. So it worked to expand the membership covered by the private Medical Benefits Fund (MBF), which the BMA had helped establish. Already active in New South Wales and Queensland, the MBF entered Victoria in 1952. Concerned about the viability of some friendly societies as agents for the medical benefits scheme, Page sought advice from two American experts, William McNay of the Michigan Hospital Service and E.A. van Steenwyck of Associated Hospital Services of Philadelphia. They found that funds in Australia were not strong enough financially and that management swallowed too much of their contributions income. Further, they thought that too many were not large enough to survive. The commonwealth sought to strengthen the system by stricter regulation of registered organizations; a fund had to have at least 1,500 members, and no more than 15 percent of income could be spent on management, while competition for members was to be controlled. Because the Menzies Liberal-Country Party government did not control the Senate (the federal upper house) for the first two years after coming to power, regulations under Labor's National Health Act had been employed to introduce pharmaceutical benefits and the pensioner medical service. Once the conservative Menzies Liberal Party-Country Party government controlled both the House of Representatives and the Senate in 1951, the BMA urged the government to pass legislation covering all of the new national health service so that a future Labor government could not easily dismantle it. The new National Health Service Act was passed in late 1953.[6]

The Menzies government's national health scheme, like the prewar national health insurance scheme and the Chifley Labor government's national health service proposals, was and remained centrally concerned with cost control. Cost containment in the 1950s and 1960s came to dominate health policy as subsequent Liberal-Country Party governments grappled unsuccessfully with the recurring problem of the BMA's recommending higher fees to its members. Private medical practitioners came to enjoy high and rising incomes in this era. Average net annual income increased from $9,016 in 1961 to $16,559 in 1971.[7] Between 1966 and 1978, net annual income grew from $12,403 to $36,889, so that by the late 1970s doctors were receiving three to four times the average income of salary and wage earners. By then they were the highest-paid occupational group in Australia.[8]

The national health service's bias toward curative medicine through the fee-for-service structure meant that prevention in general practice was neglected. A 1964 survey by the Commonwealth Health Department and the Australian College of General Practitioners reported that there was "little recognition by practitioners of the opportunities available for prevention at the clinical level" and that "most practitioners regarded prevention at all levels as the responsibility of the public health authorities."[9] Moreover, the state's underwriting of general practitioner incomes had certainly staved off the threat of group practices' taking over from solo practitioners. In New South Wales in the mid-1960s, about 40 percent of general practitioners practiced alone.

The Labor Party was slow to develop a plausible alternative to the coalition government's national health service. A basic problem was the damage caused electoraly to Labor by the 1954–55 split over anticommunism. In the 1950s and early 1960s, Labor simply talked of resurrecting the Chifley government's health plans and untying the commonwealth subsidy from voluntary insurance. In the mid-1960s, Labor briefly revisited the organizational radicalism of the wartime era. In a 1964 Victorian Fabian publication, Dr. Moss Cass, a surgeon at Melbourne's Royal Children's Hospital, proposed a salaried service and creation of medical centers in which modern primary care could be practiced. But this radical policy proposal did not survive the coalition's huge landslide victory in the 1966 federal elections. E.G. Whitlam, the new Labor leader, characteristically pragmatic in his search for electoral advantage, turned to the Melbourne University's Institute of Applied Economic and Social Research for advice and a proposal for a universal, national health insurance scheme to overcome the inadequacies of the coverage provided by the existing subsidized, voluntary insurance arrangements. The plan, based on the work of Melbourne economists John Deeble and Richard Scotton, thus eschewed potentially controversial change in the organization of medical services. It focused on the social-justice issue of access to services. Labor's universal scheme was electoraly popular, and the party did well at the 1969 elections. For some time the coalition government's voluntary scheme had been under attack for its complexity, cost and failure to provide for a significant proportion of the population, especially low-income people. Moreover, with the economy doing well, a Labor government would be well placed to introduce a new scheme. The John Gorton coalition government countered by setting up an inquiry into health insurance; the inquiry reported the voluntary scheme was "unnecessarily complex and beyond the comprehension of many"[10] and did not provide adequate rebates. Seeking to take the wind from Labor's sails, the Gorton government in 1970 offered low-income and some other groups free or subsidized insurance under the existing scheme. It also sought to streamline the scheme, introducing a schedule of most common fees and ensuring that the combined rebate from government and fund amounted to 85 percent of the schedule fee, and that the difference between the fee and the rebate was never greater than five dollars. But when it introduced higher schedule fees for specialists, general practitioners were resentful. The Australian Medical Association (AMA) was shaken by discord.

The Gough Whitlam Labor government came into power in 1972, but it was not until mid-1975 that Medibank, the universal health insurance scheme, began to operate. It had been subjected to a sustained attack in the Senate by the opposition and in the media by the AMA. Medibank included medical insurance, hospital insurance and hospital funding. Under the medical insurance provisions, all medical services carried a rebate of 85 percent of the schedule fee. The scheme was run by a single statutory body, in order to avoid the costly organizational inefficiencies of the old system of multiple private funds. With the commonwealth funding half the net operating costs of public hospitals, all residents of states that entered agreements with the commonwealth enjoyed the right to free hospital treatment by salaried or sessional doctors. Patients could choose to use their own doctors, but they would then pay for hospital accommodation (which could be covered by voluntary insurance fund membership), while rebates for medical fees were provided by Medibank. Labor did not, at that point, attack the prevailing fee-for-service system of medical services (except in encouraging the growth of salaried hospital posts, through its substantial funding of public hospitals). But the organized profession felt its autonomy threatened by the growth of institutional salaried practice and by the greater opportunity for

Table 2.1
Expenditure on Health Services in Australia, 1960/61–1972/73

	1960/61 $M	1963/64 $M	1966/67 $M	1969/70 $M	1972/73 $M
Institutional Care (Public and Private)	303	381	507	748	1,114
Other Medical Care (Government, Charitable and Private)	338	422	550	707	1,041
Public Health Services:					
Personal	18	23	30	36	89
Environmental	10	13	17	32	
Total–Public Health	28	36	47	68	89
Teaching and Research	12	16	21	30	40
Total–All Health Services	*682*	*854*	*1,125*	*1,553*	*2,284*

Source: J. Deeble, "The Health of the Nation; Who Pays?" in *The Health Problems of the Nation,* ed. J. Birman (Perth: Extension Service of University of Western Australia, 1974), 68.

government surveillance of practice made possible by the existence of a single health insurance fund. Labor did allow for the better integration of preventive and curative services, in its Community Health Program, but this was a minor part of its health policy compared with Medibank. After the Whitlam government's demise in late 1975, the program was increasingly restricted by the diminishing flow of funds from the Malcolm Fraser coalition government and by the limited commitment of state governments.[11]

In the 1960s and early 1970s, expenditure on public health as a percentage of total expenditure on health services remained fairly constant—4.2 percent in 1960–61 and 3.9 percent in 1972–73. It was small compared with expenditure on institutional (hospital) care—respectively, 44.5 percent and 48.8 percent—and on other medical care, at, respectively, 49.5 percent and 45.6 percent.[12] The details of expenditure in this period are given in table 2.1.

PUBLIC HEALTH IN THE UNITED STATES

Curative medicine and biomedical research achievements dominated the popular imagination, as well as health policy, in the United States. Like public health in Australia, public health in the United States languished, although there were exceptions. The health departments of New York and some other states made efforts to control chronic disease; also, there was a mass campaign to vaccinate against polio in the 1950s. But public health doctors were unsure about the way forward. Some saw publicly funded medical care schemes as legitimate. Others feared that this approach would marginalize prevention and health education work and that "a hypertrophied medical-care tail would soon wag the none too robust public health dog."[13] This conflict over the boundaries of public health was reflected in the question of the proper structural location of preventive medicine. Where Charles-Edward Winslow, the distinguished Yale professor of public health, saw it as part of public health, Yale's professor of preventive medicine, J.R. Paul, located it within clinical medicine. Physicians, believing that preventive medicine meant periodic personal medical examinations of individual patients, saw the reduction of chronic diseases as properly the task of private medical practitioners, not health departments: "disturbances of the climacteric, cancer, metabolic disorders, such as diabetes, cardiovascular disease" were not the proper concern of public health, and "prevention, early detection, and control of these disorders" were and would continue to be "individualistic and not en masse."[14]

Meantime, curative medicine—in the absence of a campaign by public health to promote a politically favorable public image for itself as the conqueror of infectious diseases—enjoyed a large investment of public funds. The Hill-Burton Act of 1946, which was supported by the influential American Medical Association and the American Hospital Association, provided federal funds for one-third of the costs of constructing hospitals; seventy-five million dollars a year was made available over five years. The pervasive atmosphere of anticommunism of the 1950s in any case made an extension of public services, let alone a major restructuring of the health system to integrate preventive and curative efforts, very difficult; any such proposal was easily dismissed as "socialized medicine." Whereas federal funds for medical research grew in the decade 1947–57 from $28 million to $186 million, federal grants to the states for public health contracted (even without allowance for inflation) from $45 million in 1950 to $33 million in 1959. Clinical and laboratory science received the bulk of research funds. But funding of epidemiology resulted in some very significant findings, including the connection between smoking and lung cancer, and the likely connections between elevated cholesterol and inadequate physical activity, and between arteriosclerosis and coronary heart disease.

Public health departments lacked not only funds but staff as well. One New Jersey public health officer in the late 1950s bemoaned the condition of local departments. Their work was limited to routine clinical activities, with "little or no time for community health education, the study of health problems and trends, the initiation of newer programs in diabetes control, cancer control, rheumatic fever prophylaxis, nutrition education, and radiation control."[15]

Too few graduates were coming out of schools of public health. Indeed, student numbers declined by 50 percent in 1946–56. The Senate Committee on Labor and Public Welfare in 1956 recognized that there had been a dangerous decline. Congress endorsed a traineeship program, administered by the U.S. Public Health Service, for physicians, nurses, sanitary engineers, nutritionists, social workers, dentists, health educators, veterinarians and sanitarians. Over a thousand traineeships were made available in 1957 and 1958. But a measure of the seriousness of the problem is apparent in the facts that in 1958 in excess of 2,500 public health posts could not be filled and that over twenty thousand people in government and voluntary agencies lacked appropriate training. The Hill-Rhodes Act—schools of public health had pushed hard for funding—made available a million dollars a year for training. The schools that were accredited—Berkeley, Columbia, Harvard, Johns Hopkins, Michigan, Minnesota, North Carolina, Pittsburgh, Tulane and Yale—were underfunded for teaching, and many institutions were failing to attract medical graduates. Because research was comparatively well funded, however, they were becoming more like research institutes, with growing strength in basic sciences. The price paid was that they became more remote from everyday practice and the concerns of working health departments.

In the 1960s, consciousness grew of poverty and its effects on health. In 1965, George James, the health commissioner of New York City, identified poverty as the third most significant cause of mortality in the city. The Lyndon B. Johnson administration's "War on Poverty" initiated in 1964 saw the creation of Medicare and Medicaid to underwrite the costs of health care for needy social groups. But these programs served only to bolster private medical practice and hospital care; they did not much promote preventive work. The Economic Opportunity Act of 1964 created the Office of Economic Opportunity, which supported the growth of neighborhood health centers. These offered comprehensive ambulatory services to populations lacking adequate health facilities; forty-nine such centers were functioning across the United States by 1971. The War on Poverty, like previous federal initiatives, targeted particular groups, such as veterans, migrant workers, preschool children, the aged or Native Americans. Government health programs became even more fragmented. Moreover, the practice was to establish new agencies for these purposes, with the result that established health departments were left out of the picture. The states were perceived as incapable of properly implementing progressive health and welfare measures. When in the 1960s and 1970s the problems of the natural environment became the subject of public policy, separate environmental agencies were established. Public health became institutionally isolated from environmental policy on such issues as pesticides and radiation. Always deficient in public visibility, public health was rendered less prominent than ever.

With federal funding becoming so important to them, schools of public health tailored their programs more to federal policy concerns, such as family planning, international and environmental health, and mental health. Student numbers increased, expanding by 400 percent over the period 1958–73. Graduates were joining federal and international bodies rather than local and state departments of health, and school finances were increasingly dependent on federal government largesse. Because practice still located mainly in the states, the divorce between practice and education was reinforced.[16]

PUBLIC HEALTH IN BRITAIN

The creation of the National Health Service (NHS) saw the general practitioners become independent contractors and the teaching hospitals continue as self-governing bodies. But public health doctors lost their clinical work to the general practitioners, and their authority over the municipal hospitals as well. They might have created a new role for themselves as epidemiologists and health information analysts, and as bridges connecting the three branches of the NHS. But they chose instead to take on the administration of new local government welfare and aftercare services. In this role, through the 1950s and 1960s they contended with attempts by local authorities to assert lay control over them, and with claims by subordinate professionals—sanitary inspectors, health visitors and social workers—for more autonomy. They contended too with general practitioner concerns about development of health centers and efforts to promote community care services. Moreover, by the late 1950s social medicine, social science and public health academics were proposing that medical officers of health become specialists in medical administration. They would collectively occupy a key place in health care as "health strategists," focused on the health status of populations and the planning of appropriate health services in response. The general practitioner would then integrate preventive and curative work.

The 1962 Medical Services Review Committee proposed that area health boards oversee health services, with medical officers of health becoming environmental health consultants to hospital-based departments of social health. In 1965, Sir John Reid, medical officer of health for Northamptonshire, proposed that the medical officer of health, with his or her epidemiological expertise, become a specialist on population health needs and services. In 1966, M.D. Warren of the London School of Hygiene and Tropical Medicine proposed that the general practitioner assume responsibility for preventive as well as curative medicine and that a separate specialty of medical administration be developed. The University of Edinburgh in 1959 had provided the first diploma in medical services administration. In 1965, it was proposed that the diplomas of public health and medical administration be merged as a diploma of social medicine, or community health. The Manchester diploma of public health was also reconstituted to include epidemiology and statistics, behavioral sciences, principles of administration and management and advances in medicine. The aim of these curriculum reforms was to prepare graduates to be broadly based advisers about health services rather than service managers. Meanwhile, in 1968, the Report of the Committee on Local Authority and Allied Personal Social Services recommended a unified social service department in each major local authority that would end overlap, fill gaps and generally promote community care. The expanding area of social work thus became independent of the medical officer of health's department. But in the same year, the government "green paper" (a consultative document put out by the government to promote parliamentary and community discussion and debate about some issue) on reorganization of the NHS promised public health doctors that they would enjoy a significant new role as community physicians in the reorganized NHS. Unhappily, the new role was compromised by the unresolved relationship between the executive (or management) and advisory functions of the community physician.[17]

An epidemiologist, J.N. Morris, pointing to the case of coronary heart disease, wanted cooperation between public health and clinical medicine in controlling the "diseases of affluence"; he saw the community physician offering the epidemiological information essential to effective health services. The individual would be the focus of preventive efforts, and application of epidemiological principles would reveal the social-structural and environmental factors impinging on the individual. Morris's approach was reflected in the Seebohm Committee report (of which he was a member) and in the report of the Royal Commission on Medical Education (of which Richard Titmuss, Morris's friend and colleague, was a member). The latter report (1968) identified what Morris considered the central dual functions of community physicians. Community medicine was "the specialty practised by epidemiologists and administrators of health services."[18]

Problems arose, however, in the interpretation of the role to be played by community physicians in the reorganized NHS. Medical officers of health welcomed the transformation, because it promised advancement in status for their specialty, but they do not appear to have been clear about what was involved in their new management role. Further, policy makers and academics conceived of the role rather differently. The former spoke of an integrating role for community physicians, who would connect the NHS with the local authorities and clinicians with lay administrators. The Faculty of Community Medicine (established in 1972), on the other hand, saw them as specialist advisers, utilizing their epidemiological skills and working in a complementary way with clinicians. The policy makers recognized this aspect of their work but put much weight on their responsibilities in consensus management teams. The report of the Working Party on Medical Administrators—known as the Hunter Report—in 1972 saw community physicians (or a large number of them) carrying out management duties in this way as well as acting as advisers. The community physicians, originally seen as providing information basic to the allocation of resources between hospital and nonhospital services, came to be viewed more narrowly by the management teams themselves as representatives of services in the community. Community physicians thus became involved in conflict with other doctors over resources and also grew uncertain as to whether their primary duty was to management of health services or to assessment of population health needs.[19]

PUBLIC HEALTH PROBLEMS IN THE 1950s AND 1960s

While the significance of the chronic, "degenerative" diseases was recognized as early as the 1920s, the demands of the Second World War delayed serious attempts by health authorities to do something about the new leading causes of death arising from the epidemiological transition in economically developed countries—heart disease, cancer and accidents—until the immediate postwar decades. It is possible to identify in the five decades from 1945 three main strategies employed in public health in Western countries to prevent disease and promote health: the "medical" approach, the "lifestyle" approach, and the new "public health" approach. Although they may be considered to have developed successively in this period, essential aspects of the second and third approaches have long histories. Health education, central to the lifestyle approach, goes back to early twentieth-century attempts to change the behavior of mothers in infant care, or that of tuberculosis sufferers. Emphasis on the influence of the social, economic and political environment in the new public health approach goes back to a radical tradition of public health associated with the young Rudolf Virchow and others in Germany, and Friedrich Engels in the United Kingdom, in the mid-nineteenth century.[20] Further, while this third approach has enjoyed considerable popularity since the 1980s, elements of the first two are still part of current public health practice as well.

In the medical approach, doctors are primarily responsible for prevention, and the causes of diseases are seen as biological. The medical approach involves *primary, secondary* and *tertiary* prevention. Primary prevention anticipates occurrence, in the way that immunization against poliomyelitis, measles and other common infections does. Secondary prevention involves intervention when the person does not yet know he or she has a disease, as in the case of mammography screening for early identification of breast cancer, or prenatal diagnosis of chromosomal abnormalities. Tertiary prevention seeks to minimize disability from existing disease, as in the regular use of aspirin to prevent reoccurrence of heart attack, or antihypertensive drugs for people at risk of stroke.

In the lifestyle approach, health educators (medical or nonmedical) attempt to change the individual's behavior. But, focusing too much on individual lifestyles, this approach ignores how social, economic and political factors shape the choices of individuals. It assumes that choice is both rational and free. Yet mass media, for example, impact significantly on attitudes and behavior. Moreover, in its excessive emphasis on individual responsibility, it can degenerate into blaming the victim.

The new public health approach emerged from an international movement that developed in the 1970s. The movement takes its inspiration from the World Health Organization Declaration of Alma Ata, 1978, concerning the importance of primary health care. The ideas embodied in the declaration were refined in the Ottawa Charter for Health Promotion of 1986, which came out of the First International Conference on Health Promotion, held in Ottawa, Canada.

The Ottawa conference saw social justice as a precondition of health, and advocacy and mediation as the means to achieve it. The charter called for action in the following areas: encouraging personal skills (so there would be focus on the individual as well as the social and structural); creating supportive environments; strengthening community action; making the concern of health services positive (that is, with health rather than with illness) (traditional epidemiology is concerned with prevention of ill health and clinical medicine with the cure or palliation of illness, whereas health promotion and the new public health seek to maintain or advance fitness and well-being); and building healthy public policy.

The new public health approach, then, focuses on the social, economic and policy environments, emphasizing health promotion (as opposed to health education), community participation and intersectoral collaboration. The latter would see governments, health and other departments, the private sector and nongovernmental organizations working together to construct healthy public policies. Healthy public policies may deal with other areas of policy than those traditionally associated with health—for example, transport or employment. The new public health approach seeks to modify, therefore, the social and other contextual forces that damage the health of the people. To achieve wholly its aims, the new public health would require a major social transformation such that economic and social structures, and the physical environment, produced health rather than disease.[21] In practice, it is more a beacon on the hill, drawing public health forward despite the formidable impediments posed by hostile special interests, bureaucratic inertia, and free market ideology.

THE CAMPAIGN AGAINST TUBERCULOSIS

In the 1950s and 1960s, strong emphasis was given to the medical approach to prevention, although growing stress was placed on health education. A major example of the medical approach in relation to major communicable diseases was the campaign against tuberculosis. (Another prominent case study, that of poliomyelitis, will be discussed below.)

In Australia, a national campaign against tuberculosis was initiated with the passing of the Commonwealth Tuberculosis Act, and its successive amendments in 1945–48. Mass radiography was the key to detection. Tasmania introduced compulsory surveys of the population as early as 1950;

Victoria was the last state to do so, in 1963. The campaign was an outstanding example of commonwealth-state cooperation in public health. Mortality declined very quickly from 24.8 per hundred thousand population in 1949, at the beginning of the campaign, to 2.7 in 1966, although a long-term decline had been occurring since the late nineteenth century.[22] By 1976, when the commonwealth announced it would cease to give funds to the states for the campaign, Australia had moved from a position of obscurity in tuberculosis control to one of international best practice. Morbidity, or new case discovery rates, had fallen from 49.5 per hundred thousand population in 1949 to 9.9 in 1975. In 1976 there were only six known patients in Australia who were still infectious after twelve months of treatment.[23]

The first step toward mass control took place when the Australian Army Medical Corps decided in 1939 to require all recruits to the Second Australian Imperial Force to undergo an X-ray examination. The introduction of miniature X-ray apparatus made possible screening of large populations at very small cost. The plan was put forward by Dr. Harry (later Sir Harry) Wunderly, who earlier in the 1930s had with Darcy Cowan mobilized the South Australian branch of the BMA to campaign for national TB control. A strong motivating factor in official support for mass screening of military recruits was the continuing cost of treatment for military TB cases from World War I; by 1940 it had risen to seven million pounds. The medical and economic value of the screening program was revealed by the fact that TB was diagnosed in 0.5 percent of army recruits who had already been given full clinical examinations and passed as free of the disease.

The military surveys showed the way. In 1940 the National Health and Medical Research Council proposed voluntary mass surveys of the civilian population. Both the Victorian and the New South Wales Health Departments already X-rayed citizens on a voluntary basis, as did some hospital clinics. In 1941, local government facilities at Prahran, in Melbourne, and in Adelaide became available. By 1943, however, it was clear that only coordinated and widely advertised campaigns, involving mobile visits, were likely to attract large numbers of people. It was also clear that provision of family allowances for low-income earners was essential if early institutional treatment was to be accepted by them. A meeting of commonwealth and state health ministers agreed that "an active campaign be planned in all states of the commonwealth for the full and proper treatment of tuberculosis cases and the detection of the disease in its early stages"[24] (see table 2.2).

The Tuberculosis Act of late 1945 enabled the commonwealth to make grants to the states on a pound-for-pound basis for hospital, aftercare and diagnostic facilities, and to provide allowances for those people under treatment. All this did not amount, however, to a national plan of control. After the 1946 constitutional referendum gave the commonwealth powers over medical and social services, the federal Department of Health set up a Division of Tuberculosis. Dr. Harry Wunderly, the director, presented a

Table 2.2
Estimated Tuberculosis Mortality, Australia, 1850–1990

Period	Mortality per 100,000 Population	Tuberculosis Deaths
*1850–80	120	64,000
1881–90	150	47,000
1891–1900	120	45,000
1901–10	100	45,000
1911–20	75	36,000
1921–30	60	35,000
1931–40	42	28,000
1941–50	35	23,000
1951–60	10	8,000
1961–70	3	3,000
1971–80	1	1,200
1981–90	<1	500

*Before 1875, deaths were underregistered, and disease terminology was not standardized.

Source: A.J. Proust, "The Waxing and Waning of Tuberculosis in Australia 1788 to 1988," in *History of Tuberculosis in Australia, New Zealand and Papua New Guinea,* ed. A.J. Proust (Canberra: Brolga Press, 1991), 228.

national control plan to the National Health and Medical Research Council in 1947. The states endorsed it the next year. The Tuberculosis Act of 1948 committed the commonwealth to reimburse the states for capital and maintenance spending on buildings and equipment for the diagnosis, treatment and control of TB. In addition, the commonwealth would provide income support for TB patients. The states, in return, were to provide for notification of all forms of TB, compulsory X-raying of those over the age of fourteen, compulsory examination of all contacts and suspects and isolation of recalcitrant sufferers. They were also to offer treatment free of charge to all in need of it.

In 1949, the six states signed agreements with the commonwealth. The campaign was launched amid extensive propaganda that sought to banish the stigma and fear associated with the disease. It was pointed out that not only was TB now curable but that hospitalization was not the likely death sentence of the old sanatorium days. Moreover, with the availability of income support, tuberculosis did not entail economic insecurity or the secondary stigma of pauperism. These powerful deterrents to citizen cooperation therefore no longer hampered control efforts. The states appointed full-time directors of tuberculosis, while Wunderly and his small staff in the Federal Health Department provided leadership for the national campaign. By the early 1950s, the average period in hospital for a patient had fallen from between twelve and eighteen months to between twelve and eighteen weeks.

In the twenty-seven years of the national campaign, the commonwealth spent a total of $334 million, including allowances for TB sufferers.[25]

The provision of substantial federal funds saw a considerable expansion of treatment facilities. In Queensland, for example, a new block containing eighty beds was opened at the South Brisbane Auxiliary Hospital. In 1954, prefabricated wards were set up at Chermside, where five years later the Brisbane Chest Hospital (later the Prince Charles Hospital) was opened. So speedy was the fall in incidence that TB wards in this institution were not used exclusively for TB cases. In provincial hospitals, TB annexes were constructed at Cairns, Townsville, Rockhampton and Toowoomba. In the far north, on Thursday Island in the Torres Straits, Waiben Hospital was set up for Torres Strait Islander and Aboriginal patients, while at Cherbourg a ward of forty beds was constructed for Aborigines. The Cherbourg facility, never full, became a general hospital. By the end of the 1950s enough treatment facilities for TB sufferers had been established, and more effort could be put into the other important areas of control—identification of new cases and protection of the uninfected.

In 1954 a statewide X-ray campaign supplemented skin testing of children leaving primary school. The children were given the Mantoux Test, and those reacting negatively were vaccinated with bacille Calmette-Guerin (BCG). Having started manufacture in late 1948, by the early 1950s, the Commonwealth Serum Laboratories were producing enough BCG vaccine to employ it throughout Australia. In South Australia, for example, use of the BCG vaccine was extended in 1962 from those attending the Chest Clinic to the general community. Two populations were tested and, where necessary, vaccinated: children in their last year of primary school (year seven) and national service (military) trainees. In 1952, 10.6 percent of 3,230 children of around twelve years of age and 22.2 percent of 2,212 national service trainees (eighteen-year-old males) had positive Mantoux Test results. Among the children who were tuberculin sensitive (with positive Mantoux Tests, indicating infection with the tubercle bacillus) were 8.5 percent of the Australian born and 39 percent of children born overseas. Seven years later, only 2.5 percent of Australian born twelve-year-olds, only 12 percent of national service trainees, and only 12 percent of children born overseas were tuberculin sensitive. In 1970, fewer than 1.5 percent of year-seven schoolchildren (irrespective of country of birth) were tuberculin sensitive. This declining proportion of positive children (and eighteen-year-old males) in South Australia was a good indicator of the success of the national campaign to control tuberculosis.[26] Indeed, it may be argued that BCG played a significant part in the national campaign, giving protection to adolescents, young adults, and individuals who were in particular danger in the home or work place from progressive primary tuberculosis. In addition, it bolstered resistance in young adults to postprimary infection. The Commonwealth Serum Laboratories had by 1972 made available over nine million doses of BCG. While

New Zealand, New Guinea and the Pacific Islands received some of these, the bulk was used in Australia.[27]

BCG Vaccination in Europe, Britain and the United States

First used successfully with infants in France in 1921, BCG vaccine was employed in Germany from 1925. But when seventy-two of 251 vaccinated babies died in Lubeck in 1930, its use was terminated, even though an official inquiry found that the cause of the deaths had been accidental contamination of the vaccine. Denmark, Norway and Sweden used BCG from the 1920s on an increasing scale; by 1949 it was seen in Sweden, along with general hygienic measures, as the most important protective mechanism. Yet neither Britain nor the United States had taken it up. In the 1930s, public health authorities in the former country claimed that because of memories of the nineteenth-century movement opposed to smallpox vaccination, the community would not support BCG vaccination. However, little opposition was expressed when a program was introduced in 1950. The Medical Research Council showed little interest, perhaps because in research on tuberculosis the United Kingdom was not at the forefront. Public health leaders like Sir George Buchanan, chairman of the Immunisation Committee of the Health Ministry, believed that a good system of control, using curative services and health education, already existed and that vaccination would hinder rather than promote containment. Some TB specialists saw vaccination creating a bogus sense of safety, and since many were superintendents of sanatoria, they were generally committed to the sanatorium treatment regimen—good food, fresh air and exercise. It took a crisis in recruitment of TB nurses—an estimated shortfall of almost three thousand nurses in 1949—to persuade the Health Ministry to introduce vaccination of nurses with BCG in that year. It was thought the measure would overcome anxieties about the high rate of infection among nurses and hence the recruiting problems. The next year a trial was mounted with schoolchildren. By 1953, a general program for schoolchildren was in place. This extension to a segment of the general population was undoubtedly assisted by the existence of the National Health Service and a Labor government committed to improving the health of the economically disadvantaged.

In the United States, some states had been interested in BCG vaccination; New York had opened the first vaccine clinic in 1949. However, a national program was never implemented, and interest had waned by 1959, when the focus of TB control became the new chemotherapy. American specialists in tuberculosis were committed to tuberculin testing and then treatment of people thereby discovered to be infected. Vaccination of those negatively reacting to testing would render testing ineffective for identifying foci of infection. Specialists advanced other arguments. First, evidence of efficacy from controlled trials of adequate length was not available. Also, in countries where TB rates had fallen, it was difficult to differentiate the effect of vaccination from other control measures; in countries like the Netherlands or Iceland, where the use of BCG vaccine was insignificant, TB rates had also fallen. It is interesting that in the United States, where in the 1950s public health was in retreat before the triumphant advance of curative medicine, the focus of TB control was on discovery of cases of early infection and on treatment with the new chemotherapy. The United Kingdom also was not interested in BCG vaccination until, as we have seen, a crisis in nursing recruitment required health authorities to employ the vaccine. Routine use on schoolchildren then followed, until by the late 1980s, in the face of low levels of TB, the universal school vaccination program was believed to be no longer justified.[28]

Tuberculosis Control in Britain

Tuberculosis was a significant health problem in early twentieth-century Britain. Beginning in 1911, TB dependants of workers, insured under the national health insurance scheme, qualified for treatment. After 1921, local authorities provided treatment facilities. By the late 1930s they were offering sixteen thousand hospital and sanatoria beds in England, two thousand in Wales and 4,700 in Scotland. They worked with voluntary bodies to provide clinics and aftercare. In the immediate postwar period, TB remained an important source of mortality. In 1947, the respiratory TB death rate was fifty-five per hundred thousand in England and Wales, while it was eighty in Scotland. The work of TB specialists in the new National Health Service was divided between diagnostic and curative responsibilities under a Regional Hospital Board, and prevention and care under a Local Health Authority. But regional boards commonly developed their services without much liaison with local authorities. Indeed, a 1949 investigation commissioned by the Tuberculosis Standing Advisory Committee claimed that TB specialists were not properly carrying out their work for local authorities.

The coming of the NHS saw the significant expansion of mass X-raying. Thus, in 1950–55 X-ray examinations in the Liverpool region rose from 382,000 to 937,000; in 1950–57, in the Sheffield region, it grew from 190,000 to 357,000. Efforts were especially focused on areas, like Liverpool and Glasgow, where TB prevalence was high. But while considerable progress was made in mass radiography, inertia in the treatment area—perpetuation of sanatorium treatment and thoracic surgery—retarded the campaign. Lack of nursing staff saw the closing of thousands of beds in the late 1940s. But rather than reduce the pressure for hospitals beds by more use of domiciliary care, better early diagnoses and less surgical intervention, the NHS sought to provide more beds by obtaining them from teaching and general hospitals. Further, in the early 1950s, arrangements were made with Swiss sanatoria, which had plenty of empty beds, to take English and Scottish patients.

The Swiss scheme never became substantial. Treatment outcomes were not encouraging. With patient waiting lists declining, the scheme was abandoned; only 1,025 English and 1,043 Scottish patients were treated. Indeed, by the mid-1950s, in England and Wales the waiting list had almost disappeared, and in Scotland, there was an excess of beds.

But it was the new chemotherapy that solved the problem of the immediate postwar bed shortage, by markedly cutting the period of hospitalization. It also played a very considerable part in the astounding fall in mortality in the United Kingdom, from forty-three per hundred thousand in 1950 to 1.4 per hundred thousand in 1974. It is worth remembering, however, that as in Australia, TB mortality had been declining since the nineteenth century, mainly due to a rising living standard and in particular, according to Thomas McKeown, to improving nutrition. BCG vaccination can have played no part in reducing mortality before the1950s, when it was introduced. Sanatoria and other treatment institutions had not been particularly effective in isolating active cases, because they mostly wanted to accommodate early, not chronic, cases. In addition, local authorities did not employ their compulsion powers to isolate; they simply did not have the beds, and they did not wish to become committed to material support of institutionalized patients' dependants. As late as 1941, England only had twenty-eight thousand beds for an estimated seventy-seven thousand infectious cases. Even so, it is worth noting that Sir Arthur Newsholme, the great authority on public health in the early twentieth century, believed that isolation of patients in Poor Law infirmaries played a significant part in reducing mortality from tuberculosis.

Long-standing public campaigns against spitting in public places appear not to have eradicated the practice, as public messages warning against the habit survived on a widespread scale until the 1960s. Health education aimed at improving the hygienic habits of individuals was the province of health visitors and bodies like the National Association for Prevention of Tuberculosis. It was aimed very much at wives and mothers. It is difficult to establish how effective that work was. Aftercare was another area of uncertain impact on the decline in TB. Local voluntary committees channeled income support to patients in the aftercare situation, but their capacity to do so varied across the country. Even so, Linda Bryder, a historian of tuberculosis in twentieth-century Britain, argues that what limited effect the national tuberculosis service had on TB rates until the arrival of effective chemotherapy in the postwar era came from health education and the work of the aftercare committees.[29]

From the later 1950s to 1969, when it came to a halt, mass radiography was more and more concerned with detection of such conditions as lung cancer. After 1956, the Tuberculosis Association concerned itself with other diseases. In 1968 it became the British Thoracic and Tuberculosis Association, and in 1977 the British Thoracic Association. By the mid-1960s, the focus of concern about TB had become immigrant populations; incidence (notifications) for Pakistanis was twenty-six times that of British-born, twelve times for Indians, six times for other Asians, and three times for immigrants from the West Indies. By the 1970s, incidence had climbed for Pakistanis to fifty-four times that of native-born, for Indians to twenty-seven times, and for Africans ten times. By 1986, an expert committee of the Department of Health and Social Security was proposing that vaccination efforts be directed toward high-risk groups—Asian and African immigrants, infants of Asian or African parentage and persons at risk from their work or their location overseas. Immigrants were considered to be at risk because of their generally lower socioeconomic status.[30]

Tuberculosis Control in the United States

In the 1930s, health departments had initiated mass X-ray screening, and after 1940, with the economy growing again following the Depression, the head of the National Tuberculosis Association, Kendall Emerson, could point to a renaissance in control of tuberculosis. About 1 percent of the ten million military recruits in World War II were rejected because radiography revealed evidence of pulmonary tuberculosis. In 1943, to assist the war effort, the U.S. Public Health Service created an Office of Tuberculosis Control, marking the entry of federal health authorities into control. Included in its efforts were radiographic investigations of war industries workers. The new drugs of the late 1940s and the early 1950s—streptomycin, PAS, and isoniazid—reduced the period of hospitalization. But initially they increased the importance of sanatoria, as places where the new drug therapy could be monitored. The number of sanatorium beds attained an all-time high point in 1954, when there were almost 120,000 beds.

Drug therapy became routine following the arrival of isoniazid. As evidence of resistance to this drug emerged, physicians used it in tandem with streptomycin or PAS; some used the three drugs together. Drug therapy dramatically reduced mortality. For example, in Washington State the mortality rate in Seattle and King County combined dropped in 1948–54 from 35.1 to 6.2 per hundred thousand population, and this fall mirrored a national decline. However, prevalence did not decline so much, partly because chronic cases could not be rehabilitated, and in part because more determined screening campaigns unearthed cases that would otherwise have been missed. With the decline in TB, "phthisiologists" began to call themselves "chest physicians," to reflect the fact that their field of specialization went beyond tuberculosis to embrace other forms of lung disease and respiratory conditions, like asthma.

While the general mortality from TB fell notably in the face of the new drugs, death rates among the socially disadvantaged—the poor, racial minorities and the homeless—continued to be between three and five times those of the general population. Thus, in 1948, where white males and females had death rates of 33.3 and 15.4 per hundred thousand respectively, those for nonwhites were 92.1 and 65.4.

In 1945–60, even as antibiotics promised to bring TB under control—at a conference in Harriman, New York, in 1959 it was said that widespread use of chemotherapy as a public health measure made the elimination of tuberculosis a real possibility[31]—some health professionals resurrected the concept of TB as a social problem with medical aspects, a concept popular in the late nineteenth and early twentieth centuries. Microbiologist René Dubos in particular saw as the basic answer to TB not better drugs or vaccines but better housing and nutrition, and full employment. But his emphasis on social justice and economic well-being was a minority viewpoint. The majority of those working in tuberculosis control cleaved to the narrower, medical approach to prevention and containment, stressing the need to ensure that poor patients stayed in the hospital and completed their courses of antibiotics. In the 1970s a new drug, rifampin, helped keep TB rates falling. Directly observed therapy (DOT), whereby outreach workers supervised outpatients in the taking of medication, was introduced as a strategy to achieve patient compliance where compliance was otherwise difficult to obtain.

The white plague—tuberculosis—struck back, first in New York City. Incidence, which had declined to 17.2 per hundred thousand in 1979, climbed consistently to fifty-two per hundred thousand in 1992. In the country as a whole, the increase began in the mid-1980s. New cases rose from 22,101 in 1985 to 26,673 in 1992. Moreover, the disease became more drug resistant. A New York study in 1991 found that TB in 19 percent of patients was resistant to both rifampin and isoniazid, the least toxic and most effective of the available drugs. Florida as well as New York saw drug-resistant variants of the disease; they produced 80 to 90 percent mortality in patients with human immunodeficiency virus (HIV).

Perhaps the most significant negative influence on the TB rate in the 1980s was the emergence of HIV/AIDS. Not only were those with suppressed immune function more susceptible to TB, but diagnosis and treatment of TB were more difficult when the person had HIV/AIDS. Other negative influences on the TB rate were the growth of poverty; the lack of appropriate public health facilities—sanatoria, clinics or screening programs—in many parts of the United States; and immigration from economically underdeveloped countries where TB was prevalent.

More funding, including federal funding, became available, and health departments built up tuberculosis divisions again. They used incentives to get uncooperative patients to take regular medication—noncompliance has been blamed for the development of resistant strains of TB. Incentives like subway tokens, food coupons, and above all DOT have been employed before the last-resort measure of detention, which in any case requires due legal process.

Introduced in Denver, Colorado, in the 1960s and 1970s, DOT (much of which takes place with the voluntary participation of patients) sees the patient take medication under the supervision of an outreach worker in a medical or community setting. Treatment-completion rates have been so high in some DOT schemes that compulsory institutionalization has in many places almost disappeared. But in part the effectiveness of DOT derives from the existence of the ultimate sanction of detention. In places, like New York, with many noncompliant patients, detainees come from the socially disadvantaged ranks—ethnic minorities, the homeless, those with HIV/AIDS, and drug users. In such circumstances, the possibility of discrimination and punitive practice is very real. Indeed, some jurisdictions, using criminal not civil law, may detain patients in prisons when secure hospital facilities are not available.

While contemporary tuberculosis workers may urge action to better the social conditions of patients—housing for the homeless, for example—the social improvement they envision is of a limited kind compared with earlier advocacy of wholesale social and economic reform to alter the underlying conditions producing TB among the poor. Contemporary strategies concerning the social problems of patients are aimed at enabling them to complete medical treatment. DOT best represents this narrower, medical approach to control, aiming simply to improve the patient's quality of life by eradicating his or her tuberculosis. It is not intended to reduce homelessness, poverty or drug abuse. The former head of the New York City Tuberculosis Control Bureau, T.R. Frieden, pragmatically observed, "If the health department can successfully treat his tuberculosis, he [the patient] may still be HIV infected and still have problems with drugs and homelessness, but he will never have tuberculosis again—and that is one less thing for him to worry about."[32]

Nationally, incidence fell from 26,673 new cases in 1992 to 21,327 in 1996. In New York, where there had been 3,811 new cases in 1982, there were only 2,053 in 1996. This recent decline in incidence has coincided with the widespread use of DOT and other treatment incentives. At the same time, however, social problems that promote the spread of TB have not been reduced. So long as the decline continues, then, it appears that control may be possible through a medical approach and without resort to more basic social and economic improvement of the living conditions of the disadvantaged.[33] But the longer-term situation does not look so optimistic, in the light of the fact that drug-resistant tuberculosis could not be held in check in the former Soviet Union, even when authorities followed WHO advice to use DOT. Moreover, by 1999 multidrug-resistant tuberculosis was present in over a hundred countries.[34]

CONTROL OF POLIOMYELITIS

Control of poliomyelitis is the other great historical example of the medical approach to prevention. Endemic in unsanitary communities, the disease became epidemic as sanitation improved and populations, now lacking acquired immunity, were exposed to the virus at older ages.[35] A London physician, Michael Underwood, as early as 1784 described a disease of children that was probably poliomyelitis. However, it was not properly described clinically until Monteggia (1813) and Heine (1840) did so. Jacob Heine, a German orthopedic surgeon, was one of the first to recognize that the locus of the problem lay in the central nervous system. Although small outbreaks of polio were reported in many countries from 1830, only when larger epidemics occurred in Scandinavia from the 1860s did doctors discuss whether the disease was communicable. Until the later nineteenth century, when it became clear that adolescents and young adults could be struck down, the disease was considered to be one of infants and young children; the term "infantile paralysis" had been used.

In 1890, international attention was focused on polio when a Stockholm pediatrician, Oskar Medin, discussed at the International Medical Congress in Berlin a Swedish outbreak of 1887 involving forty-four cases. In 1894, the first reported epidemic occurred in the United States, in southern Vermont; it involved 122 cases. In 1884–1907, seventeen epidemics occurred in various parts of the country, the most severe in 1907, when in New York alone 2,500 cases occurred. In 1905, Sweden had an epidemic involving 1,031 cases. Ivor Wickman, Medin's student, concluded from study of the epidemic that cases that did not develop paralysis were important in the spread of the disease. He determined the length of the disease's incubation period. Six years later, an epidemic of unprecedented size took place; 3,840 cases were officially recorded. Sweden acquired the unhappy reputation of being a breeding ground for polio epidemics, a reputation the United States was soon also to acquire.

Karl Landsteiner in Vienna in 1908 successfully transferred the disease from a human being to a monkey but was unable to transfer it from that monkey to others. It fell to Simon Flexner, head of the Rockefeller Institute for Medical Research, who had begun to investigate polio as a result of the 1907 epidemic, to pass the disease from human to monkey and then from monkey to monkey, thus showing experimentally that it was indeed an infectious disease. He also showed that the pathogen was a filterable virus, not a bacterium or protozoan. However, so little was understood about viruses at this time that apart from their ultramicroscopic size, their differences from bacteria were not appreciated.

From 1909 to 1915, the annual incidence rate (reported cases) in the United States did not rise above 7.9 per hundred thousand, but in the 1916 New York City epidemic incidence reached 28.5. Quarantine and restrictions on travel were unpopular and difficult to sustain. Quarantine was all the more difficult to enforce when the definition of what constituted a case of polio was unclear. The 1920s saw efforts in the United States and other parts of the Western world, like Australia, to use therapeutically serum developed from polio sufferers who were in the convalescent stage. Later work showed it was not beneficial, but it appeared at the time to be useful, because the natural history of the disease is such that only a few who experience "pre-paralytic polio" develop paralysis. As incidence in the United States grew, polio came to be seen as a major national health problem. The United States in the interwar period became preeminent as a research center. Australian researchers made some contribution to knowledge of polio. F.M. (later Sir Macfarlane) Burnet and Jean (later Dame Jean) Macnamara (a pediatrician who was the key Australian supporter of the convalescent serum treatment) showed experimentally that two antigenically different strains of polio virus existed. These became known as Type I and Type II. Later, a third type was identified.[36]

Poliomyelitis in the United States and the United Kingdom

President F.D. Roosevelt, himself a sufferer from the disease, played a central part in the establishment of the National Foundation for Infantile Paralysis. While polio was not a large contributor to mortality, the fact that it could leave its mainly child victims seriously disabled made the attempt to control it a very popular cause. The annual March of Dimes brought in more funds by way of donations than any other medical cause received. These funds very largely went into support of medical research. In early 1954, a vaccine developed by Jonas Salk (building on the work of J.F. Enders and others) was the subject of a huge double-blind trial involving hundreds of thousands of children across eleven states. When epidemiologists released the successful results, the news was widely welcomed by the public and the media. Although some experts thought it premature, the National Institutes of Health (NIH) supported immediate release of the vaccine. In April 1955 Mrs. O.C. Hobby, Secretary of Health, Education and Welfare, licensed six pharmaceutical companies to distribute the vaccine. Within a short time, cases of polio among vaccinated children appeared—seventy-one cases of paralytic polio and eleven deaths. Investigation identified vaccine made by Cutter Laboratories as the main source of infection. Further testing ensued, and the Salk (inactivated virus) vaccine was generally employed by 1960. But work was proceeding on an attenuated virus, oral vaccine. Following trials in 1961, a vaccine developed by Albert Sabin was licensed for general use. In the 1960s the oral vaccine was employed in immunization campaigns throughout the country. By 1974, nationwide there were only seven cases reported. Two decades later so thoroughly had polio been banished that health authorities in the United States, as in Australia, were having to promote immunization, as some parents had become complacent about the disease.[37]

Historically, Britain had been slower than other Western countries to adopt immunization measures against diphtheria and tuberculosis. This was in part the legacy of a strong antivaccination movement dating from the nineteenth century. When it became available in 1955, after polio epidemics in 1947 and 1950, Salk vaccine was to be used to protect children under eleven years and hospital staff at risk of infection. Keen to avoid spending dollars on the Salk vaccine at a time of a dollar shortage, the government wanted to use a British vaccine, which was also supposed to be safer. But production of the home product was delayed. By mid-1957, the existing program had immunized as few as one million of seven and half million children under eleven years. The advent of a new epidemic that year forced the government to purchase Salk vaccine from North America despite the fact that the Medical Research Council had not yet tested its safety. An immunization program would be provided for the population below fifteen years of age, mothers, and some high-risk groups. Further purchase of Salk vaccine became necessary when British supplies continued to be delayed and public pressure mounted for extension of the campaign to persons aged fifteen to nineteen years. Perceiving that its aim of immunizing 50 percent of the target populations was unlikely to be achieved by mid-1958, the government had to order more vaccine from North America, even though imports remained unlicensed by the MRC.

Progress was being made with protection, however, and a national publicity campaign got under way in November 1958. By the close of that year, 60 percent of those under fifteen years had been given at least two injections. By 1960, 75 percent of those under sixteen years had received the same. The program was enlarged in early 1960 to include the population under forty years. By 1961, all age groups could be accommodated. The effectiveness of the immunization program is reflected in the fact that reported polio cases were over three thousand in 1957 but a mere 250 in 1960.

However, polio flared up again in some areas in 1961. In the same year, following endorsement by the MRC, the government agreed to distribution of the Sabin oral vaccine. Demand for immunization was rising. In October 1961, use of the Sabin vaccine having gone well in a campaign in Hull, the health minister announced that Sabin would replace Salk across the country. In the 1970s, public confidence in whooping cough vaccination fell as disputes among experts about the safety and efficacy of vaccination against this disease were publicized in the mass media. Vaccination coverage, which had been 79 percent in England in 1973, declined to 31 percent in 1978, and was as low as 16 percent in Wales. Uptake of other infant immunizations declined, including that for polio, which fell by more than 30 percent. The incidence of polio increased in 1976 and 1977.[38]

Poliomyelitis in Australia

Cases of Landry's paralysis (considered to be due to the polio virus) were reported in Australian medical journals at Maclean, NSW, in 1887; Sydney in 1890; and Port Macquarie, NSW, in 1893. The first reported epidemic of poliomyelitis (fourteen cases) took place at Port Lincoln, South Australia, in 1895. With one exception, all patients were older than three years, the oldest being twenty-six years. A larger epidemic began in Sydney in summer 1903–4 and spread through NSW, Queensland, Victoria and South Australia. An extensive epidemic occurred in Victoria in spring and summer 1908, with six deaths recorded, and smaller outbreaks occurred in Bendigo (Victoria), Ballina and Sydney (NSW), and in Tasmania in 1909. The year 1915 was one of heavy incidence in Queensland (332 cases); 1916 in NSW (311 cases); 1918 and 1925 in Victoria (303 and 139 cases); 1919 and 1924 in Queensland (119 and 112 cases); and 1921, 1923 and 1924 in NSW (184, 104 and 108 cases).[39]

Two large epidemics occurred in Australia in the twentieth century, the smaller in the late 1930s and a longer-lasting one in the 1940s and 1950s. The first epidemic began in Melbourne in June 1937 and spread throughout Victoria over the next nine months. Well over two thousand cases and more than a hundred deaths were reported in that state. Western Australia was hardly affected, while Queensland and South Australia experienced an increase in incidence but nothing like that experienced at the same time by NSW and Tasmania. Health authorities had to deal with the epidemic with very limited means. Sufferers were isolated and cared for in infectious-diseases hospitals; respirators were provided for those with severe respiratory paralysis.

But while it was clear that carriers in the community as well as patients with acute illness in hospitals were capable of spreading the disease, the mode of spread was not known. No drug cure existed. Attempts were made to prevent unnecessary movement by, and assembly of, people. Heads of households were required to report cases. But these precautions were largely forlorn hopes. Many citizens became alarmed at the helplessness of health experts in the face of the epidemic spread of the disease. States considered unilateral closure of borders. For instance, South Australia contemplated closing its border with Victoria, the worst-hit state, not even considering the constitutionality of this action. It did not proceed, because of the likely adverse effect on social and economic intercourse and because it was hoped that the epidemic might be contained by the lesser measure of isolating sufferers and their contacts. However, interstate visits by schoolchildren in either direction between South Australia and Victoria were prohibited.

The last great epidemic occurred in 1949–56, during which time a total of sixteen thousand cases were reported. Prior to 1949, cases in a single state had exceeded a thousand on only one occasion, in 1937 in Victoria, when 1,369 cases were recorded But in 1951, when the epidemic was peaking, three states—NSW, Queensland and South Australia—reported more than a thousand cases each. The epidemic was different in its sheer size; it was nationwide in extent. It clearly required a national response. The NHMRC set up a Poliomyelitis Committee, which made recommendations to the commonwealth government concerning a national approach to the epidemic, including commonwealth provision of allowances and rehabilitation for those suffering from the crippling effects of the disease (see table 2.3). Commonwealth-state cooperation was important in bringing this last major epidemic to an end and in bringing polio under control.

A massive immunization program began to be prepared late in 1955, the commonwealth supplying, free of charge, Salk vaccine to the states. Actual mass immunization began in mid-1956. The vaccine was produced at the Commonwealth Serum Laboratories at Melbourne from the close of 1955 under the strictest conditions, overseas misadventures in the production of the vaccine having indicated the potential for tragedy. The states organized their own immunization campaigns, although the NHMRC set down priorities in populations to be immunized: until 1958, persons under fourteen years of age, pregnant women, and those at high risk from contact. Subsequently, all persons fifteen to forty-four years of age were included. In prewar years the health authorities had been disappointed by the poor community response to diphtheria immunization, but people now needed no convincing about polio immunization. In South Australia, for example, by 1961 an estimated 78 percent of those aged under fourteen years and 46 percent of those fifteen to forty-four years had undergone a course of three Salk injections. Reported polio cases in Australia fell from 1,194 in 1956, the last year of the great epidemic, to one in 1966. In Queensland, a small epidemic broke out in 1961–62, with 178 cases being reported. Several people who had been vaccinated became paralyzed. Type 3 polio virus was later implicated in the outbreak. The National Poliomyelitis Surveillance Committee found inadequate the potency of the Type 3 component of the existing vaccine, and the deficiency was corrected. From 1967, in any case, the oral Sabin vaccine replaced the injected Salk vaccine. Between 1965 and 1970, only six confirmed cases of polio were reported nationally.[40]

No case of polio due to a wild virus (as opposed to a vaccine-associated case) was reported in Australia after 1986. But Australia is vulnerable to imported wild virus, so high immunization coverage is critical. In 1988 WHO set the target of global eradication of polio by 2000. In 1994, the Pan-American Health Organization certified North and South America free of polio. The same year, in the Western Pacific Region of WHO (of which Australia is a member), a total of 699 cases were reported in China, Cambodia, Laos, Vietnam and the Philippines. In winter 1994–95, China immunized more than eighty million children, and the last case of indigenous, wild polio occurred there in 1994.[41]

The dramatic impact that vaccines have had on the incidence of polio and other common infections can been seen in table 2.4.

Table 2.3
Polio Cases in Australia, 1929–66

Year	NSW	Vic	Qld	South Aust	West Aust	Tas	NT	ACT	Australia
1929	240	144	22	8	10	12	–	–	440
1930	30	93	4	15	4	113	–	1	260
1931	106	276	45	27	–	8	–	–	462
1932	382	27	284	18	2	3	1	–	717
1933	12	16	11	13	3	1	–	–	56
1934	91	182	16	4	5	32	–	–	330
1935	181	64	21	18	7	4	–	1	296
1936	22	7	13	5	3	–	–	–	50
1937	70	1,369	19	85	15	299	–	–	1,857
1938	687	807	162	284	47	707	1	3	2,698
1939	33	42	23	4	5	1	1	–	109
1940	11	19	44	63	2	–	–	–	139
1941	–	–	–	1	–	–	–	–	1
1942	34	23	7	3	18	7	–	–	92
1943	–	–	–	2	–	–	–	–	2
1944	15	9	7	2	5	3	–	–	41
1945	668	238	299	9	5	3	–	3	1,226
1946	656	247	149	66	2	98	–	5	1,223
1947	83	126	19	55	2	1	–	2	288
1948	91	56	37	89	311	7	1	1	593

1949	183	761	20	582	61	36	–	5	1,648
1950	789	202	106	972	59	51	–	27	2,206
1951	1,526	433	1,030	1,456	94	171	8	17	4,735
1952	415	335	159	709	37	100	–	1	1,756
1953	635	251	198	392	45	111	1	1	1,634
1954	562	572	140	174	434	10	–	26	1,918
1955	222	235	190	182	33	7	4	1	874
1956	240	251	112	122	401	55	–	13	1,194
1957	58	13	24	16	8	6	–	–	125
1958	23	60	5	10	2	–	–	–	100
1959	16	30	4	1	3	–	–	–	54
1960	9	23	6	10	4	36	17	–	105
1961	201	50	141	44	2	11	1	–	450
1962	177	20	38	17	4	–	1	2	259
1963	3	19	1	8	5	–	–	–	36
1964	1	6	–	–	–	–	–	–	7
1965	3	–	–	–	–	1	–	–	4
1966	–	–	1	–	–	–	–	–	1

Source: A.J.G. Buxton, "Poliomyelitis in South Australia 1937–1956" (Honors dissertation, History, University of Adelaide, Adelaide, 1977), 84.

Table 2.4
Vaccine Efficacy in the U.S. as Assessed by Comparing Maximum Morbidity Levels before Vaccine Availability and Levels Some Years after Compulsory Vaccination

	Before Vaccination		After Vaccination		
Infections	Cases	Year	Cases in 1992	Cases in 1996	% Decrease in Disease Incidence
Polio (paralysis)	21,000	1952	4	0	99.98
Measles	894,000	1941	2,237	500	99.75
Mumps	152,000	1968	2,572	600	98.31
Pertussis	265,000	1934	4,083	6,400	98.46
Diphtheria	207,000	1921	4	1	99.99
Hib	20,000	1984	1,412		92.94

Source: G. Ada, "The Efficacy and Safety of Vaccines," *Nature and Society Forum* (April–May 1998): 10.

THE SECOND EPIDEMIOLOGICAL REVOLUTION

In Australia, as in other economically advanced countries, public health began to respond to the diseases of "affluence"—chronic, noncommunicable diseases—in the 1950s and 1960s. Where sanitary hygiene had been concerned with cleanliness, the "new hygiene" was concerned with diet and physical activity. Knowledge about the "new hygiene" came from the work of chronic disease epidemiologists.[42] Health authorities sought to apply public health preventive approaches to other health problems of the "affluent society"—to traffic accidents, alcohol and other drug dependence and tobacco smoking.

In Britain, epidemiology of noncommunicable disease had advanced in an academic setting. In the United States, it was located also in federal, state and local health departments. Its strong growth in these countries at an earlier stage than in other parts of Europe owed something to the long existence of epidemiology in Britain, and something also to the opportunities for the cooperation of epidemiologists and biostatisticians provided by institutions like the London School of Hygiene and the American schools of public health. In England, Major Greenwood brought out in 1935 his *Epidemics and Crowd Disease*. This book discussed cancer as well as TB and other infectious diseases. Indeed, the study of TB, with its chronic nature, enabled the concern of epidemiologists to move more easily from communicable to noncommunicable conditions. In the United States, Joseph Goldberger of the U.S. Public Health Service, who had carried out distinguished studies of yellow fever and typhus, concluded in 1915 that pellagra was a noncommunicable, diet-deficiency disease, not an infection, as had been widely believed. In 1937, lack of nicotinic acid was found to be the specific vitamin deficiency involved. The 1930s also saw the development of the epidemiology of fluoride and dental disease.

Although as early as the 1920s, public health experts were aware that noncommunicable diseases were becoming more important as infections receded as causes of illness and death, only in the postwar period did epidemiologists seriously address the problems of this second "epidemiological revolution." In the prewar era, diseases like heart disease and cancer were considered to be the unavoidable results of aging. They were truly degenerative conditions. But the postwar studies of heart disease and lung cancer pointed up their environmental causes, which were potentially preventable.

Two lots of studies were particularly influential: those in England in the 1950s and 1960s by Richard Doll and A.B. Hill on the association between smoking and lung cancer; and the Framingham study of heart disease in the 1940s and 1950s in the United States. The English studies found that the probability of smokers getting lung cancer was greater than that of nonsmokers; that the probability of heavy smokers getting lung cancer was greater than that of light smokers; that the probability of nonsmokers developing lung cancer was very small; but that most smokers did not get lung cancer. Smoking was thus a weakly sufficient cause of lung cancer, not a necessary or a strongly sufficient one. The investigators in the Framingham study, in identifying hypercholesterolemia and hypertension as factors increasing the risk of coronary heart disease, were similarly talking about multiple weakly sufficient causes.

The authors of the first modern book on epidemiology in the era of diseases of affluence, *Epidemiologic Methods*, published in 1960, introduced the idea of "webs of causation" as a concept better fitted to contemporary reality than "chains of causation." René Dubos in 1959 expressed the same idea in relation to infectious disease, where parasites and hosts mutually adapt and disease disturbs that ecological equilibrium: "Most disease states are the indirect outcome of a constellation of circumstances rather than the direct result of single determinant factors."[43] Just as Thomas McKeown did, he pointed out that mortality had declined in the West well before the germ theory and, certainly, before antimicrobial drugs: "In truth the mortality of . . . infections had begun to recede in Western Europe and North America long before the introduction of specific methods of therapy, indeed before the demonstration of the germ theory of disease."[44]

In the 1960s and 1970s in the Western world, modern technology came to be seen by many, in the light of its use in the Vietnam War and its deleterious effects on the natural environment—the first phase of the "green" movement flourished then—as a threat to the future of human kind. Some saw technology as actively dealing out death, through such means as environmental carcinogens; some saw people using it to kill themselves as in traffic accidents; and some blamed it for failing to deliver cures to cancer and heart disease. Within epidemiology and public health, the question of the causes of mortality was opened up again. Since most discussants agreed that medical care had little effect on mortality, the focus was the relative contributions of the environment and individual behavior. Medical care could have a major effect on mortality rates only when an effective therapy for a very common death-dealing disease spread quickly through the medical care system, as was the case with antibiotic treatment of tuberculosis in the 1950s; or when an effective therapy for a broad range of common diseases spread quickly, as with antibiotic treatment of a number of infectious disease in the late 1930s and the 1940s. The argument involved, on the one side, those who stressed social and economic factors and, on the other, those stressing lifestyle factors. All agreed that the causality was multifactorial in nature.

The "determinists" (as Kunitz calls them) saw society as the cause of disease and identified macro-factors like poverty, unemployment, loss of social support networks due to urbanization and uncontrolled technological development. Marxists sheeted home these factors to the ultimate cause, capitalist organization of the economy. Dubos brought an evolutionary perspective to bear, pointing out that to their biological peril, humans are not adapted to the contemporary technologically driven, "Faustian" civilization of mastery over nature. The "voluntarists" saw the cause in the individual's loss of control over his or her behavior. The solution lay in assumption of moral responsibility. Thomas McKeown in the 1970s provided the voluntarists with a historical account of the mortality decline in the West, an account that supported their propositions. Exogenous social and economic influences on mortality had so waned that endogenous factors subject to the individual would now largely determine morbidity and mortality. He identified the main influences on mortality in order of significance from the eighteenth century as environmental (nutrition and hygiene), behavioral (control of reproduction), and medical (immunization and therapy). But, he said, behavioral influences were now relatively more significant than environmental ones. The emphasis on individual behavior began to take on a distinctly moralistic, judgmental and politically conservative tone in some quarters. John Knowles, president of the Rockefeller Foundation, asserted: "Prevention of disease means forsaking bad habits which many people enjoy . . . it means doing things which require special effort—exercising regularly, going to the dentist, practicing contraception, ensuring harmonious family life, submitting to screening examinations. The idea of individual responsibility flies in the face of American history which has seen a people steadfastly sanctifying individual freedom while progressively narrowing it through the development of the beneficent state."[45]

The voluntarist emphasis on individual responsibility and behavior change was especially welcome to many Western governments, which were keen to contain the escalating costs of health care. The Lalonde Report of 1974, *A New Perspective on the Health of Canadians,* saw improvement in health status coming mainly from "improving the environment, moderating self-imposed risks and adding to our knowledge of human biology." But from the specific recommendations, it was clear that the emphasis would be on the reduction of self-imposed risks.

In the United States, under the administration of President Jimmy Carter disease prevention became an important theme of health policy. Surgeon General Julius Richmond aimed to change habits deleterious to health: smoking, drinking, poor diet, sedentary lifestyle and lax safety practices. Michael McGinnis, head of the new Office of Disease Prevention and Health Promotion, produced *Healthy People,* published as the Surgeon General's 1979 Report on Health Promotion and Disease Prevention which became the bible of the health promotion movement, and *Objectives for the Nation,* published in 1980, which set national health goals and targets for each age group of the population. Joseph Califano, secretary of health, education and welfare, in the foreword to *Healthy People,* highlighted the emphasis on individual behavioral change: "You, the individual can do more for your own health and well-being, than any doctor, any hospital, any drug, any exotic medical device."[46] In the United Kingdom, the Wilson Labor government published a consultative document, *Prevention and Health: Everybody's Business,* in 1976. Dr. David Owen, Minister of State (Health), said that the objective in publishing it was "changing public attitudes so that the National Health Service is not seen as the sole provider of health in this country, but that each of us should develop a responsibility for our (sic) own health."[47] The Treasury viewed the document as signaling greater commitment in health policy to containment of spending. Ten years later, a junior health minister in the Thatcher Conservative government, Edwina Currie, could explain why health in the north of England was worse than in the South in the following way: "We have problems here of high smoking and alcoholism. Some of these problems are things we can tackle by impressing on people the need to look after themselves better. That is something which is taken more seriously down South. There is no reason why it cannot be taken seriously up here."[48]

One drawback with the voluntarist, or individualist, position is that when a public health problem is approached in individualist terms (as lung cancer has been combated by trying to counsel individuals to stop smoking) rather than in population terms (by influencing price through punitive taxation and controls on advertising), the numbers reached are comparatively small (the comparative success of public health action against smoking in affluent countries has encouraged the tobacco industry to target markets in developing countries, where no such impediments exist). Further, antismoking educational campaigns in developed countries have influenced the educated, middle classes more than the poor, arguably because the former, with more sense of personal control over their lives, can choose more easily other ways of dealing with stress. In any case, the individualist and population-based (or sociostructural) explanations of disease causation can be viewed as applying at different levels of analysis. Disease occurs at different levels of life organization: populations, individuals, organs, tissue, cells, and molecules. Accordingly, disease causes can be analyzed at different levels: socioeconomic factors, individual lifestyle, the organ burden of a carcinogen and DNA adducts. Thus, factors in developing countries producing high mortality in childhood can be identified at the proximate tier—the immediate biomedical conditions that result in death (the interaction of malnutrition and infection); at the intermediate tier—child-care practices and other ways of behaving that expose children more to factors at the proximate point; and the ultimate tier—the social, economic and cultural processes and structures that produce unequal distribution of the basic necessities of food, shelter and sanitation.[49]

Approaches to the problem of levels of organizations may be divided into two kinds, reflecting two different conceptualizations of scientific knowledge: the bottom-up, reductionist and positivist approach; and the top-down, realist and structuralist approach. The first identifies the most basic components of a disease process, using information at this level to attain understanding of higher levels of organization. Thus, molecular epidemiology works from the molecular level to health policy. It focuses on individual, specific risk factors, and considers the randomized clinical trial the gold standard for study design. But it does not use theory distinctively related to disease as it happens at the population level. In other sciences, no attempt is made to work from the most basic level; for example, in meteorology, weather prediction is not based on measurement of individual molecules. Chaos theory alone rules out this approach, on the ground that small inaccuracies may give rise to massive effects in nonlinear systems. The top-down approach implies a structural model of causation. Where positivism is concerned with patterns of events, this approach is concerned with the structures that cause these events. Populations are not simply aggregations of discrete individuals. Each population has a history, a culture, a social and economic organization that impacts upon how and why individuals are exposed to particular factors. Understanding of disease causation in a population requires understanding of the local context, not just identification of universal relationships. Qualitative and historical studies are needed to supplement quantitative, epidemiological study.

In a population, usually, a continuum of disease risk exists; it may be more effective to make small improvements in the health of a "sick population" than try to treat or prevent illness in "sick individuals." Since group variables may be significant apart from individual level variables, ecological studies may be required. The deficiencies of ecological analysis apply only when there is extrapolation down from the population to the individual level. The randomized clinical trial may be inappropriate when historical and social context needs to be considered. Attempting to control the conflation of causes of disease by eliminating the influence of all but one cause destroys consideration of the historical and social context. It also eliminates the multiple moderating influences that make up true causation.[50]

Control of Chronic Diseases

Although American public health authorities began to appreciate the importance of heart disease and cancer as causes of death and disability in the prewar period, they were reluctant to trespass on what they considered the preserves of private medicine, and they did little preventive work. Some of the larger health departments set up cardiovascular and cancer diagnostic units. A New York City clinic in 1947 offered a cancer diagnosis center, and some venereal disease (VD) clinics from 1956 offered routine testing for cervical cancer. Health departments also supported health education work in these areas carried out by private cancer and heart disease associations. In the United Kingdom, the epidemiological transition was in progress by the 1920s. Coronary heart disease (CHD) and cancer between them produced by 1921 the same mortality as infectious disease. Ten years later they were the major causes of adult mortality. In England and Wales, in 1922–84, life expectancy at birth for males rose from 55.6 to 71.6 years, and for females from 59.6 to 77.6 years. But this notable increase was due largely to a decline in infant mortality. For males aged forty-five, the increase in life expectancy in this period was a mere 3.5 years, while for females it was 6.7 years. Increases in the burden of chronic diseases, particularly CHD and cancer, were responsible for constraining the improvement in middle-age life expectancy. Indeed, in the 1930s, life expectancy of males aged forty-five years declined.[51] In Australia an epidemic of cardiovascular disease deaths began in the mid-to-late 1920s. Mortality increased quickly up to the mid-1950s; then the trend flattened—increasing slowly in males but falling slowly in females—till 1970, after which mortality for both sexes declined quickly. Female cancer mortality hardly changed between the 1900s and 1990. The stasis was the result of that fact that declines in stomach and uterine (including cervical) cancer were canceled out by increases in cancer of the lung, colon, pancreas and ovary. Male cancer mortality increased slowly to 1950 and then increased in a sustained way to the mid-1980s, after which it plateaued. It began to decrease in the late 1980s. The increase in male cancer mortality from the 1900s to 1990 is almost wholly due to increase in lung cancer deaths.[52]

Cardiovascular Disease

Russian work in the early twentieth century on animals fed diets heavy with saturated fat and cholesterol showed that such food produced fatty deposits in the linings of arteries—atherosclerotic lesions—and that increased blood cholesterol levels were associated with these lesions. But if fed diets heavy with unsaturated fats, animals developed little atherosclerosis. Many later studies confirmed the relationship between cholesterol and atherosclerosis. But thrombosis that causes clinical complications and CHD does not necessarily follow on atherosclerosis, so the incidence of clinical CHD is determined by factors producing atherosclerosis and factors producing thrombosis. As the wealth of Western countries increased in the twentieth century, so too did the incidence of CHD rise. It seemed to be a disease of affluence. Mortality rose markedly as per capita incomes rose after the Second World War. But in 1970–85 in England and Wales, and other West European countries, mortality declined quite sharply, although economic growth continued. Similar declines took place in other economically advanced countries like the United States, Australia, New Zealand, Canada and Japan.[53] The determinants of variations in CHD mortality are still open to debate. I will discuss the respective roles of culture, genetics, health care, nutrition, smoking and socioeconomic factors later; I turn now to the collective response to the fast-rising CHD mortality in the 1940s, '50s and '60s.

In 1945 in the United States, publicly donated funds for control of heart disease (three cents for each case) were miniscule compared with those raised for poliomyelitis (ninety-four dollars), tuberculosis (twenty-two dollars) and cancer (eight dollars). By the late 1940s, the American Heart Association (AHA) was running a powerful publicity campaign. Newspapers, radio and magazines were identifying heart disease as a major health problem. The AHA was able to provide fifty million dollars for research in 1948–60. Federal funds were also forthcoming. In 1948, the National Heart Institute (which became the National Heart and Lung Institute in 1969, and the National Heart, Lung and Blood Institute in 1977) was established. Its funding increased at a steady pace until the 1960s. At a time of strong support for medical research, in 1954–61, funding grew from fifteen to eighty-seven million dollars. By the middle to late 1950s, the print media were widely reporting claims about the relationship between high blood cholesterol and heart disease. A New York nutritionist was reported in *Time* magazine in 1956 as saying, "No prudent person who has had, or wishes to avoid, coronary heart disease should eat a high-fat diet of the type consumed by most Americans."[54]

The emerging issue of cholesterol and heart disease reinvigorated the war between manufacturers of butter and margarine. At the end of 1959, the FDA publicly stated that a causal relationship between CHD and blood cholesterol levels had been established. A year later, the AHA somewhat reluctantly supported dietary changes to reduce cholesterol levels in high-risk patients as a means to prevent heart attacks. The AMA Council on Foods and Nutrition made similarly cautious recommendations, warning that dietary changes should only be made under medical supervision. In mid-1964, the AHA publicly recommended that the whole population lower its fat consumption, while at the close of 1965 the AMA Council on Foods and Nutrition recommended to physicians that modification of diet be viewed as a means of prevention for young men vulnerable to coronary heart disease. The AMA admitted that there was still no "definitive proof" of the cholesterol hypothesis. Both the AMA and the AHA were basing their stands on epidemiological data suggesting a relationship between cholesterol levels and risk of heart disease. The long-running Framingham Heart Study used cholesterol levels to group subjects, then compared rates of heart disease in different groups so that relative risk for different levels could be calculated. By 1962, as a result of the study findings, it was being widely asserted that as levels of serum cholesterol grew from low to high, risk increased more than five times, and that a 1 percent difference in serum cholesterol was associated with a 2.66 percent difference in risk at all levels of serum cholesterol.

Researchers were eager to carry out a large-scale, definitive study to test the cholesterol hypothesis, but a National Heart and Lung Institute task force was against a purely dietary study, proposing instead a multiple-risk-factor intervention trial—MRFIT—to test whether reduction of smoking, high blood pressure and high cholesterol would bring down CHD mortality. Planning of the MRFIT study commenced in 1971, and the results were published in 1982: mortality in the intervention and control groups did not differ. But this "disappointing" result was explained by risk-factor change in the control group—the men in both groups had changed their behavior, and this reduced risk of heart attack. Concurrent with the MRFIT study was the Lipid Research Clinics Coronary Primary Prevention Trial (LRC-CPPT). The principal investigator was quoted as saying in 1984 that the trial had indisputably shown that lowering cholesterol with diet and drugs could reduce the risk of heart disease and heart attack. High-risk subjects—middle-aged males whose cholesterol levels placed them in the top 5 percent of the population distribution—had been chosen for the intervention group. But to establish a substantial difference in cholesterol levels of the control and intervention groups (after intervention), the investigators decided against relying on diet change to lower cholesterol in the intervention group and instead to employ cholestyramine, a cholesterol-lowering drug. At the conclusion of the trial those taking the drug manifested less heart disease, but the statistical difference between the intervention and control groups was only marginally significant.

The LRC-CPPT investigators, having decided that the cholesterol-lowering effect of diet change alone would be inadequate for the trial, nonetheless argued that their results supported the use of dietary treatment in most age groups. They proposed that the population over two years of age reduce dietary fat consumption and that the estimated 25 percent of the national population with cholesterol levels placing them at moderate to high risk of heart disease follow medically supervised diets (with or without drugs). A National Cholesterol Education Program was launched. Awareness of the relationships between dietary fat, cholesterol and heart disease has now become widespread in the United States, as in other affluent countries. From the late 1970s, the well-to-do middle classes were caught up in a healthy-lifestyle movement, whether as aficionados of jogging, aerobic and weights workouts, or the Pritikin or other special diets. Health policy makers, as we have seen, eager to contain the rocketing costs of health care, were only too pleased to reinforce the idea of lifestyle modification to control chronic diseases and therefore supported individual responsibility for prevention of CHD through cholesterol reduction.[55]

Inspired by the example of the AHA—a body of cardiologists from 1924 and, as we have seen, a community organization from 1948—and by the Canadian Heart Foundation (1956), a small group of Sydney doctors, lawyers and businessmen met in July 1958 with the trustees of the R.T. Hall Trust (which had funded TB treatment since 1909 but was looking for a new role, with TB fast receding as a health problem), the NSW health minister and the chairman of the NSW Health Commission. The group decided to invite other states to join them to form the National Heart Foundation of Australia. Dr. (later Sir) Kempson Maddox, a Sydney cardiologist, had already persuaded the trust to provide funds for a foundation that would promote better treatment and prevention of heart disease. As a first step, Dr. Paul White, an eminent Boston cardiologist and leading member of the AHA, had been invited in June to Australia to lecture for the Cardiac Society of Australia and New Zealand (established in 1951 as the Australasian Cardiac Society). There he had publicly urged establishment of an organization to control heart disease. He also had won the support of the prime minister, Robert Menzies.

Early in 1959 the prime minister opened a meeting of state delegates, chaired by Professor A.H. Ennor of the Australian National University's John Curtin School of Medical Research. The meeting resolved that there should be a National Heart Foundation (NHF), with divisions in each state and headquarters in Canberra. From the outset the NHF had a threefold objective: funding of research and research training, education of the community and of doctors, and a rehabilitation program to reduce unnecessary cardiac invalidism. (Special clinics were created for the latter purpose; they were phased out in the 1970s as their approach was adopted by mainstream health services.)[56] Almost $4.7 million was raised in the first public appeal; the bulk of it was invested. A second appeal for funds was made in 1969, and $1.7 million was received in donations. Continuous fund-raising began in 1970. Research was by far and away the main area of foundation expenditure, with education and rehabilitation bringing up the rear. By the late 1960s, two-thirds of the budget (about four hundred thousand dollars per annum) was being spent on research. Grants-in-aid had been made to 134 research projects for periods between one and eight years; six senior research fellows, twenty-two research fellows, seventeen overseas research fellows and forty-two research assistants were funded; and forty-three overseas travel grants and twenty other travel grants were provided. By 1975, $600,000 was being spent on research grants and $315,000 on education and rehabilitation, of which education received about two-thirds. The foundation's total annual expenditure rose from $257,000 in 1962 to $3.3 million in 1979.[57]

The foundation followed a medical approach to prevention, the primary target being high-risk cases. Its community education program encouraged regular visits to the doctor for routine health assessments and urged high-risk patients to modify their risk factors, under medical supervision—through weight reduction, increased physical activity, reduction of blood lipids, reduction of blood pressure and cessation of smoking. From 1962 to 1988, a news bulletin, *National Heart News*, was produced three to four times a year for health professionals and the community. In 1966, the NSW division initiated "Heart Week" involving a week-long radio, television, newspaper and periodical campaign with a scientific and educational exhibition in the Sydney town hall at its center. So successful was the program that it was taken up nationally from 1968. The foundation also sponsored occasional publications like the cookbook *Polyunsaturated Cookery,* launched by the prime minister's wife, Mrs. Margaret Whitlam, in 1974. After 1973, when a decision was made to increase community education about risk-factor reduction and other matters, expenditure on education was increased to provide for "education officer units" in the state and national divisions. That account rose from $111,000 in 1973 to $884,000 in 1980. In 1982 Ross Hohnen, secretary of the Australian National University, reviewed the educational activities of the foundation. After pointing out that the history of health education in Australia had been one predominantly of brief initiatives with no long-term commitment of resources, little attempt to evaluate results and no follow-up, he claimed the foundation's promotional activities had been so successful that they had encouraged governments themselves to expand health promotion programs.[58]

In the course of the 1980s, the foundation conducted three risk-factor-prevalence surveys. They revealed declines in smoking and high-blood-pressure prevalence, as well as the fact that hypertension was better controlled. But the third survey, in 1989, showed no significant decline in blood cholesterol levels, despite the intense education programs run by the foundation and other bodies over a considerable period of time. Physical activity was found to have increased, but so had body weight in men and women. Indeed, the lack of improvement in lipid patterns may reflect the increase in the numbers of overweight people. Australia's meat consumption remained high in the postwar era, in line with historical trends and despite massive immigration from parts of the world where meat was traditionally a much smaller aspect of diet. Apparent annual consumption of meat per capita was virtually the same in 1976–79, at 100.6 kilograms, as in 1936–39, at 101.5 kilograms. Since 1981–82, however, high beef prices had pulled consumption down. Where poultry had been in the nineteenth and earlier twentieth centuries expensive, mass production from the 1960s made it relatively cheap protein food, with consumption per capita rising from 5.2 kilograms in 1964–65 to twenty-one kilograms in 1984–85. The ratio of saturated to polyunsaturated fat in beef is four to one, where in chicken it is almost one to one. Consumption of fish (which has much less fat than does beef) increased from 2.7 kilograms per capita in 1936–39 to 3.7 kilograms in 1984–85. Cheese, which represents another alternative to red meat as a source of protein, became more popular, partly because immigrants introduced a great variety of cheeses other than the traditional cheddar. Where in 1936–39 apparent annual consumption per capita was a mere 2 kilograms, in 1984–85 it was 8.1 kilograms.

Australians were great consumers of butter before World War II, in 1936–39 consuming per capita 14.9 kilograms of butter but only four hundred grams of table margarine. In 1963, the first polyunsaturated margarine, "Miracle," was marketed; it was intended particularly for cardiac patients. Once South Australia permitted uncontrolled production of margarine from 1976, quotas on production, which the dairy industry had so tenaciously defended, were no longer operative. By 1984–85, apparent annual per capita consumption of butter had fallen to 3.9 kilograms, while that of table margarine (mostly polyunsaturated) was 6.7 kilograms, and of other margarine 2.3 kilograms. A 1975 survey of households in Sydney and Melbourne found that 66 percent believed margarine was good for their health, while only 55 percent thought butter was so. The meat pie, with its poor-quality meat and heavy saturated fat and salt content, had been a traditional Australian fast food. In the 1950s the Chiko roll (meat, barley, vegetables and onion in pastry, deep fried) became a popular competitor food. But from the late 1960s, American fast-food companies colonized the local market—from 1968 Kentucky Fried Chicken, and from 1971, Pizza Hut and McDonald's. The salt content in their products was high. Fat was the source of 30–40 percent of energy in a pizza, 42 percent in a hamburger, and 55 percent in Kentucky Fried Chicken. These fast-food chains did introduce some changes after nutritionists' criticisms of their products. Salads were provided at Pizza Hut; McDonald's fortified its flour with thiamin, riboflavin, niacin and iron, and its outlets made available orange juice and whole-wheat buns. In the course of the 1980s, in urban areas, eating habits changed quickly. Where at the start of the decade perhaps 25 percent of each dollar spent on food went to pay for carry-outs and meals consumed outside the home, by 1986 30 percent was going for food not prepared at home.[59]

Among Australians aged between twenty and sixty-nine years, in the period from the late 1960s to 1993 CHD mortality declined by 66 percent and stroke mortality by more than 70 percent; for those over seventy years, the figures were 49 percent and 54 percent respectively. These impressive drops appear to have been the result of declines in both incidence and case fatality rates. WHO's Multinational Monitoring of Trends and Determinants in Cardiovascular Disease (MONICA) study has centers in Perth and Newcastle. Perth data for 1971–88 suggest that declining incidence alone accounted for declining CHD mortality until 1976, after which case survival rates also contributed to the fall. Newcastle reported falling male incidence in the latter half of the 1980s but also falling total case fatality and in-hospital case fatality of patients who survived at least one hour from onset of symptoms. Thus prevention and treatment contributed to the decline in CHD mortality, although the precise contribution of each is unclear. Even more unclear are the precise respective contributions of health promotion and education, and lifestyle modification, on the one hand, and clinical interventions on the other. Thrombolytic therapy and prescription of aspirin regimens became considerably more common in 1984–90. By the end of this period about one-third of patients were undergoing the former. Where 4,235 coronary bypass operations and eleven angioplasty procedures were performed in Australia in 1980, 14,600 operations and 8,300 procedures were carried out in 1993.

In international comparative terms, Australia was doing reasonably well. In 1993, for twenty-eight countries with the highest CHD death rates for twenty-five to seventy-four-year-olds, that country was located among the lower 50 percent of countries, lower than the United Kingdom, the United States and New Zealand, but much higher than France and Japan. For stroke mortality, Australia was located among the lowest-ranking countries of the group, although well above Switzerland. There is room for improvement from other perspectives as well. Heart attack and stroke combined account for twice as many premature deaths as lung and breast cancer combined; five times as many as traffic accidents. Moreover, CHD mortality disproportionately impinged on the socially and economically disadvantaged, being higher for the less educated and for blue-collar workers than for the better educated and for white-collar workers. Cardiovascular mortality rates among young and middle-aged Aboriginal adults were between ten and twenty times those of non-Aboriginals.[60]

Variations in CHD mortality thus occur between socioeconomic groups within countries. But they also occur between countries. Differences in heredity partly explain differences among individuals within a national population—not, however, substantial differences between populations. The fact that CHD mortality declined in the United States by 48 percent in 1970–85 indicates that social and cultural rather than genetic factors have impact on CHD; gene frequencies would not change at such a pace. Quality medical care may help improve CHD death rates and may explain some of the variation among First World countries; where Japan and Britain in 1990 spent 6.5 and 6.1 percent of gross domestic product on health care, the United States spent 12.4 percent, and Canada and a number of European nations spent 8 to 9 percent. Yet the countries spending much more than Japan reported greater CHD incidence and lower life expectancy. Moreover, Japan, which at the start of the 1950s had the highest mortality (of a group of countries including the United States and England/Wales) from causes susceptible to medical interventions, manifested the greatest decline by 1980. But it also manifested by the late 1960s a marked decline from causes not susceptible to medical measures. Quality medical care, therefore, does not account for this marked and speedy fall in mortality.

Greater intake of polyunsaturates in the United States from the 1960s (and in Britain from the 1970s) may well have contributed to the fall in CHD mortality. High intake of saturates may have underpinned the great prevalence of CHD at mid-century. However, since saturated fat consumption may well have been high in the United States for a previous half-century, other factors operating in combination may have been necessary to produce the epidemic of CHD peaking around mid-century. Increased prevalence of smoking appears to be one such factor, especially as lung cancer rose at the same time as CHD did. Certainly, smoking was very prevalent in Japan in the late 1980s. But offsetting that was a low fat diet. In Japan, the ratio of polyunsaturates to saturates was one to one; in Britain one to three; 25 percent of the Japanese diet but 42 percent of the British was fat. Diet thus balanced smoking, but other factors have to be invoked to account for the substantial 38 percent decline in CHD in Japanese men in 1970–85.

Life expectancy in Japan outstripped Britain's in the two decades from 1965 at the same time as the former's economic performance raced ahead of that of Britain—high economic growth but low inflation and little unemployment. But superior economic growth may not be a sufficient explanation. Rather, as Wilkinson has shown from an international perspective, the correlation between life expectancy and income is firmer with measures of national income distribution than with per capita gross national product alone. Among the countries of the Organization for Economic Cooperation and Development (OECD), Japan enjoyed not only one of the largest gross national products but manifested the narrowest differentials between people at the top end of the income ladder and those at the lower end. The history of CHD in Japan suggests that lifestyle factors, such as nutrition and smoking, impact on CHD mortality, but in ways importantly influenced not only by national income but by narrow national income inequalities. In a later chapter I will return to the concern of contemporary public health workers with socioeconomic inequalities and health status.

Smoking and Lung Cancer

Male cancer mortality in Australia increased slowly from the 1900s to 1950, when a sustained linear increase began that lasted to the mid-1980s. The increase over the whole period was almost wholly due to increased lung cancer mortality. There was a plateau until the late 1980s, when it began to fall. Lung cancer remained in the 1990s the leading cause of cancer death in males, even though the death rate had fallen from a peak in the early 1980s of seventy per hundred thousand to fifty-six per hundred thousand. Male lung cancer mortality will very probably continue to fall, because of declining male smoking rates in the 1980s and 1990s. Since the 1960s, female lung cancer mortality has continued to rise, although the rate of increase has appeared to be slowing in recent years. Lung cancer has become the third most common cause of cancer mortality among women.[61]

Cancer mortality was also increasing in the United States in the first half of the twentieth century, rising from forty-eight thousand deaths in 1900 to 170,000 in 1950. Deaths reached 462,000 in 1985. Moreover, lung cancer deaths were growing more quickly than those from other cancers. They increased from 2.3 percent to 4.5 percent of cancer deaths in 1930–40; by 1950 they accounted for 15 percent. Cigarette consumption per adult per year was increasing as well. It rose from 1,485 in 1930 to 3,552 in 1950 in the United States, and from 1,380 to 2,180 in Britain. Consumption of tobacco per capita per year in Australia rose from 1.19 kilograms in 1903 to 1.59 kilograms in 1930, then dipped (because of the Depression) to 1.27 kilograms in 1934. It was 1.41 kilograms in 1945. It rose to 2.36 kilograms in 1955, peaked at 2.49 kilograms in 1960, and remained at 2.40 kilograms in 1970. Consumption of tobacco per adult per year declined by 48.7 percent between 1965 and 1993, from 3.35 kilograms to 1.72 kilograms. There was in the course of the century a trend toward preference for cigarettes over other forms of tobacco use in Australia. As a proportion of the weight of tobacco consumed, cigarettes were 10.9 percent in 1903, 28.3 percent in 1920, and 29.6 percent in 1930. These are factory-made cigarettes; the percentages would be much greater if figures on cigarettes rolled by smokers from cut tobacco were available. By 1967, factory-made cigarettes (and cigars) constituted 87.5 percent of tobacco consumed, with hand-rolled cigarettes making up 11.5 percent and pipe tobacco 1 percent. Where Australian consumption of tobacco per adult had been below that of Britain in the Depression years of the 1930s, it surpassed that of Britain in the affluent 1950s and 1960s. In a rank order of forty-seven countries, Australia was the eighth-largest consumer of tobacco per adult in 1965, climbing to seventh in 1973.[62]

Early Opposition to Tobacco Use

The Rev. Samuel Wesley had outlawed snuff and tobacco in his 1744 *Directions to the Band Societies,* but the Society of Methodists subsequently refrained from a general prohibition, although candidates for the ministry were supposed not to smoke. However, mainstream Christian churches in nineteenth-century Australia accepted that those who wished to smoke could do so. In the half-century beginning in the 1880s, perhaps the most prominent critics of smoking were members of the temperance movement. The Women's Christian Temperance Union (WCTU), translated to Australia from the United States in the 1880s, organized the first widespread antismoking campaigns in the 1890s, following the creation of an Anti-Narcotics Department by Jessie Ackermann, a visiting American temperance activist. The American WCTU had supported a Department for the Overthrow of the Tobacco Habit from 1895, and its publications were available in Australia. As well as seeking to educate the public and requiring from its members pledges not to smoke, the WCTU lobbied in all colonies and states to have antismoking legislation introduced. They began in South Australia in the mid-1890s. In the 1900s the WCTU argued against smoking on the grounds that it retarded growth in young people and promoted bad character traits. By the 1930s it was running arguments on both health and eugenic grounds: the adverse effect on the unborn child of women's smoking, and the weakening of the health of the future mothers of the "race." Other temperance bodies, like the Independent Order of the Good Templars, the Rechabites, and the Band of Hope, also campaigned against tobacco. Influenced by legislation passed in many American states in the 1890s, New South Wales passed juvenile-smoking legislation. Western Australia was the last state to do so, in 1917.

Cigarette smoking had become more popular after World War I, and temperance now faced the formidable task of attacking adult as well as juvenile smoking. In the 1920s, Methodists and Anglican evangelicals mounted a new campaign, led by Robert Hammond, a longtime Anglican clergyman of inner-city Sydney. The attack was multipronged, focusing on the cost, the dirtiness of the habit, and its aggravation of moral depravity and criminal tendencies. Young, sexually emancipated women smokers of the 1920s, "flappers," were particular targets. But Hammond went further, condemning smoking as harmful to health. Drawing on international literature like J.D. Rolleston's article in the *British Journal of Inebriety,* Hammond in 1932 discussed smoking and cancer. His ally, Francis Molesworth, a chemist, established the Non-Smokers League of Australia in 1933. This organization campaigned unsuccessfully to have smoking banned on public transport and in restaurants. Hammond was also allied with the Methodist-based Christian Anti-Smoking League, which was set up in 1936 and distributed antismoking leaflets to an apathetic, even hostile, public over the next two decades. By the 1940s, all drive had gone out of the temperance antismoking crusade. When the "crusade" was revived in the 1950s, it was led by health professionals. Yet historical associations with the moralism of the temperance movement served to give antismoking efforts a "killjoy" flavor. As the *Medical Journal of Australia* recognized in 1950, "fear of the label of 'crank'" initially discouraged medical opposition to smoking.[63]

In 1939, F.H. Muller had published the results of a case control study in Germany that showed an association between smoking and lung cancer. In the interwar period, studies in the United States and Britain also pointed to the involvement of tobacco in the aetiology of lung cancer. In 1931, in the United States, Frederick Hoffman had shown a connection between smoking and cancer, but his only response was to advise moderation in smoking. In 1938 Raymond Pearl showed that when the mortality of smokers and nonsmokers was compared it was clear that the former died earlier, but he did not offer an explanation. Surgeons Michael Bakey and Alton Ochsner connected smoking with lung cancer. Laboratory work done on animals showed that the constituents of tobacco were carcinogenic. However, conflicting results marked the research until 1950, when a series of epidemiological studies in the United States and Britain provided convincing evidence of an association between smoking and lung cancer. From being 1.1 percent of all cancers in the United States in 1920, lung cancer had risen to 2.2 percent in 1930 and 10 percent in 1956. In England, the incidence of lung cancer had increased thirty-eightfold between 1920 and 1954. In 1950, three successive reports of case control studies—the first by R. Schreck and others, the second by E.L. Wynder and E.A. Graham, and the third by M.L. Levin and others—provided evidence of the aetiological role of smoking in lung cancer. Indeed, a fourth study, a British one by Richard Doll and Austin Bradford Hill, gained in credibility because of the consistency of its results with those of the three American studies. This study, together with Doll's and Hill's national cohort study of doctors, proved to be a major force in shifting the paradigm on which epidemiological study of chronic disease was based from an intrinsic to an environmental causal model.

Doll and Hill showed that among doctors studied, the cancer death rate per hundred thousand population was, for nonsmokers, seven; for pipe smokers, thirty-eight; for pipe and cigarette smokers, sixty-eight; and for cigarette smokers, 125.[64] At the end of 1959, a WHO study group chaired by Doll concluded that "the sum total of the evidence available today was most reasonably interpreted as indicating that cigarette smoking is a major causative factor in the increasing incidence of human carcinoma of the lung." It rejected criticism of the evidence as not casting serious doubt on smoking as a causal factor.[65] By 1962 the Royal College of Physicians in Britain, and by 1964 the surgeon general in the United States, were publicly stating that smokers ran a great risk of serious ill health. In the course of the 1960s, tobacco control became part of the political agenda; a battle developed between the pro-tobacco cohorts—tobacco companies, tobacco producers, some government agencies and some consumers—and the antitobacco cohorts—health professionals, consumer pressure groups, and other government agencies. As in the case of alcoholic-beverage control, governments were pulled in opposite directions. On the one hand, they had a duty to promote the health of the people and protect them from dangerous substances. On the other, they enjoyed substantial revenues from taxes on tobacco products; in addition, politicians were sensitive about alienating

Table 2.5
Six Leading Multinational Tobacco Companies—Sales and Cigarette Output

Company	Sales in 1989 (U.S. dollars, million)	Cigarette Output in 1988 (billion)
Philip Morris	39,069	555
British American Tobacco	23,529	575
R.J. Reynolds	15,224	285
Imperial Tobacco	9,900	43
American Brands	7,265	90
Rothmans International	2,210	220

Source: J. Goodman, *Tobacco in History: The Cultures of Dependence* (London: Routledge, 1993), 11.

tobacco producers and people employed in that economically significant industry. Tobacco growing in the United States was very extensive; five hundred thousand people were employed in tobacco growing in 1987. Five of eight multinational tobacco companies were American, the rest European (see table 2.5). Their sales were huge.

Very large revenues flowed to governments from taxes on tobacco products: in 1983, in Britain, over eight billion dollars; in Germany, about seven billion; and in the United States (1986), $9.4 billion. Tobacco companies vigorously criticized the evidence that smoking was dangerous to health. They sought to cast the issues in terms of individual choice and freedom from authority.[66]

Official Action in Britain

In Britain the first government statement on the subject was issued by the Conservative health minister, Ian Macleod, in 1954. It stressed the problems of interpreting the data on smoking and lung cancer. The tobacco industry, which criticized the argument for causality, called for more research and gave the Medical Research Council 250,000 pounds for the purpose. The MRC report of 1957 concluded that given the epidemiological and laboratory evidence, smoking caused lung cancer. The *British Medical Journal* endorsed the position editorially. The government was forced into a response. A junior health minister stated that any health education program would be run by local government. This meant, in effect, that the government would leave it to the informed individual to protect himself or herself.

When by 1959 smoking prevalence continued to rise despite education, ministers considered but did not accept the idea of a special grant to promote public education through the Central Council for Health Education. The stand of those keen to see vigorous official action—such as the chief medical officer, Sir George Godber; the Central Health Services Council, and the Standing Medical Advisory Committee—was vindicated by the publication in 1962 of the report *Smoking and Health.* The report, which received a huge amount of publicity, declared that smoking was a major cause of lung cancer, bronchitis and, probably, heart disease. It proposed, besides public education, limits on tobacco advertising, tighter restrictions on sales to underage people, product modification to reduce harmful constituents, establishment of antismoking clinics and imposition of increased taxes on cigarettes. The MRC strongly endorsed the report. Ministers were divided, like their departments. Treasury maintained opposition to increased taxes and supported a libertarian position on intervention, whereas the Health Ministry wanted some restriction on cigarette advertising as well as more health education campaigns. Ministers could agree only to increase health education activities. The appearance of the U.S. surgeon general's report on smoking and health in 1964 forced the Conservative government to consider control measures introduced in America, like prohibition of TV advertising of cigarettes and restrictions on smoking in public places. Such action was rejected as involving too many difficulties in implementation. A private member's bill to require health warnings on cigarette packets was also rejected.

Harold Wilson led Labour into government in October 1964, ending thirteen years of Conservative rule. Labour only had a small majority of five seats in the House of Commons but went on to win a substantial majority in the general election of March 1966. Kenneth Robinson, whose father, a general practitioner in the north of England, had died prematurely, had been appointed health minister in the first Wilson government and had concentrated on health policy since entering Parliament in 1949. But health policy was not high on the agenda of the government, and Robinson was not now a member of the cabinet. In November 1968, the Departments of Health and Social Security were amalgamated under Richard Crossman, as secretary of state for social services. Robinson went to a junior ministerial post in housing and local government.

The tobacco industry had voluntarily restricted advertising on television before 9 P.M. since 1962. However, Robinson wanted a complete ban; the chancellor of the Exchequer opposed a ban. Treasury influence in the 1960s and 1970s in preventing introduction of really rigorous controls and largely confining government intervention to health education should not be underestimated. The tobacco tax represented a valuable economic regulator, because demand for tobacco was very inelastic. The health benefits of tobacco control had real economic costs, including larger pension outlays as retired people lived longer, smaller tax income, and more unemployment. Robinson managed to get a legislative ban on televised advertising in 1965. He was initially unable to get ministerial support for further restrictions but was then authorized to state publicly that legislation would be introduced banning cigarette coupon-gift schemes and restricting other promotions; limiting various types of advertising; and restricting spending on advertising. Having obtained grudging endorsement of legislation from his colleagues, he found progress stopped by Crossman, although publicly the government continued to maintain that it would legislate to limit advertising and promotion, and might support warning notices on cigarette packs. Unable to proceed in new directions, the health authorities pushed health education.

The Wilson Labour government lost the general election of 1970, an election in which the NHS did not figure as an important subject. Sir Keith Joseph, the new Conservative secretary of state for social services, responsible for the Department of Health and Social Security, wanted legislation that would include warnings on packs and advertisements; details of the chemical constituents of cigarettes on packs; and restrictions on sale of loose cigarettes, on vending machines, and smoking in public places, if the tobacco companies would not voluntarily accept such proposals. Treasury managed to prevent extra taxes on tobacco, proposed in an effort to reduce consumption.

The cause of the antismoking movement was advanced by the establishment of the pressure group "Action on Smoking and Health" (ASH) in 1971. The strength of the cause was growing among members of Parliament. Ministers were not keen, however, to endorse the legislative option, urging instead more discussions with the industry. The industry agreed that a warning that smoking can damage health should appear on packs, posters and advertisements; in turn, the government agreed it would not legislate, although it would press on with education and publicity opposed to smoking. When industry and independent experts could not cooperate on the task of deciding acceptable tar and nicotine levels and other technical questions, an Independent Scientific Committee on Smoking and Health was created to carry out the work.

Labour formed a minority government in early 1974 and remained in office until 1979. Barbara Castle, the new Labour secretary of state for social services, was a smoker, but Dr. David Owen, minister for state for health affairs, was strongly committed to further action against smoking. In early 1975 the industry rejected Owen's proposals for a levy on their profits to fund health education, restrictions on sports sponsorships, and abandonment of cinema advertising and coupon use. But it agreed to negotiate about stronger health warnings and information on tar content on packets, and it accepted control of its advertising code by the Advertising Standards Authority. Owen was eager to introduce legislation on sale, advertising and labeling, especially in the light of the introduction of tobacco substitutes. However, his colleagues insisted on continuing negotiations with the industry. These continued, with no significant outcomes.

David Ennals, the secretary of state from 1976, and R.D. Moyle, Owen's successor, came under growing pressure for more substantial action from the

Social Services and Employment Sub-Committee and bodies like the Royal College of Physicians and ASH. Yet again, ministers would not support legislation. Ennals had to negotiate from a weakened base. He won industry's agreement to the Independent Scientific Committee's voluntary overview of tobacco substitutes and additives; however, since both smokers themselves and antismoking groups rejected the latter "solution" to the health risks of smoking, it proved an empty gain. A small victory was industry agreement to a somewhat stronger warning on packets about damage to health and to voluntary reduction of advertising and of production of cigarettes with high tar content. The government promised a three-year moratorium on additional antismoking measures. The white paper "Prevention and Health" included a mere two of the Social Services and Employment Sub-Committee's proposals concerning smoking and health: restriction of sports sponsorship and nonsmoking areas in public locations.

Apart from government calls for voluntary curbs on smoking in public places in England and in Scotland, the antismoking movement was left to fight the tobacco industry on its own. The difference in resources was marked. Where about 330,000 pounds was spent on health education campaigns in 1975, seventy million pounds was spent by the tobacco industry on promotion. With the cost to the NHS of smoking-related morbidity at about a hundred million pounds per year by the end of the 1970s, however, the government was nudged forward by the growth of community support for stronger control measures. The results of a poll run by the *Sunday Times* published in early 1980 showed that 73 percent of people supported prohibition of advertising of cigarettes.[67]

Official Action in the United States

In the United States a study group on smoking and health had been set up in 1956 by the Public Health Service in cooperation with the American Heart Association and the American Cancer Society. Three years later, in an article in the *Journal of the AMA*, Surgeon General Leroy Burney stated, "The weight of evidence at present implicates smoking as the principal etiological factor in the increased incidence of lung cancer."[68] In 1962, Surgeon General Luther Terry established an Advisory Committee on Smoking and Health, which in just over a year reviewed about seven thousand expert publications put out since 1950. This was as much a political as a scientific exercise, because the tobacco industry had for some time dismissed the epidemiological evidence as "merely statistical" and unconfirmed by laboratory findings. Public health authorities saw that the epidemiology had to be accepted in medical and scientific circles as well as by the public. The committee was careful to acknowledge the complex questions around the issue of causality: "No member . . . used the word 'cause' in an absolute sense. . . . Although various disciplines and fields of scientific knowledge were represented among the membership, all members shared a common conception of the multiple etiology of biological processes. No member was so naïve as to insist upon mono-etiology in pathological processes or in vital phenomena."[69]

The 1964 Surgeon General's report found that for male smokers lung cancer mortality was 1,000 percent greater than for nonsmokers, while coronary heart disease incidence was seventy times greater. In the twenty-five years that followed, national smoking behavior was transformed—42 percent of American adults smoked in 1964, but only 26 percent did so in 1989. It was widely believed in the 1960s that having become informed of the dangers, Americans would quit or not take up smoking. However, the 1965 federal Cigarette Labeling and Advertising Act, which created the National Clearinghouse on Smoking and Health to promote health education, restrained the required warning on packs. Reliance on individual responsibility after education was a significant factor limiting official action. Further, the powerful tobacco lobby, particularly that of the tobacco growers, worked to minimize regulation. The influence of television was becoming enormous in the 1960s, as coverage of such events as John Kennedy's assassination and the Vietnam War attested. Not only were the advertising resources of the tobacco industry very great, but the Federal Trade Commission's capacity to require accountability was limited by inadequate regulations. Nonetheless a consumer lawyer, John Banzhaf III, who founded ASH, was able to exploit the fairness doctrine in the courts to win extensive free time for antismoking advertisements. Ultimately, the tobacco industry agreed to legislation prohibiting broadcast advertising. By the 1970s the federal government had in place antismoking measures—funding for education, warnings on packs and bans on broadcast advertising. These, however, were balanced by support for the tobacco industry through subsidies. Moreover, the tobacco industry was able to use effectively the high American valuation of individual freedom; government support for education was acceptable, but restrictions on behavior were not.

The emergence in the 1980s of data on the health dangers of "involuntary" or "passive" smoking proved to be a powerful counter to this individualism, and communitarian values were revivified. The 1986 *Surgeon General's Report* endorsed the material on passive smoking. Where only ninety local communities then had restricted smoking in public places, 320 had done so by 1988. From early 1990, a virtually complete ban on smoking on domestic aircraft was introduced. The appeal to the libertarian ethic and to freedom of choice was further undermined by the growing evidence of the addictive nature of smoking. The 1988 *Surgeon General's Report* raised the issue of addiction, which made more difficult the industry's established stance on smoking as an individual responsibility. It also fueled the case for compensatory damages to be paid by tobacco companies for disease and death associated with smoking. By 1990, cigarette smoking was estimated to be costing fifty-two billion dollars a year for health care and lost economic productivity. In addition to the economic cost, there was the human cost—about 390,000 deaths each year attributable to cigarette smoking.

The emphasis on individual risk and responsibility is at odds with the evidence that smoking is a socioeconomic and cultural phenomenon that is not simply a product of individual choice. Between 1974 and 1985, smoking prevalence among college graduates declined from 28 to 18 percent, whereas among those without a degree the fall was only from 36 to 34 percent. Also, in 1985, where 29 percent of whites were smokers, 35 percent of blacks smoked.[70]

Official Action in Australia

In the 1950s, the Australian medical profession was not united about the health risks of smoking. The *Medical Journal of Australia* in 1956 pointed out that lung cancer and heart disease were associated with smoking, and most medical practitioners advised against smoking. A year earlier, Sir Macfarlane Burnet, an internationally renowned medical scientist, drew attention to the health risks of smoking. Yet Sir Herbert Schlink, chairman of the Royal Prince Alfred Hospital, Sydney, and a senior medical "statesman," declared that the connection between lung cancer and smoking had not been proven. By the 1960s, however, doctors themselves were giving up smoking, advising patients not to smoke, and collectively calling for education and control measures. Surveys of doctors in 1964 and 1970 showed that cigarette smokers had declined from 26.8 to 20.5 percent and that nonsmokers had increased from 56.5 to 67 percent. A 1976 survey showed cigarette smokers to have declined further to 14 percent, while nonsmokers were 76 percent. In 1970, 35 percent of doctors routinely encouraged patients not to smoke; in 1976, 66 percent did so.

In October 1962, the Australian Medical Association (AMA), the Royal Australasian College of Physicians (RACP), the Royal Australasian College of Surgeon (RACS), the Australian College of General Practitioners and the Anti-Cancer Council of Victoria expressed support for the report of the Royal College of Physicians on smoking and health. They urged the federal government to introduce a health education program and to restrict advertising of tobacco products. In May 1962, the NHMRC had recommended that the commonwealth and states aim ultimately to prohibit all tobacco advertising and, in the meantime, prohibit advertising directed at younger people; that the states initiate publicity campaigns and health education to reduce smoking; that the states prohibit smoking in places subject to health and related legislation; and that the commonwealth, the Commonwealth Scientific and Industrial Research Organization and the tobacco industry together work out measures to reduce risks. In March 1964 the prime minister, Sir Robert Menzies, stated that the commonwealth and states had agreed that the best approach was education of the young and were ready to launch a campaign.

Health education remained the focus of government attention in the 1960s, despite growing demand from health professionals that wider action be taken.[71] In October 1965, the Australian Cancer Society brought together representatives of the AMA, RACP, RACS, Australian College of Pathologists, National Heart Foundation and National Tuberculosis and Chest Association to call upon the federal health minister. They proposed that the government restrict cigarette advertising, obtain survey information on the smoking behavior of young people, initiate an antismoking campaign, and support research on the cancer-causing capacity of tobacco. The commonwealth government, unlike the British government, refused to ban television advertising. Instead, it accepted a proposal, originating with the Federation of Commercial Television Stations, for a voluntary industry code on responsible advertising, which came into operation in 1966. The *Medical Journal of Australia* concluded in 1967 that this "pretentious" code was, when closely analyzed, "not worth a row of beans."[72] It called for the commonwealth to ban immediately all television advertising.

In the growing antismoking movement, two of the more influential organizations were the Victorian Anti-Cancer Council (ACC) and the Australian Council on Smoking and Health (ACOSH). Set up in 1936 to support research, the Victorian ACC, which relied upon public appeals and private donations, was independent of government funding. Its annual income rose from just under twenty thousand dollars in 1957 to $1.1 million twenty years later. The best endowed of the antismoking bodies, it was more prominent than the Australian Cancer Society, which had been formed in 1961 as a federation of state bodies. The Australian body carried out educational work, publishing eighty thousand copies of *Smoking and Your Health* in 1963 and providing schools with copies of *Smoking and You* in 1966. It also lobbied governments to educate the community and to control advertising.

Dr. Cotter Harvey, a NSW specialist in chest diseases, had first been convinced of the health risks of smoking after listening to Dr. Alton Ochsner at the 1948 conference of the American Thoracic Society. He set up ACOSH in 1966, in part inspired by the example of the Interagency Council on Smoking and Health, established in the United States in 1964. Like the Interagency, ACOSH brought together government agencies and health pressure groups. The NSW Health and Education Departments had representatives on ACOSH. Commonwealth departments were not represented. But medical bodies like the AMA and health pressure groups like the National Heart Foundation were the core of ACOSH, which, unlike the temperance bodies of the earlier antismoking movement, was secular and medical in outlook. ACOSH established state branches in Tasmania (1966), Western Australia (1971) and South Australia (1973) but did not bother in Queensland, because the Health Education Council there was already working hard on smoking and health, or in Victoria, where the ACC already occupied the field.

Cotter Harvey was a determined lobbyist, even in the face of government passivity. In late 1971 he headed a deputation of thirteen medical and three national health bodies to ask the federal Liberal health minister to introduce measures called for in WHO resolutions of May 1970. Unable to advance the cause of tobacco control, he resigned from the Liberal Party, blaming lack of progress on its unwillingness to alienate the tobacco industry.

While state and federal governments, then, were reluctant to go beyond education campaigns, some local authorities took action. Bankstown Municipal Council in Sydney in 1968 erected posters warning of the risks of smoking. Ten years later, the NSW Local Government Association supported North Sydney Council's ban on a large neon advertisement for cigarettes in its area. Sydney City Council refused to allow advertising on council property.[73]

Although community opinion in the course of the 1960s was increasingly ready to accept that smoking was a health risk, leading Liberal-Country Party government figures remained unconvinced. The federal treasurer, Billy Snedden, wanted proof in 1971 that smoking caused heart disease and lung cancer. Other Liberals, while ready to accept that smoking was dangerous to health, saw it as a matter of education and individual responsibility, not restrictive legislation. They were in any case reluctant to pay the political price of antagonizing the tobacco lobby.

Concerned about survey evidence of smoking by schoolchildren, the NHMRC in 1969 proposed warnings on cigarette packets, control of advertising, and a national campaign about the dangers of smoking. Dr. Gwyn Howells, the commonwealth director general of health from 1973, spoke out more than his predecessor had about the health risks, addressing the issue at length in his annual report of 1974–75. The Senate Standing Committee on Social Welfare, in an initiative unusual for inquiries into drug abuse at this time, investigated tobacco and alcohol—the legal drugs—in its inquiry into drug abuse problems in Australia in the late 1970s. In 1980, the Fraser Liberal-National Party government decided to implement some of the committee's recommendations: to seek to reduce tobacco consumption per head; to lower tar and nicotine yields and to have tar and nicotine content stated on packets (introduced in 1982); and to control smoking in commonwealth offices and public places. It did not implement proposals to reduce consumption by 2 percent per year for five years, to increase taxes to discourage smoking, or to control corporate and perimeter advertising and sports sponsorships. Nor did it withdraw funding from research into tobacco cultivation.

Except for 1972–75, when the Whitlam Labor government was in office, conservative governments were in power at the federal level from 1949 to 1983. The AMA, though known for its own generally conservative approach to politics and social affairs, had become frustrated by the reluctance of conservative administrations to advance tobacco control. In 1979, the AMA not only supported the proposals of the Senate Select Committee but advanced some of its own—prohibiting vending machines, taxing cigarettes by tar content, levying a tax on cigarettes to finance a public education campaign, prohibiting sales to children, and making the cost of cigarette promotion no longer tax deductible.

Some individual doctors protested smoking by defacing billboards advertising cigarettes. Thus, Dr. Josephine Kavanagh, a Melbourne radiologist, was fined for writing on a Marlboro poster, "coffin nails" and "Come to Cancer Country." In 1979, the Movement Opposed to the Promotion of Unhealthy Products (MOPUP) was established at the University of Sydney, with some prominent medical and political figures as members. It called for prohibition of all advertising and sports promotion. MOPUP members were involved in a successful complaint to the Advertising Standards Council that the appearance of actor Paul Hogan (who enjoyed high regard among children) in advertising of Winfield cigarettes breached the voluntary advertising code. Billboard Utilizing Graffitists Against Unhealthy Promotions (BUGA UP) was started by a graphic artist, Bill Snow, in 1979; its members defaced poster advertisements for a range of "objectionable" products, including cigarettes. Billboards with advertisements involving the "Marlboro Man," a cowboy figure, had the slogan "The World Is My Ashtray" attached to them. The Outdoor Advertising Association mounted an advertising campaign against the Billboard Utilizing Graffitists, branding them as criminals, but the courts generally dealt sympathetically with members of BUGA UP who came before them. With Cotter Harvey's retirement, ACOSH declined in the late 1970s, although the South Australian branch was reactivated in 1980 and induced the State Transport Authority to end advertising on its buses, trains and billboards. In 1982 a private member's bill prohibiting advertising of tobacco products almost passed through the lower house of the South Australian Parliament.

Medical and lay groups in the antismoking movement continued to pressure governments and to transform public perceptions of smoking. In Sydney, the Non-Smokers Movement, established in 1977, was particularly interested in controlling smoking in public venues. It persuaded the NSW government to ban smoking in elevators and to allow taxi drivers to prohibit smoking in their cabs.

For many years, the NSW railways set aside only 25 percent of cars as nonsmoking. In 1973, the number was raised to 50 percent, and four years later, no smoking at all was permitted. Other states pursued the same path. Where in 1974 Australia's international airline, Qantas, had no nonsmoking area, by 1978 it allowed smoking in only 40 percent of seats. Ansett (then a leading internal airline) went from no nonsmoking seats in 1972 to 70 percent ten years later. Individual states undertook education of the public;

Western Australia ran a campaign as early as 1957. School education programs became common in most states during the 1960s. But the federal Liberal-Country Party government refused in 1964 to provide funds for public education, arguing it was a state responsibility.

Some in the extraparliamentary Liberal Party were becoming dissatisfied with the lack of action by Liberal administrations. In 1972, some Liberal backbench members of the federal Parliament pressured the McMahon government to introduce new measures. Legislation was passed requiring television and radio advertisements to carry a three-second spoken warning that smoking is a health hazard. Responding to longtime recommendations by the NHMRC and the Conference of Federal and State Health Ministers, the McMahon government also provided in 1972 half a million dollars per year for three years for an antismoking media campaign. In these years, tobacco companies were spending about eleven million dollars a year on advertising.

By the beginning of 1974, when the national campaign had reached the halfway point, just over 69 percent of people knew of the campaign. National surveys showed that smokers who in the previous year had tried to give up smoking had increased from 61 in 1972 to 67.2 percent in 1974. Various local initiatives were also taking place across Australia. ACOSH and Rotary sponsored a "No Smoking Week" in 1973 in the large country center of Bathurst, NSW. They were following the lead of campaigners in Longnor, England, in 1970, and Mauriac, France, in 1972. The NSW health authorities in early 1979 initiated a healthy-lifestyle campaign in some northern country centers. Lismore had community and media programs; Coffs Harbour, media; and Tamworth acted as a control. Although cigarette advertising had increased markedly in Lismore, by 1981, the year the campaign ended, the number of smokers had declined in Tamworth by 4.5 percent, in Coffs Harbour by 8 percent, and in Lismore by 12 percent. In 1983 the first mass media QUIT campaign took place. Western Australia, NSW, Victoria and South Australia ran campaigns each year, using media-based and other strategies. Paid television advertising formed much of the mass media effort, but radio was also used, especially to reach non-English-speaking people. Efforts more recently have become directed at specific populations like Aborigines, Torres Strait Islanders, and non-English-speaking immigrants.

Tobacco consumption (annual per adult), which had risen from 1.8 kilograms in 1945 to 3.5 kilograms in 1960, declined by 48.7 percent between 1965 and 1993, falling from 3.35 to 1.72 kilograms. But from 1965 to 1975, annual consumption continued virtually unchanged. This plateau was probably a reflection of the lack of government action. Certainly, after 1977 (the year after a national ban on radio and television advertising) the average annual drop was 2.5 percent, and from 1983, when the first mass media QUIT campaign began, the fall increased to a mean of 3.1 percent per year.[74]

According to a Gallup poll in 1962, 21 percent of people supported absolute prohibition of cigarette advertising. Ten years later, the number had climbed to 39 percent. Not only did the federal government fail to keep up with public opinion, it failed to keep pace with other Western countries. As we have seen, Britain banned advertising of cigarettes on television as early as 1965. The United States followed in 1971, West Germany in 1973, Norway in 1975 and Australia in 1976. In 1972 Labor, as the opposition, had failed to have a ban introduced, but in government it legislated to end advertising. Its successor, the Fraser Liberal-National Party government, resisted the tobacco lobby's push to negate the ban. While direct advertising on radio and television was phased out in 1976–77, "incidental" advertising (television reporting on sporting or cultural events sponsored by a tobacco company) continued, although sponsorship bans have much reduced this indirect form of advertising. Advertising in the print media was prohibited in legislation of 1989. Remaining forms, like billboards and illuminated signs, were prohibited from the end of 1995. A 1969 poll had revealed 80 percent support for health warnings on cigarette packets, and in the same year the Health Ministers' Conference agreed to the proposal. But NSW, where about 60 percent of cigarettes were made, had held back; Sir Robert Askin, the premier, would not heed the advice of his health minister, A. H. Jago. Victoria and Western Australia, however, decided to proceed. In late 1972, NSW finally passed the requisite legislation. Victoria, Tasmania, South Australia, Western Australia and the two territories required warnings from the start of 1973, while NSW and Queensland required the same from mid-1973. Tobacco was heavily taxed, at 50 to 60 percent of the retail price; governments refused to risk the wrath of the electors by adding a health tax to an already heavily taxed product.

The Australian Labor Party Conference in 1977 committed the party in office to imposing differential taxes on low- and high-tar cigarettes. The AMA urged in 1982 a drastic increase in excise, the revenue from which would be used for health promotion purposes. But in this era even Labor governments were reluctant to take this path to reducing consumption, because it would penalize disproportionately low-income earners or threaten jobs in the tobacco industry. In 1987, the Victorian Labor government imposed a wholesale tax on tobacco products to fund programs of the Victorian Health Promotion Foundation, VicHealth, promoting health and preventing disease and disability. Governments in some other jurisdictions followed suit: Foundation SA (South Australia) in 1988, the Australian Capital Territory Health Promotion Fund in 1989, and Healthway in Western Australia in 1991. These bodies were intended to provide funds for sponsorship of sports and cultural activities, replacing tobacco companies. Two years after VicHealth entered the field, sport in Victoria had become almost free of tobacco company sponsorship. The main football codes in Victoria and Western Australia followed smoke-free policies at venues, while community support for smoking restrictions at cultural and other sports venues was increasing.

The smoking rate of adult males has consistently declined, from 75 percent in 1945 to 28 percent in 1992. The decline for adult women is not nearly so impressive—an estimated 26 percent in 1945, rising to 33 percent in 1976, from when there was a slow decline to 24 percent in 1992. The National Drug Strategy from the mid-1980s helped promote the visibility of smoking as a health issue, but most campaigns have been at the state level; and legislative and regulatory interventions have not in the main sprung from a coordinated, national policy. As we have seen, a range of nongovernment and government organizations have acted at national, state and local levels. Health professionals, especially doctors, have played a leading part in the long campaign to educate the public and persuade governments to take action.[75]

Traffic Accidents

Traffic crashes are responsible worldwide for around one million deaths a year, not a large source of mortality compared with heart disease or cancer. In economically advanced countries like the United States or Australia, the largest amount of mortality relates to young men, a fact associated with the frequency of risk taking, such as drinking and driving, and with the level of car ownership in this subpopulation. The risk of death has declined over the last three decades, in part at least because of public health and safety measures, as well as better vehicle design, road improvements and more effective trauma management. Control of speeding, better pre-licence training, drunk-driving measures (especially random breath tests), and compulsory seat-belt wearing have been reinforced by health education and mass media campaigns.

In 1965, the *Medical Journal of Australia* said that traffic accidents had reached "alarming proportions." Deaths rose from twenty-five per hundred thousand population in 1952 to a peak of 30.4 in 1970 but fell to 19.1 in 1985. They fell further to 11.1 in 1994. The decline from 1970 took place in the face of a virtual doubling of the amount of road travel, and it occurred particularly rapidly in the early 1990s. Indeed, in 1989–94 road deaths fell 31 percent. Alcohol abuse was a major factor in the deaths on the roads. L.R.M. Drew proposed in the late 1970s that about 50 percent of deaths over the previous twenty-five years had been alcohol related.[76]

Australia is approximately the size of mainland United States (without Alaska), but it has only 8 percent of the population of America. Very dependent on road transport, Australia possesses an extensive road system, the maintenance of which is supported by comparatively few taxpayers. Moreover, historically, Australian culture has tolerated heavy consumption of alcoholic beverages. The decline in road traffic accidents in the last three decades has been in a period of both economic growth and some recession, so that the decline has not been primarily due to a fall in travel consequent on reduced economic activity. The public health and safety measures taken by federal and state governments must be credited with a good deal of the responsibility for lowering the death rate over the last thirty years.

As early as the late 1930s, drunk driving was beginning to be seen by health and legal professionals in Australia as a problem. In 1942, the NSW branch of the BMA convened a symposium on "driving under the influence [of alcohol]." Speakers included a barrister, a police sergeant, and a psychiatrist from Royal Prince Alfred Hospital, Dr. John McGeorge. McGeorge pointed out that reliable medical diagnosis of "under the influence" was difficult. Indeed, "a correct diagnosis can be reached only after considering a combination of several observations, including the general demeanour, the state of the clothing, the manner of walking, sitting down and rising, the ability to pick up small objects from the floor and the presence of hiccup." In the same year, a Brisbane doctor, N.M. Gutteridge, asked if the world war was being waged to keep Australia safe for the breweries, given the privileged position the alcohol industry had in government eyes because of the revenue it generated for the state, and the discreet donations it was making to party funds. He called for public education about the effect of alcohol on driving efficiency and asked whether it would be too much to expect of the "social sense" of the alcohol industry that it help with educating the public.[77]

Per capita consumption of alcohol rose steeply from the end of the Second World War to the early 1950s, more slowly from then to the early 1960s, and steeply again from the early 1960s to the early 1970s. Individual doctors in the 1950s pointed to the mounting drunk-driving problem in Australia. F.S. Hansman pointed out that in 1951 for forty-nine of the largest cities in the world, the average mortality rate from traffic accidents was 9.13 per hundred thousand population. Melbourne and Sydney headed the list, with rates of 22.4 and 21.7 respectively.

In the period from 1950 to the late 1970s, per capita consumption of alcohol and the death rate of males fifteen to twenty-four years old from motor vehicle accidents correlated closely, although other factors were influential, such as the fact that a growing number of young males were obtaining access to vehicles. There was a plateau in death rates that began a few years before the fall in per capita beer consumption. This probably reflected the introduction of compulsory use of seat belts as well as improvements in roads and vehicle designs. The downturn in death rates took place earlier among thirty-five to fifty-four-year-old males than in twenty-five to thirty-four-year-olds and teenage males, perhaps because the younger age groups would more likely be driving older cars, lacking newer safety features, and would be more

Table 2.6
Alcohol Consumption and Motor Vehicle Accident Rates, Australia, 1977

State/Territory	Alcohol, gms Daily per Person	Motor Vehicle Accidents per 100,000 People
NT	25.3	596
WA	16.2	520
NSW	13.3	564
Vic	12.4	388
Qld	11.9	360
SA	12.0	621
Tas	10.4	390
Australia	13.0	480

Source: A.J. McMichael and A.J. McLean, "Alcohol and Road Accidents in Australia: Corroborative Population-Based Evidence," *Community Health Studies* 4(3) (1980): 283.

likely to ride motorcycles, the use of which had become popular again in the 1960s.

Three jurisdictions were above the national average for alcohol consumption: the Northern Territory, Western Australia and NSW. Except for South Australia, the accident rate correlates with per capita daily alcohol consumption (see table 2.6). The accident rate for South Australia reflects different criteria applied to accident reporting and the fact that this state is the most urbanized.[78]

The federal Liberal-National Party governments of this era were not prepared to employ alcohol taxes to fund measures to reduce consumption in the interests of preventing traffic accidents. (As we have seen, they were equally reluctant to use tobacco taxes to finance measures to reduce consumption.) When the Liberal treasurer, William McMahon, was asked in 1968 to lower excise taxes on low-alcohol beer to reduce road casualties, he said he would look into the matter. Nothing happened, and the matter was raised again in federal Parliament in 1979 and 1982. The treasurer, John Howard, replied in 1982 that where excise had been lowered overseas, consumers showed no greater preference for low-alcohol beer. Likewise, in 1980, the federal government rejected a Labor proposal that in the Australian Capital Territory, where it had jurisdiction, a low or nil blood alcohol level be required of learner drivers and those driving paying-passenger or heavy commercial vehicles.[79]

Australia pioneered interventions to reduce traffic accidents. Within Australia, Victoria often led the way. In 1971, this state introduced legislation on compulsory use of seat belts, and within a year all states and territories had introduced such legislation. By the end of the 1970s, a number of European countries, the Soviet Union and some Canadian provinces had introduced compulsory seat-belt measures. The Victorian legislation followed rather than preceded achievement of community consensus in favor of the initiative. In contemporary educated, rights-conscious society, consensus about the need for such coercive measures must exist, or they may prove counterproductive, creating widespread contempt for the law. In 1963, the Bolte Liberal government in Victoria appointed a senior barrister, P.D. Phillips, royal commissioner to investigate the liquor law. Rather predictably, Phillips delivered a report that proposed liberalization of licensing laws. Legislation was introduced providing for 10 P.M. closing (to replace long-standing 6 P.M. closing) of licensed establishments. This was to apply from the beginning of February 1966. Phillips believed that total consumption of alcohol would not increase because of an extension of trading hours and that the number of traffic accidents would not grow. However, the change of closing time did alter the temporal distribution of accidents. Casualty-producing accidents doubled between 10 and 11 P.M., and halved between 6 and 7 P.M.

Victoria was the first jurisdiction to introduce compulsory use of the breathalyzer. The Phillips inquiry recommended that it be made illegal to drive with a blood alcohol level above 0.05 grams per hundred milliliters, and the measure was introduced in 1966. From 1974 all traffic-accident casualties entering hospitals in Victoria had to be blood-tested. South Australia had introduced the measure a year earlier. In 1976 the random breathalyzer testing of drivers by police was introduced in Victoria. NSW, Queensland and Tasmania followed Victoria in choosing the 0.05 blood alcohol level in the early 1980s. Other states and territories chose the 0.08 limit. Random breathalyzer testing (RBT) was introduced in the Northern Territory in 1980, in South Australia in 1981, in NSW in 1982, and in Tasmania and Western Australia in 1983. Queensland adopted it in 1986. Alcohol-related fatalities declined 36 percent in NSW and 42 percent in Tasmania in the three years after RBT was introduced. In 1982–85, all states adopted the blood-alcohol level of 0.02 or zero for new or young drivers.[80]

These measures were expanded over time. In 1976, it became a legal requirement that children and babies be effectively restrained in motor vehicles. Recent use of seat belts has been estimated to be 96 percent for front seats and 86 percent for back seats. The mandatory use of bicycle helmets was brought in between 1990 and 1992. Large-scale media campaigns were used to educate people before compulsion was introduced. Among Victorian children, use rates increased from 65 percent before compulsion to 77 percent (1992) after its introduction, and among adults from 36 percent (1990) to 84 percent (1992).

As for RBT, high visibility and heavy penalties appear to be behind its success. In 1993–94, Queensland had the greatest percentage of positive RBTs, 2 percent of drivers, while Victoria had the smallest, 0.15 percent. NSW and South Australia were 0.66 and 0.62 percent, respectively. Heavy penalties—loss of license and steep fines—have reduced drunk driving. Highly visible speed cameras on roads have been used to deter as well as detect, as with RBT. The success of anti-drunk-driving measures is shown by the fact that nationally, the percentage of fatally injured drivers and motorcyclists with a blood alcohol concentration of 0.05 or over fell from 44 in 1981 to 30 in 1995. But there have been marked differences between the jurisdictions. In the Northern Territory, known for its high consumption of alcohol, the percentage fluctuated from 77 in 1981 to 33 in 1988, to 77 in 1993. Moreover, the impact of speed-reduction measures may not be as great as would be liked. In a survey in the mid-1990s, 78 percent of respondents admitted they occasionally exceeded speed limits by ten kilometers per hour or more, although they strongly supported strict enforcement of speed limits in urban areas.

Federal and state governments have since the late 1980s put much funding into mass media campaigns pointing up the risks of speeding, drunk driving, and failure to wear seat belts. Indeed, since the 1992 National Road Safety Plan, while there are differences between the states in resources committed and in approaches, all accept that RBT, mass media campaigns, and control of speeding should be the primary foci in road safety. The federal Office of Road Safety in 1990–94 spent just under ten million dollars on maintaining a national database for road statistics and on research into behavioral issues, road engineering and vehicle safety standards. A number of research centers in the states have contributed to evaluation of road safety campaigns and development of best-practice principles. The Monash University Accident Research Centre, set up in 1987, has helped make Victorian evidence-based practice an exemplar in road safety for the other states. The Road Accident Prevention Research Centre, University of Western Australia, established in 1989, receives its funds from the Western Australian Health Department; South Australia has the Road Accident Research Unit at the University of Adelaide, which as early as the mid-1970s was receiving funding from the Federal Transport Department to investigate alcohol's role in road accidents. This is now funded by the NHMRC. Victoria is also host to the Australian Road Research Board, which is funded by the federal and state governments.

The safety of road vehicles themselves has increased in the last two decades or so. Features like air bags, antilock brakes, and ergometrically designed interiors are fast becoming standard in new vehicles. A set of safety standards, the Australian Design Rules, are being applied to Australian-made and imported vehicles to enhance crash-reduction safety and occupant protection. Design rules include minimum head-restraint heights on front seats and minimum side-door strength, energy-absorbing steering columns, and antiburst door locks and hinges. Road engineering improvements, including widening, intersection changes, and in urban areas, traffic-calming devices, have contributed importantly to the decline in mortality and morbidity.

Improvement of locations with bad accident records has been a particularly effective intervention. When Victoria spent an additional seventy-five million in 1992–94 to get rid of such locations, an estimated 4.8 percent decline in serious crashes resulted.

A multipronged approach to road safety has, historically, been the key to reduction of mortality and morbidity. A combination of legislation, publicity and strict enforcement has worked well. In Victoria, for example, in April–June 1990 the publicity campaign based on the slogan, "Don't Fool Yourself—Speed Kills," was run in concert with a speed-camera program. Melbourne saw a decline of 20 to 30 percent in casualty crashes in this period. Education and publicity campaigns were employed prior to legislation about seat-belt wearing, bicycle helmets and drunk driving. As far back as 1981, publicity campaigns concerning bicycle helmets were run in Victoria. In addition, subsidies for helmets and school education programs on bicycle safety were provided. The result was that 60 percent of children voluntarily wore helmets. Such a degree of acceptance made feasible introduction of compulsory use, after which compliance climbed to between 70 and 80 percent.

However, the number of road accidents remained unacceptably high. Recently the Australian Transport Council adopted the National Road Safety Strategy 2001–2010 and Action Plan 2001 and 2002. The aim of the Strategy is to bring down road deaths per hundred thousand population by 40 percent. The strategy and the action plan are complementary, the first setting objectives and the second detailing action by which to attain these objectives. Responding to the fact that alcohol abuse is a significant factor in 27 percent of fatal accidents, the action plan includes the following measures: extension of publicity and enforcement campaigns; punishments in drunk-driving cases proportional to the danger created; implementation of measures arising from the Australian Optimal Rural Drink Driving Enforcement Program; promotion of low-alcohol and nonalcoholic drinks and "responsible serving" in bars; introduction of alcohol ignition interlocks as options in sentencing regimes; promotion of voluntary fitting of alcohol interlocks; and encouragement of intelligence-based enforcement practices.[81]

Alcohol and Other Drugs

Historical trends in alcohol consumption in Australia reveal that consumption has tended to rise in times of economic prosperity and fall in times of economic contraction. The early colonists had a huge reputation for drinking to excess. But when viewed comparatively, their behavior does not seem so unusual. The colonists' consumption in 1800–20 was similar to that of their kin in Britain. It was probably somewhat larger by the 1830s, but it was significantly smaller than that of the U.S. population. In 1860–1900, Australian colonists consumed more wine than the people of the "Mother

Country," about the same volume of spirits, and a great deal less beer, although in the late nineteenth century Australia became the beer-drinking country of today. If we trace the long-term trend in per capita consumption of alcohol, there was from about 1855 a downward movement that reached its nadir in the economic depression of the early 1930s. It then rose steadily until the 1980s, when it declined somewhat.[82]

The earliest attempt to control inebriety was the moral one advanced by the temperance movement that spread from Britain (which had received it from the United States) to the Australian colonies. As early as the 1830s, Governor George Gipps agreed to be patron of the Sydney Temperance Society. Temperance grew stronger in the late nineteenth century, holding Australasian conventions in 1880 and 1888. The recurrent theme, in Australia as in other parts of the Western world, of press comment, sanitary inquiries, and pronouncements of clergy, charities, and the temperance movement itself was that a basic cause of poverty was the moral disorder represented by excessive drinking. When appeals to individual conscience proved inadequate, temperance sought legal restrictions on the sale of liquor. Despite some success, opening hours remained long in the nineteenth century, and even where Sunday closing of hotel bars was achieved, the law was often flouted. The greatest success was the attainment of 6 P.M. closing in South Australia, NSW, Victoria and Tasmania in 1916, an achievement much assisted by the widespread belief that more controls on liquor would assist the war effort. After the war, the temperance movement lacked the political support needed to win its ultimate goal—prohibition. But it was entrenched enough to defend 6 P.M. closing for another half-century.[83]

In the first half of the nineteenth century, doctors in Europe and the United States—Thomas Trotter, Benjamin Rush, von Bruhl-Cramer, Lippich, Magnus Huss—developed the disease concept of alcoholism. Where Trotter saw it as a psychosis with physical effects, von Bruhl-Cramer as a physical disease of the nervous system, and the French psychiatrist, Esquirol as an impulsive monomania, Huss offered a strictly clinical view, defining it as a disease, corresponding to chronic poisoning. With alcoholism now identified as a disease, doctors in England campaigned for establishment of retreats where treatment might be carried out. Donald Dalrymple, proprietor of Heigham Lunatic Asylum, was much impressed by cure rates—33 to 50 percent—claimed by American retreats. On entering Parliament in 1870, he introduced a private member's bill to license the few existing retreats and to provide public funds for new ones. Members concerned about freedom of the individual or the interests of the liquor trade blocked passage of legislation for some years. In 1876, the Society for Promoting Legislation for the Control and Cure of Habitual Drunkards was formed, with Norman Kerr, a public health doctor, as president. The 1879 Habitual Drunkards Act licensed retreats but was permissive concerning treatment. Kerr labored for some years to have provision introduced for compulsory treatment. The 1898

Inebriates Act provided for this, but only where a person pleaded guilty to drunkenness, or was convicted, four times. Criminal cases were treated in government reformatories, while noncriminal cases continued to be treated in licensed retreats.

In Australia, as early as 1872, Victoria enacted legislation providing for medical treatment of inebriates. A Melbourne doctor, Charles McCarthy, influenced by his reading about the Binghampton Inebriates Asylum in the United States, had pressed publicly between 1859 and 1871 for a retreat. He was instrumental in the opening of the Northcote retreat after the passing of inebriates legislation in 1872. While South Australia passed an Inebriates Act in 1874 and in 1881, and Victoria the Inebriates Asylums Act in 1888, it was only the 1890s and early 1900s that saw considerable legislative action: the Inebriates Hospitals Act of 1892 in Tasmania; the Inebriates Institutions Act of 1896 in Queensland; the Inebriates Act of 1900 in New South Wales; the Inebriates Act, 1904, in Victoria; the Inebriates Act, 1908, in South Australia; and the Inebriates Act, 1912, in Western Australia.

In late-nineteenth-century Australia, fundamental changes were occurring in both the prison and psychiatric hospital systems. In NSW, Frederic Norton Manning, the dominant figure in Australian psychiatry at this time and first inspector general of the insane (1878–97), modernized the state lunacy system, while Frederick Neitenstein, comptroller general of prisons from 1895, modernized the prison system. Under Manning's leadership, doctors consolidated their control of the lunatic asylums, and inebriety came to be seen as a disease to be treated, not a crime to be punished. Under Neitenstein, prisons became "hospitals for moral disease" devoted to "treating" criminality. There was also a strong practical incentive for trying to end the revolving-door cycle of habitual drunkards who kept returning to prison. A therapeutic approach to inebriety might reduce chronic overcrowding of prisons.

In the first flush of official enthusiasm for the disease concept, an effort was made to make available specialized treatment facilities. But government support was quite inadequate. Enthusiasm waned, in part because "cures" were notoriously difficult to obtain. Nonetheless, a South Australian royal commission investigating "drug cures" used at the Caulfield Institute for Alcoholism, Melbourne and the Central Methodist Missions in Melbourne and Sydney reported in 1906 that they were effective in the majority of cases. It also supported use of hypnotic suggestion as treatment. More than thirty years later, the senior psychiatrist at Brisbane Hospital, John Bostock, claimed that the sheet anchor of treatment was suggestion and persuasion, whether through hypnosis or counseling, although relapses were common.

Governments relied much on charitable organizations to provide treatment facilities. The Victorian government established Lara, a retreat for male inebriates, but females had to use the Salvation Army facility, Brightside, which received some government funding. Facilities could be grim, applying strict discipline to keep the inebriate "dry" rather than genuine therapy. In NSW, some noncriminal cases were treated in a Salvation Army licensed home, while individuals who could afford it were treated in private hospitals. Criminal inebriates were housed in a facility set up by the Prisons Department. From 1915 to 1929, voluntary cases were also treated under Prisons Department auspices. With the closure of this facility, long-stay patients were accommodated in state psychiatric hospitals. Successive heads of the psychiatric services protested about the inappropriateness of the arrangement, but it continued well into the second half of the twentieth century. Of the other states, Queensland is perhaps closest to NSW in the custodial character of public facilities. Inebriates were sent to the isolation of Stradbroke Island, where in the Dunwich Benevolent Asylum they were housed with the aged and the mentally infirm poor. A combination of strict patient control, rest, nourishment, manual labor and moral exhortation was employed to "cure" the disease. Reasons of cost deterred the state government for many years from transferring the institution to the mainland. When Dunwich was closed in 1946, the successor institution for inebriates was opened in a section of the Marburg prison farm.[84]

The 1950s and 1960s were years of economic prosperity and rising consumption of alcoholic beverages. Although the later 1970s were years of restricted economic growth, alcohol consumption continued to grow, from 8.3 liters per capita in 1970 to 9.7 in 1976. It remained at 9.7 liters in 1982 but subsequently declined, reaching 8.5 liters in 1990 and 7.65 liters in 1995. In 1961, the *Medical Journal of Australia* noted that Australia had an estimated three hundred thousand "problem" drinkers, while alcohol was costing the country four hundred million dollars a year in accidents, lost production and institutional care. Doctors themselves were showing renewed concern with treatment. New services were being set up in hospitals like the Royal Brisbane Hospital, St. Vincent's Hospital in Sydney, and the Alfred and the Royal Melbourne Hospitals. Langton Clinic was opened in Sydney in 1959, Wacol Clinic in Brisbane in 1965 and St Anthony's Hospital in Adelaide in 1968. There was a spate of new legislation, and the central argument advanced by sponsors of the old Inebriates Acts was paraded again—alcohol abuse was a disease to be cured, not a crime to be punished.

In 1961, the South Australian government introduced the Alcohol and Drug Addicts (Treatment) Bill. The minister for education in his second-reading speech asserted firmly that "imprisonment has no curative value." He indicated that treatment centers, unconnected with prisons and psychiatric hospitals, would be set up. In the early 1960s, the Queensland government amended the Liquor Acts to make available sixty thousand dollars a year for treatment and education. A few years later it amended the Inebriates Act—the first discussion of it in the Parliament in seventy years—to permit voluntary admissions to the Wacol Clinic. Victoria also introduced modern legislation. The Alcoholic and Drug-Dependent Persons Bill provided for voluntary treatment and outpatient care. Tasmania passed the Alcohol and Drug Dependence Act in the 1960s and by the early 1970s had a specific Alcohol and Drug Dependence Service. The Western Australia government decided to bring in new legislation in the early 1970s and established an Alcohol and Drug Authority. The Byford center was transferred from the control of the Inebriates Board to that of the new authority. NSW was somewhat slower to create a special service. In 1977 the newly elected Wran Labor government created an interim Drug and Alcohol Authority under the health minister's control but in 1980 turned it into a statutory body. The new authority advised on education and treatment programs, and it administered grants for voluntary organizations working in education and treatment.[85]

Voluntary organizations have played a significant part in the rehabilitation of alcoholics, as indeed in other areas of health. The early involvement of the Salvation Army and the Methodist missions has been noted. Modern self-help groups continue the tradition of nonmedical involvement. One of the most famous self-help bodies in the field of drug dependence is Alcoholics Anonymous (AA), which was started in 1934 by an American businessman who was grappling with his own alcoholism. AA spread quickly from America to Australia, reaching Sydney in the 1940s. By the 1950s, groups existed in towns and cities throughout the country. The group employs a disease concept of alcoholism. Nonetheless, spirituality lies at the heart of AA; the alcoholic must take responsibility for his or her actions and not assume a dependent role in relation to those providing medical care. Health professionals thus are not seen as playing primary roles in the healing process.

Nongovernment organizations not only involved themselves in treatment and rehabilitation but assumed a substantial educative role in relation to governments, employers, unions and the community. In the 1950s and early 1960s, NSW, Victoria and South Australia saw establishment of foundations having this broad brief: the Foundation for Research and Treatment of Alcoholism and Drug Dependence of New South Wales in 1956, and the Victorian Foundation on Alcoholism and Drug Dependence in 1959. South Australia followed in 1963 with the South Australian Foundation on Alcoholism and Drug Dependence. By the mid-1970s, a federal body—the Australian Foundation on Alcoholism and Drug Dependence—was in existence. Further state and territory foundations were also being established. The foundations promoted the concept of alcoholism as a treatable disease, encouraging governments and the community to support creation of public facilities offering effective treatment and preventive strategies.[86]

By the 1970s, in Australia and overseas, not only was the effectiveness of treatment being questioned but a population-based, preventive approach was being advocated as an alternative to the historical emphasis on an individualistic, curative approach. The *Lancet* pointed out in 1977 that one could discern "the deposits . . . of a sequence of therapeutic fashions—the residues of almost forgotten enthusiasm for inpatient psychotherapy units, for group processes and the therapeutic community, for family therapy, and later for community psychiatry."[87] The Western Australia Honorary Royal Commission on treatment of alcohol and drug dependence observed in 1973 that one of the key factors blocking progress in treatment was the fact that "at present, there is no clearly superior or successful treatment method."[88] An American study of the same period analyzed twenty-two studies that evaluated treatment outcomes. The authors found that no statistically significant differences in outcomes existed where treatment settings were comparable, even when different methods were used—drug therapy, hypnosis, group therapy, aversion therapy, imprisonment and probation. The authors of an officially commissioned 1979 review of alcohol policies in Britain stated that there was no known, single, best method of treatment and that individuals were known to have recovered without treatment, as a result of life changes at work or in the family. They pointed out that alcohol provided social benefits as well as imposed costs—export income and employment, and annual government revenue of two billion pounds. Any alcohol policy had to include economic and fiscal objectives aimed at containing total consumption, not simply deal with the health-related consequences of alcohol abuse. Preventing consumption from rising would prevent alcohol-related disabilities from increasing.[89]

From the late 1960s, WHO research and policy on alcohol problems broadened from concern with treatment to containment of consumption. A team of Finnish researchers, Kettil Bruun and colleagues, asserted: "Alcohol control measures can be used to limit consumption; thus, control of alcohol availability becomes a public health issue."[90] In 1972, Bruun, on a visit to Australia, suggested that policy here should involve attempts to influence overall consumption by price manipulation and control of advertising. The problem was that with a free enterprise economy and a culture tolerant of heavy drinking, policy change would be so fraught with political and ideological difficulties that governments would hesitate to act. As long ago as 1979, Professor R.E. Kendell of Edinburgh pointed out how the dogma of the disease concept stood in the way of the more effective approach of reducing consumption by price increases or restriction of availability. The latter was, he argued, a political, not a medical problem, and also an educational one, in that public opinion had to support policy change.

By the middle to late 1980s, a consensus was established among experts in Australia and overseas that fiscal measures and reduction of availability, supplemented by mass education campaigns, was the royal road to victory in the war against alcohol abuse. In its 1987 report on the health consequences of alcohol abuse, the Royal College of Physicians in London urged the British government to reduce overall alcohol consumption over the next decade to about five liters per capita, using price manipulation; and to halt liberalization of licensing laws. It also recommended advertising controls, a tougher approach to drunk driving, support for research and education and creation of a single official agency to coordinate policy.

Apart from the question of political will to impose potentially unpopular consumption control policies, the task of influencing public opinion was daunting. A health education budget of one to two million pounds was a puny weapon against the alcohol industry's hundred million pounds for advertising. Moreover, national governments would have to do battle with transnational corporations with production and market strategies geared to operations in a global market having an estimated value of $170 billion at this time. Another difficulty was that in postwar decades public awareness was focused to a great extent in Australia, as in other Western countries, on illegal drugs. A British commentator noted, "It is extraordinary that a statistic of one million or more 'alcoholics' in Britain raises hardly a murmur, yet panic ensues when the number of drug addicts reaches 50,000."[91] In Australia too by the later 1980s experts on alcohol abuse saw reducing gross consumption as a primary means of reducing health-related alcohol problems. One Sydney expert, Dr. Alex Wodak, called upon doctors, as the group best acquainted with the ill effects of greater consumption, to resist fiercely contemporary government and industry efforts to promote consumption in the name of employment and the growth of the tourism industry.[92]

Before looking at the development of a national policy on alcohol and other drug abuse, we will trace the history of government and community responses to use of illegal drugs in Australia. In the nineteenth century, the Poisons Acts of the different colonies (which were modeled on British legislation) controlled sale of drugs. Drug use, including recreational use, was a matter of personal choice. The purpose of legislation was not to prevent addiction or recreational use; it was to trace poisoners and prevent serious accidents by ensuring proper labeling. Thus the 1876 Sale and Use of Poisons Acts in NSW and Victoria identified certain drugs that could be sold only by a pharmacist or doctor and that required explicit labeling. Sales were otherwise not restricted. Medical prescriptions, homeopathic compounds and patent medicines (which commonly contained opiates or alcohol) escaped these requirements. Purchasers of drugs known to be used in deliberate acts of poisoning, like arsenic and strychnine, were required to give details of name, address, occupation and intended use of the drug. They had to be at least eighteen years of age and, if unknown to the vendor, had to have a witness present known to both parties. Opium, opium preparations and cocaine were not included in this category. In NSW, however, laudanum did fall into that category, because there lawmakers believed it was used in intentional poisoning cases often enough for purchase to be restricted.

A campaign against opium smoking had been building strength since the 1870s. Since the vast majority of smokers were Chinese, the issue had got caught up in anti-Chinese and Asian immigration restriction agitation. The

NSW premier, Joseph Carruthers, claimed in the early 1900s, "There are only about 200 white smokers in the Commonwealth, and . . . they are confined in nearly every case to the wives of Chinese, and to abandoned women of the lowest class. The habit is not on the increase."[93] Assisting the emergence of state prohibition of opium use in the early twentieth century was the progressivist emphasis on the physical health and purity of the nation and race (discussed in *The People's Health,* volume 1). Coupled with this was the widespread political faith, especially in Liberal and Labor circles, in legislative intervention to produce social change and promote nation building (again noted in the companion volume to this study). I have in volume 1 noted the growth of more interventionist public health and pure food legislation in the early 1900s, as well as venereal disease legislation establishing compulsory treatment; as that arch-progressive and national hygienist J.S. Elkington put it, "Serious acceptance of a doctrine of national physical morality will cause preventable disease to be regarded as somebody's crime."[94]

Prime Minister Alfred Deakin persuaded the states to accept the revenue loss resulting from a federal prohibition on importing of smoking opium, and in 1905 the ban was put in place. The states then legislated to outlaw smoking, sale, preparation and possession of opium. The prohibition law impinged almost exclusively on Chinese residents; all 216 persons prosecuted in 1926 for preparation were Chinese. Restrictions were progressively tightened, first in Victoria and then in other states. The Victorian Poisons Act, 1920, extended coverage to cocaine, synthetic cocaine, heroin, Indian hemp (cannabis), morphine and other opium derivatives. The Poisons Act of 1925 made possession unlawful; it became punishable by a fine of a hundred pounds or one year in prison. Returned soldiers were reportedly using cocaine in 1919. The press made much of its use in the 1920s in Sydney and Melbourne by prostitutes and criminals. But at the height of the moral panic, as few as twenty-eight people in 1928 and thirty-four in 1929 were prosecuted in NSW. Even so, with the commonwealth having ratified the 1925 Geneva Convention (which strengthened international control of the drug trade), NSW was under pressure to follow Victoria and prohibit (except when used in prescriptions) the sale, use and possession of opiates and cocaine. It did so in the 1927 Police Offences Amendment (Drugs) Act.

In the United States, the Treasury Department had used the 1914 Harrison Act as part of a campaign to eradicate addiction. In 1919 the Supreme Court found that medical use of heroin to alleviate addicts' withdrawal symptoms was not allowed by the act. In 1925 the finding was overturned, but the Federal Bureau of Narcotics was influential enough to contain the reversal's consequences. In the United Kingdom, in contrast, reaction to the Rolleston Report of 1926, which saw addiction as a disease, ensured that doctors could keep addicts on maintenance supplies of heroin or morphine. The "British system" continued into the 1960s. In Australia, heroin (like morphine) was heavily used by doctors for chronic and acute pain, and for maintenance of addicts. Per capita consumption of heroin in Australia in the early 1930s was triple that of Britain, and for cocaine, double what was consumed in Britain. In 1931, the Australian rate of consumption was 3.1 kilos of heroin per one million population, and in 1946, 2.42 kilos, 4.3 in 1949, and 5.25 in 1957—the last the largest in the world at the time. There was some cocaine use by the "criminal classes," and a few Chinese opium smokers remained. But in the interwar period, and until some time after World War II, addicts were mainly middle-class people, including a high proportion of health professionals.[95]

Even during the Pacific War, American prohibitionist policy continued. In 1943 a statement was issued of the U.S. intention to end smoking of opium in all areas liberated from the Japanese, including British colonies where opium smoking had been tolerated. The new defense dependence on the United States meant that Australia supported the American government in this matter. In the 1950s in America, Cold War anticommunism became caught up with the antidrugs campaign. Internationally, the long-term prohibitionist policy of the United States was enjoying increasing success. The 1953 Opium Protocol, which Australia and twenty-six other countries ratified, ensured that international law applied to the legal trade in opium, from the growing of poppies to medicinal use. Harry Anslinger, long-time head of the Federal Bureau of Narcotics and also American representative on the United Nations Commission on Narcotic Drugs, not infrequently claimed that the People's Republic of China was pursuing a policy of trafficking in heroin to obtain foreign exchange, but also to weaken the health and morale of Western countries.

Although there was almost no illegal use of heroin in Australia, in contrast to the United States, the Australian government was very concerned about its international reputation for very high per capita consumption, which was due to common medical use for pain control, plus use in very small amounts in proprietary medicines. Although the NHMRC, the RACP and the College of Obstetricians and Gynaecologists advised against prohibition of heroin—the BMA Federal Council agreed to it—the federal government banned the importation of heroin in mid-1953. The states fell into line by late 1953, prohibiting manufacture. NSW and Western Australia went farther and prohibited possession, making heroin completely illegal. In Britain, medical and other public opposition to prohibition—heroin addiction there too was an insignificant problem—ensured that use under medical prescription continued. Opposition to the ban from some doctors, especially in Victoria, remained strong in the later 1950s. Since some Victorian hospitals had supplies of heroin dating from before the ban on importation and manufacture, heroin continued to be employed sometimes for intractable pain in the 1960s. But even in the states where it could still be legally administered, the bans meant that supplies were not to be had.

In the course of the 1960s, illegal drug use increased markedly, especially in NSW, as the rebellious baby-boomer generation discovered "alternative" lifestyles. Cosmopolitan Sydney, with its strong trade and tourist links with Asia and the Pacific, was at the forefront of these changes. Arrests for cannabis possession increased in NSW 1,000 percent in 1966–69. Young American servicemen, on rest and recreational leave from Vietnam in Sydney in the late 1960s, brought with them an influential culture of high use of cannabis and heroin. Politicians reacted with a sense of urgency and some anxiety to what they saw as this new threat to the moral integrity of the young. Cannabis, made a prohibited import in NSW in 1956, became a prohibited drug in 1966. Law enforcement, particularly against the trafficker, was on the increase at federal and state levels. The Liberal minister for customs and excise from 1970 to 1972, Don Chipp, pushed strongly for greater resources for his department. He opposed law reform to decriminalize use of cannabis. The addict was an object of pity; the drug pusher was evil and deserved to feel the full weight of the law. In 1970, the NSW Liberal government targeted traffickers, legislating to make dealing in a drug of addiction illegal. All states now punished trafficking as a separate offense.

Drug policy became a point of debate between the two sides of politics. Moreover, cannabis, the most controversial drug, was becoming ever more popular among young people, with convictions in NSW rising from fifty-seven in 1966 to 4,300 in 1977. In 1979, the conservative National Party government in Queensland considered whether to exploit politically Labor's perceived identification with a "soft" approach to illegal drug use. The Queensland Labor Party was committed to decriminalization of the personal use of marijuana; the NSW Labor Party believed it should be approached in a different way from the opiates, and Victorian Labor saw criminalization under existing state law as misguided. But once in power, Labor became defensive, not wishing to be seen by electors as soft on drugs. In early 1977 the new Labor premier of NSW, Neville Wran, made clear publicly that his government had no intention of legalizing the personal use of marijuana.[96]

In 1971, the federal Liberal-Country Party government provided the states with five hundred thousand dollars for drug education work, as a result of urgent recommendations by the 1969–71 Senate Select Committee on Drug Trafficking and Drug Abuse. The committee had decided that alcohol and tobacco were indeed drugs but that to investigate them adequately would delay its report on the "growing social problem" of abuse of narcotics, hallucinogens and pharmaceutical products. It did, however, note that alcohol and tobacco were the most widely used drugs in Australia.[97] The federal government had established the National Standing Control Committee on Drugs of Dependence in 1969 to deal with legislation, law enforcement, treatment and education. The committee was dominated by the Department of Customs and Excise, with its approach of law enforcement and suppression. Sir William Refshauge, commonwealth director general of health, 1960–73, hardly attended meetings because of Customs' growing influence on drug policy. The national drug education program was described by a Commonwealth Health Department officer as low key and intended to bring about long-term behavior change. A 1982 evaluation of the program made a very limited claim for success. As early as 1972, Chipp, the minister for customs and excise, admitted that the primary objective of the program was to educate the community about illegal narcotic drugs.[98]

Between 1969 and 1980, five major official inquiries took place into the nonmedical use of drugs. Only one, the Senate Standing Committee on Social Welfare inquiry, 1974–77, chaired by Liberal senator Peter Baume, a physician, looked at alcohol and tobacco. But all were concerned with illegal drug use. Official and community preoccupation with illegal drugs was patent, as Baume himself recognized: "We're big on heroin and hashish policy—we're weak on policy to deal with the legal drugs, as if being legal was in itself complete justification for laissez faire policies."[99] The Baume committee (with two senators dissenting, but with bipartisan agreement) had recommended that personal use of cannabis not be a criminal offense; the only penalty would be a pecuniary one. Moreover, it had clearly pointed out the health and social effects of drugs were not connected with their legal status: "Abuse of opiates and other narcotics is serious but alcohol and tobacco are abused by a greater number of people and at greater social and economic cost."[100]

Like the Baume inquiry, the South Australian Royal Commission into the nonmedical use of drugs, chaired by Professor Ronald Sackville, took a broad approach to the "drug problem," going well beyond the received wisdom and criticizing the law enforcement approach. On cannabis, it proposed that cultivation for personal use, small-scale free distribution to adults, and use in private be made legal. The inquiry had been set up in 1976 by the Dunstan Labor government because of disagreements within the state party about reform of the law on cannabis. Sackville himself was skeptical about the enduring belief that criminal sanctions would substantially reduce use of illicit drugs, as well as about the efficacy of a more recent panacea, drug education. Evidence showed that drug education programs did not significantly modify behavior. Equally, treatment alone was not the answer. The Sackville commission's work was subject to much media and political discussion, most of it focused on its proposals concerning cannabis. The controversy worried the new Labor premier, Des Corcoran (Don Dunstan had retired because of ill health). It was made clear there would be no reform of the law on cannabis. Moreover, the Labor government did not attempt to have the report debated in Parliament, nor was any ministerial statement made concerning the government's attitude to its recommendations.

Two and a half years after the Baume committee report, the federal Fraser Liberal-National Party government announced in 1980 its support for the committee's recommendation that a health-oriented national strategy concerning the dangers of alcohol, tobacco, analgesics and illegal drugs be developed. In its health-oriented alcohol policy, the government indicated that it supported overall reduction of consumption. But it did not commit itself to concrete goals or specify definite strategies. Even where it accepted the committee's recommendations to use fiscal measures to reduce consumption, it remained vague, simply saying when taxes on alcohol were being determined, health considerations would be taken into account.[101]

Members of the federal Labor Party had at times been ready to criticize mainstream drug policy. Dr. Neal Blewett, who became federal health minister when Labor came to power in 1983 and remained in that office till 1990, had supported reform of the law on cannabis as early as the 1960s. Just following his appointment as health minister, Blewett spoke on television about his approach to cannabis. He evoked such a large critical reaction that in order to push for change on more important health issues, he henceforth avoided this controversial policy area.

With a high level of community anxiety about organized crime and drug trafficking, the federal government created in 1984 the National Crime Authority, basically a permanent royal commission on organized crime. The first chairman was Justice Donald Stewart, who as royal commissioner inquiring into drug trafficking had reported in 1983 on the collapsed Nugan Hand Bank and its connections with Terence Clark's drug trafficking syndicate. In the middle of the 1984 election campaign, the Labor prime minister, R.J.L. Hawke, promised, if returned to office, to launch a National Campaign against Drug Abuse (NCADA). A special premiers conference on drugs convened by the reelected Labor government formally established NCADA in April 1985. At the drug summit the states and the commonwealth agreed to "do everything possible to combat the growing problems of drug abuse and addiction in Australia."[102] A workshop for professionals brought together by Neal Blewett prior to the summit proposed that alcohol and tobacco be a major concern of any national campaign. Yet, while the summit accepted that the campaign would encompass legal drugs, it agreed that the focus should be on illegal drugs.

The campaign channeled considerable new funds into research, treatment and education. In 1985–88 the commonwealth and states provided $110 million through NCADA for new and existing activities: seventy-seven million dollars for treatment and education in the states and territories; twenty-six million dollars for national education and research projects; and $7.5 million for drug law enforcement. Toward the end of this triennium, a task force appointed by the federal health minister to evaluate NCADA's performance identified certain policy issues that it believed would preoccupy policy makers into the 1990s. These included the facts that long-established organizations in the field of rehabilitation and their methods were being challenged by a more professional constituency impatient with established approaches; that a conflict existed between influential voices that wanted the emphasis to be placed on illegal drugs and those drawing on epidemiological evidence showing that legal drugs, especially alcohol and tobacco, produced most of the drug-related ill health and deaths, as well as most of the social problems; that while harm minimization was the agreed objective of NCADA, disagreement existed between those interpreting this to mean promotion of efforts to reduce drug use and so the amount of harm, and those focusing on minimizing harm and not being concerned about the level of drug use.[103]

A draft national alcohol policy was put together in 1984 by the National Standing Committee on Alcohol for the Standing Committee of Health Ministers. After NCADA came into existence in 1985, drafting was taken over by the Alcohol Subcommittee of the Standing Committee of Officials, reporting to the Ministerial Council on Drug Strategy. Blewett released the draft for public discussion at the close of 1986. A revised draft (after public submissions) was put to the ministerial council. The general objective of harm minimization was widely accepted, but the alcohol industry saw reduction of per capita consumption as state interference in what should be individual responsibility for alcohol use. Health professionals responded that the evidence showed that as per capita consumption grew so did indices of harm, and that treatment and education might change the heavy drinker's behavior but the majority of alcohol-related problems, produced by the less heavy drinkers, would continue. The industry's view that health education alone was adequate ignored environmental determinants like price and availability and the extent to which education had to compete with widespread advertising encouraging greater consumption. The wine industry was unhappy about the idea of a price rise, claiming that an increase would not cut the consumption level of heavy drinkers but would cause drinkers to substitute "unhealthy" alternative alcoholic beverages for "healthy" wine. The professionals replied with evidence indicating that heavy drinkers did cut consumption in the face of price rises and that it was the amount of alcohol (in whatever form consumed) that determined the extent of harm. Further, the overall fall in consumption of alcohol in recent years, not the greater consumption of wine, had been responsible for a reduction in health problems.

When in early 1988 health ministers considered the draft policy, Dr. John Cornwall, the minister for health in South Australia, the leading wine-producing state, expressed reservations about those areas dealing with availability, pricing and advertising. He said his government saw alcohol in a different light from tobacco—if used in moderation, it believed, alcohol was not harmful. South Australia had no intention of restricting sponsorship or advertising. The new minister, Frank Blevins, a year later confirmed South Australia's great reluctance to restrict advertising and its opposition to basing taxation on volume of alcohol, which would damage the wine industry greatly. In March 1989 the Ministerial Council on Drug Strategy accepted a modified version of the draft national policy. The health minister of South Australia had successfully moved that two sections of the draft as presented be taken out. The federal health minister had pointed out the inconsistency of differential taxation, accepting the basis of alcoholic content for beer but rejecting it for wine. Government supervision of advertising had also been rejected in favor of voluntary codes of practice.[104]

Leading professionals in the field of alcohol and health were unhappy about the compromises made in the final policy document. Professor David Hawks, director of the National Centre for Research into Prevention of Drug Abuse, Perth, pointed out that while the draft made sure that individual responsibility was supported by various controls, the final policy emphasized education and treatment, which were more acceptable to the alcohol industry. In the area of pricing and taxation, the specific aim of relating tax to alcohol content, thus favoring lower-alcohol drinks, had disappeared, whereas the more general aim of assessing the impact of excise changes on incidence and prevalence of alcohol problems had remained. Concerning availability, the earlier objective of increasing the effectiveness of existing licensing laws had become ensuring effective policing. Both the draft and final documents criticized certain marketing and advertising practices. However, the final document omitted specific references to the targeting of youth and women, increasing use of lifestyle advertising, and sponsorship of sporting and cultural activities. Also omitted were support for an independent body to oversee advertising, for a levy on alcohol sales to finance education about responsible use, and for exclusion of all advertising where the audience included a substantial percentage of children. Gains had nonetheless been made, Hawks acknowledged: governments had publicly committed themselves to the aim of harm minimization; they had accepted that harm arose from normal consumption as well as from heavy drinking; and they had recognized that attention to advertising, availability and pricing was as important as support for education and treatment.[105]

As we have seen, the first evaluation of NCADA took place in 1988. The second was in 1992, and it recommended that NCADA be continued as the National Drug Strategy (NDS). It identified a number of deficiencies in NCADA: a lack of strategic goals, failure to establish a partnership between health and law enforcement, obstacles to innovation, inadequate community consultation, and failure to meet the needs of special population groups. The Ministerial Council on Drug Strategy in 1992 agreed to raise the share of NDS funding for law enforcement to 10 percent over three years. In addition, the commonwealth created the National Drug Crime Prevention Fund. The NDS Plan of 1993–97 stated a number of goals and targets for its five years of duration. To achieve the primary aim of harm minimization, three goals were to be pursued: minimization of the level of illness, disease, injury and death from abuse of alcohol, tobacco, and pharmaceutical and illegal drugs; minimization of drug-related crime and violence; and minimization of personal and social disruption, and of quality-of-life and economic losses. The key targets were: reduced injuries, violence and loss of productivity; further reduction in the prevalence of smoking and the beginning of smoking habits, especially among the disadvantaged and young people; reduction in the inappropriate use of drugs by young people; reduction in the misuse of prescription drugs; reduction in the prevalence of trafficking in and use of illegal drugs; and prevention of the spread of the hepatitides, HIV/AIDS and other infections from unsafe injecting of illegal drugs and from unsafe sex associated with intoxication.

The largest source of funding was the commonwealth. Federal funds (which were matched by the states and territories) expanded from twelve million dollars in 1985 to $20.7 million in 1996–97. The commonwealth also provided funds for national programs such as the two national drug and alcohol research centers, one in Sydney and one in Perth. These outlays amounted to $66.4 million in 1993–97. From the end of 1991, recoveries under the Proceeds of Crime Act of 1987, the Customs Act of 1901 and the Crimes Act of 1914 were forwarded to the Confiscated Assets Trust Fund. The fund provided over $7.6 million to the Federal Health Department (it also provided funds for law enforcement projects via the federal Attorney-General's Department) for drug education and rehabilitation. About 33 percent of projects funded under the commonwealth-states matched-funding program and 50 percent of national programs were prevention initiatives: public awareness campaigns like "Speed Catches Up with You" (amphetamine use), "Alcohol and Violence Tears You Apart" (moderation in drinking), and reducing youth smoking; National Initiatives in Drug Education to train schoolteachers and then parents and community and industry groups; a range of prevention programs for Aboriginal and Torres Strait Islander people, including a joint project with the Northern Territory government to prevent petrol sniffing.

In 1995, 18,124 Australians (13,163 males and 4,961 females) died from tobacco-related disease, 3,642 (2,440 males and 1,202 females) from alcohol-related conditions, and 778 from illegal drug use. About 175,000 Australians were hospitalized for illness resulting from tobacco, alcohol or illegal drug use. Drugs caused more mortality and morbidity than homicide, accidental falls, HIV/AIDS, and breast and cervical cancer combined. The economic cost of prevention, treatment, loss of productivity, property crime, theft, accidents and law enforcement was more than eighteen billion dollars a year, and this did not include social consequences like family breakdown and the suffering experienced by those who abused drugs themselves and by others. The economic costs (1992) of tobacco use amounted to $12.7 billion, or 67.3 percent of all costs related to drug abuse.

Between 1985 and 1995, when NCADA and NDS were functioning, the prevalence of males smoking fell from about 40 to 30 percent, while female prevalence declined only from about 30 to 26 percent. The prevalence in males has been falling since 1945, so not too much can be made of the impact of the national campaigns. But, in addition, community perceptions and attitudes significantly changed over the decade, probably further evidence of the impact of the campaigns. Where in 1985 about 6 percent of adults believed smoking was the most serious drug problem, 23 percent thought so in 1995; 81 percent believed that regular exposure of nonsmokers to smoke—passive smoking—might result in future health problems. Attitude and perception change is clear in the case of alcohol as well. In 1985–95, the percentage of adults seeing alcohol as the key drug problem increased from 7 to 14, and adolescents seeing alcohol this way increased fivefold, to 11 percent. A majority of the population in 1995 endorsed various preventive initiatives—no TV advertisements until after 9:30 P.M. (76 percent); increasing the legal age for drinking (53 percent); stricter enforcement of the law prohibiting service for drunken patrons (92 percent); and provision of only low-alcohol drinks at sporting events (74 percent). Probably too much should not be made of the effect of the national campaigns on the downward trend in per capita consumption, because the trend began (in the early 1980s) before NCADA commenced (in 1985), and similar trends took place in many countries. A trend toward more responsible drinking in 1988–95 was not solely due to the national campaigns, but it represents some further probable evidence of harm minimization resulting from the government efforts. By 1995, 73 percent of people drinking were moderate drinkers, while heavy drinkers had fallen to 14 percent and binge drinkers to 6 percent. The proportion of adolescents who were nondrinkers rose by 9 percent, and those who were moderate drinkers by 5 percent.

Pharmaceuticals are not perceived by the community as a significant component of the "drug problem." Fewer than 3 percent of people surveyed saw pharmaceuticals in this way—14 percent when specific pharmaceuticals were included. In 1993–95, people fourteen years of age and older using tranquilizers or barbiturates for nonmedical purposes declined by 33 and 25 percent, respectively. However, most of the preventive effort was channeled through the National Pharmaceutical Strategy rather than NDS.

Of the illegal drugs, cannabis is the most often used: 31 percent of people have ever used it, while 13 percent had used it in the year before the 1995 survey. Fewer than 10 percent ever used hallucinogens or amphetamines, and far fewer ever used heroin or cocaine; 2 percent reported using ecstasy or other designer drugs. But use of illegal drugs is greatest among people under thirty-five years of age, while males are more likely to experiment or sustain use. As we have noted, far fewer deaths result from illegal drug use than from tobacco or alcohol, but the people who do die from drugs are usually considerably younger—36.7 years of potential life lost on average, compared with 4.7 years for a tobacco-related death. Apart from overdoses and injection of impure substances, needle sharing is a major source of harm, because of the risk of the spread of HIV, hepatitis and other viruses. By mid-

1995, 940 males and 186 females had been infected with HIV where the injection of drugs was a factor in transmission. The estimated cost of illegal drug use—lost productivity, treatment and law enforcement—in 1992 was $1.68 billion; this figure did not include the cost of property crimes committed by addicts to pay for drugs. Moreover, 11 percent of all prisoners are drug offenders, while an indefinite proportion of the rest committed crimes to pay for, or while under the influence of, drugs.

The NDS (including NCADA) appears to have had no moderating effect on consumption of cannabis. For persons aged twenty to twenty-nine years and for adolescents, consumption increased 5 percent between 1988 and 1995. The high sampling variability of general-population surveys for infrequent events like illegal use of drugs other than cannabis meant that consumption trends for other drugs cannot be conclusively established. Another index of harm involves trends in HIV cases involving injecting drugs. These fell from eighty-four in 1990–91 to fifty-seven in 1995–96. The achievement must be attributed at least as much to the National HIV/AIDS Strategy as the NDS, but the latter probably played some part in harm minimization in this area. Arguably, another achievement in harm minimization has been the greater emphasis in law enforcement on drug trafficking rather than possession. In 1985–94, the number of persons in prison for trafficking increased, while the number of those there for possession declined.

The concept of harm minimization was central to the NDS. It meant the reduction of harm associated with tobacco, alcohol and other drug use; it did not necessarily involve reduction in rates of use, as such. This plus a number of other features of the Australian NDS made it internationally noteworthy. These features included a comprehensiveness under which legal, as well as illegal, drugs were addressed; a balanced approach by which prevention, treatment, research and education all received support and effort was put into both supply and demand-reduction strategies; and the building of partnerships between health, law enforcement, education, nongovernment organizations and private enterprises. Unlike national drug strategies in a number of other countries, the NDS was not limited to illegal drugs. This comprehensiveness brought various benefits, including appreciation of the features common to addiction and to treatment for various psychoactive substances, as well as more balanced attention to the various psychoactive substances, legal and illegal. The NDS was able to foster a more tolerant setting for debate about appropriate approaches by supporting interventions that ranged from a focus on abstinence to harm reduction. It facilitated public discussion of radical interventions like the proposed heroin trial in the Australian Capital Territory, and it modestly supported bodies representative of drug users.

The NDS was successful in targeting certain high-risk groups—Aboriginal and Torres Strait Islander peoples (32 percent of projects), young people

(30 percent), women (29 percent) and criminal offenders (29 percent). But little was done for the homeless, people with physical or intellectual disabilities or women and older people at high risk of misuse of pharmaceuticals. A special characteristic of the NDS was the emphasis on health rather than law enforcement activities. This distinguished it from national drug strategies in many other countries, where, while little evidence of effectiveness exists, the emphasis was on supply reduction through law enforcement. In the NCADA phase of the NDS, almost no funds were provided for law enforcement, because prior to 1985 so much of the effort to contain drug misuse had been directed to law enforcement activities. NCADA set out emphatically to redress the balance. The 1992 evaluation of the NDS proposed greater funding for law enforcement. Subsequently, 10 percent of matched funds plus the National Drug Crime Prevention Fund were pledged for law enforcement work. By 1997, some states and territories had not yet reached the 10 percent level of spending.

The NDS put much effort into supporting prevention. In this it was departing from the usual order of priorities, in which, as Smart has noted, "prevention is usually a poor stepsister to treatment and enforcement effort when it comes to alcohol and drug problems."[106] The NDS also strongly supported research as the basis for the entire strategy. Research supported by the NDS—whether in the two national research centers or through individual projects—has turned Australia into one of the leading producers of research on alcohol and other drugs in the world. Treatment, like prevention, has proven to be cost effective—one dollar spent on treatment in the United States is estimated to save the health care system seven dollars. But according to Professors Eric Single and Timothy Rohl, independent experts who reviewed the NDS in the late 1990s, the NDS should be directing its energies to development of new treatments rather than putting so much support into established treatment services. If the NDS meant to make itself redundant, effort should have been going into education and training of medical and other professionals so that mainstream health and social services, along with the specialized facilities like detoxification centers and dedicated treatment centers, would prevent and treat drug-related disorders. The guiding principle of harm minimization proved influential in bringing about a more consistent national approach to drug problems. Inadequate coordination of strategic planning between commonwealth and states, however, led to a situation where despite agreement to give high priority to prevention, at least 50 percent of funds eventually went to established treatment facilities. Also, lack of coordinated planning created difficulties concerning accountability, as strikingly evidenced by the incompleteness of central records of projects funded through the NDS.

The National Drug Strategic Framework 1998–99 to 2002–2003 includes four complementary strategies covering alcohol, tobacco, illicit drugs and drug education in schools. At the midpoint in its life, the strategic framework has recognized that more emphasis must be placed on prevention. Under the framework, prevention is one of eight priority areas. Preventive action is to apply equally to harmful drug use, supply of drugs and drug-related harm.[107]

As this chapter has shown, the "diseases of affluence"—cancer and cardiovascular disease, alcohol and other drug dependence, and traffic accidents—simply would not, unlike bacterial infections, retreat in the face of the magic bullets of curative medicine. Preventive strategies and control of risk factors seemed to offer more effective firepower. Moreover, with national governments in Australia as elsewhere spending great and increasing sums on treatment and rehabilitation, the less costly path of prevention appeared even more attractive. In the following chapter, we examine the rise and fall of a major commonwealth initiative in preventive policy—the Community Health Program. The strength of private, fee-for-service medicine was to restrict the chances for success of this publicly funded, national exercise in integrating organizationally preventive and curative services, although other factors contributed importantly to its decline and fall.

NOTES

1. I. Chapple, "Metamorphoses in Medicine: A View from General Practice," *Medical Journal of Australia* 161 (1994): 45; J.A. Gillespie, *The Price of Health: Australian Governments and Medical Politics 1910–1960* (Cambridge: Cambridge University Press, 1991), 240.

2. Sir Theodore Fox, "The Antipodes: Private Practice Publicly Supported," *Lancet* 1 (1963): 875–79.

3. Ibid., 875.

4. Quoted in S. Sax, *A Strife of Interests: Politics and Policies in Australian Health Services* (Sydney: George Allen and Unwin, 1984), 59.

5. Quoted in J.A. Gillespie, *The Price of Health: Australian Governments and Medical Politics 1910–1960* (Cambridge: Cambridge University Press, 1991), 254.

6. Sax, *A Strife of Interests,* 59–66; Gillespie, *The Price of Health,* 256–78.

7. M.C. Brown, *The Financing of Personal Health Services in New Zealand, Canada and Australia* (Canberra: Australian National University, 1977), 147.

8. R. Taylor, "Income from Private Medical Practice in Australia 1966–1978: An Analysis of Taxation Statistics," *Community Health Studies* 8(1) (1984): 1–9.

9. Quoted in Gillespie, *The Price of Health,* 282.

10. Quoted in S.J. Duckett, "Structural Interests and Australian Health Policy," *Social Science and Medicine* 18(11) (1984): 960.

11. Gillespie, *The Price of Health,* 281–85; Duckett, "Structural Interests and Australian Health Policy," 959–61.

12. J. Deeble, "The Health of the Nation: Who Pays?" in *The Health Problems of the Nation,* ed. J. Birman (Perth: Extension Service of University of Western Australia, 1974), 69.

13. Quoted in E. Fee, "The Origins and Development of Public Health in the

United States," in *Oxford Textbook of Public Health,* vol 1., ed. W.W. Holland, R. Detels and G. Knox (Oxford: Oxford University Press, 1991), 13.

14. Quoted in ibid., 13.

15. Quoted in E. Fee, "Public Health and the State: The United States," in *The History of Public Health and the Modern State,* ed. D. Porter (Amsterdam, Atlanta: Editions Rodopi B.V., 1994), 254–55.

16. Ibid., 252–59; J. Duffy, *The Sanitarians: A History of American Public Health* (Urbana: University of Illinois Press, 1990), 294–97; E. Fee, "The Origins and Development of Public Health in the United States," 15–18.

17. J. Lewis, "The Public's Health: Philosophy and Practice in Britain in the Twentieth Century," in *A History of Education in Public Health,* ed. E. Fee and R.M. Acheson (New York: Oxford University Press, 1991), 217–25; W.W. Holland and S. Stewart, *Public Health: The Vision and the Challenge* (London: Nuffield Trust, 1998), 114–17.

18. Quoted in Holland and Stewart, *Public Health,* 117.

19. J. Lewis, "The Origins and Development of Public Health in the UK," in *Oxford Textbook of Public Health,* vol. 1, ed. W.W. Holland, R. Detels and G. Knox (Oxford: Oxford University Press, 1991), 31–32; Holland and Stewart, *Public Health,* 117–19.

20. E. Fee, "Public Health, Past and Present: A Shared Social Vision," in G. Rosen's, *A History of Public Health* (Baltimore: Johns Hopkins University Press, 1993), xxvii.

21. G.R. Palmer and S.D. Short, *Health Care and Public Policy: An Australian Analysis* (South Melbourne: Macmillan Education Australia, 1994), 206–15; G. Macdonald and R. Bunton, "Health Promotion: Discipline or Disciplines?" in *Health Promotion: Disciplines and Diversity,* ed. R. Bunton and G. Macdonald (London: Routledge, 1992), 8–17; A. Tannahill, "Epidemiology and Health Promotion: A Common Understanding," in *Health Promotion. Disciplines and Diversity,* ed. Bunton and Macdonald, 100.

22. "The Control of Tuberculosis in Australia," *Medical Journal of Australia* 2 (1960): 225; "Tuberculosis and Complacency," *Medical Journal of Australia* 2 (1967): 459–60; "Compulsory Mass X-Ray Surveys: The Future," *Medical Journal of Australia* 2 (1971): 61–62.

23. T.C. Boag, "Australia Wins Fight to Control Tuberculosis," *Health* 26 (1976): 8–12.

24. Quoted in C. Thame, "Health and the State: The Development of Collective Responsibility for Health Care in Australia in the First Half of the Twentieth Century" (Ph.D. dissertation, Australian National University, Canberra, 1974), 111.

25. Ibid., 180–14; Boag, "Australia Wins Fight to Control Tuberculosis," 8–12.

26. R. Patrick, *A History of Health and Medicine in Queensland 1824–1960* (St. Lucia: University of Queensland Press, 1987), 218; P. Woodruff, *Two Million South Australians* (Kent Town: Peacock, 1984), 101–2.

27. P. Woodruff, "BCG Vaccine: Its Use in South Australia," in *History of Tuberculosis in Australia, New Zealand and Papua New Guinea,* ed. A.J. Proust (Canberra: Brolga Press, 1991), 162.

28. L. Bryder, "BCG Vaccination: Comparative Perspectives," in *New Perspectives on the History of Medicine,* eds. H. Attwood, R. Gillespie and M. Lewis (Parkville: Medical History Unit, University of Melbourne, 1990), 194–99; J. Duffy, *A History*

of Public Health in New York City 1866–1966 (New York: Russell Sage Foundation, 1974), 551–52.

29. C. Webster, *The Health Services since the War,* vol. 1, *Problems of Health Care: The National Health Service before 1957* (London: Her Majesty's Stationery Office [hereafter HMSO], 1988), 7–8, 321–24; L. Bryder, *Below the Magic Mountain: A Social History of Tuberculosis in Twentieth-Century Britain* (Oxford: Clarendon Press, 1988), 227–61; L.G. Wilson, "The Historical Decline of Tuberculosis in Europe and America: Its Causes and Significance," *Journal of History of Medicine and Allied Sciences* 45 (1990): 367.

30. Bryder, *Below the Magic Mountain,* 262–65.

31. B.H. Lerner, *Contagion and Confinement: Controlling Tuberculosis along the Skid Road* (Baltimore: Johns Hopkins University Press, 1998), 60.

32. Quoted in ibid., 173.

33. Lerner, *Contagion and Confinement,* 35–40, 56–61, 70–77, 165–73; S.M. Rothman, *Living in the Shadow of Death: Tuberculosis and the Social Experience of Illness in American History* (New York: Basic Books, 1994), 250–52.

34. L. Garrett, *Betrayal of Trust: The Collapse of Global Public Health* (New York: Hyperion, 2000), 575–76.

35. B. Feery, "Impact of Immunization on Disease Patterns in Australia," *Medical Journal of Australia* 2 (1981): 175.

36. S. Benison, "Poliomyelitis and the Rockefeller Institute: Social Effects and Institutional Response," *Journal of History of Medicine and Allied Sciences* 29 (1974): 74–75; E.H. Ackerknecht, *History and Geography of the Most Important Diseases* (New York: Hafner, 1965), 80–83; M. Burnet, *Walter and Eliza Hall Institute 1915–1965* (Carlton: Melbourne University Press, 1971), 132–34; A.J.G. Buxton, "Poliomyelitis in South Australia 1937–1956" (honors dissertation, history, University of Adelaide: Adelaide, 1977), 3–8.

37. F. Mullan, *Plagues and Politics: The Story of the United States Public Health Service* (New York: Basic Books, 1989), 133–34; P. Starr, *The Social Transformation of American Medicine* (New York: Basic Books, 1982), 346–47; Duffy, *The Sanitarians,* 282–83.

38. C. Webster, *The Health Services since the War,* vol. 2, *Government and Health Care: The National Health Service 1958–1979* (London: HMSO, 1996), 128–31, 680.

39. J.B. Cleland and E.W. Ferguson, "Acute Anterior Poliomyelitis, Including Landry's Paralysis," in *Report of Director General of Public Health, New South Wales, 1913* (Sydney: Government Printer, 1913), 262–64; J.H.L. Cumpston, *Health and Disease in Australia: A History,* ed. M.J. Lewis (Canberra: Australian Government Publishing Service [hereafter AGPS], 1989), 326.

40. A.J.G. Buxton, "Poliomyelitis in South Australia 1937–1956" (honors dissertation, history, University of Adelaide, Adelaide, 1977), 18–22, 62–64, 80–81; Woodruff, *Two Million South Australians,* 82–87; Patrick, *A History of Health and Medicine in Queensland 1824–1960,* 239–40; L.S. Ibels, P. Berriman and E. Davis, "Poliomyelitis: Still with Us," *Medical Journal of Australia* 1 (1971): 593.

41. A. Herceg and R. Hall, "Polio Vaccination and Polio Eradication," *Medical Journal of Australia* 163 (1995): 399–400; G. Ada, "The Efficacy and Safety of Vaccines," *Nature and Society Forum* (April–May 1998): 8.

42. J. Powles, "Professional Hygienists and the Health of the Nation," in *The*

Commonwealth of Science: ANZAAS and the Scientific Enterprise in Australia 1888–1988, ed. R. MacLeod (Melbourne: Oxford University Press, 1988), 292–307.

43. Quoted in S.J. Kunitz, "Explanations and Ideologies of Mortality Patterns," *Population and Development Review* 13 (1987): 387.

44. Quoted in ibid., 388; Mullan, *Plagues and Politics,* 68–70; R. Beaglehole and R. Bonita, *Public Health at the Crossroads: Achievements and Prospects* (Cambridge: Cambridge University Press, 1999), 95–97.

45. Quoted in Kunitz, "Explanations and Ideologies of Mortality Patterns," 393.

46. Quoted in Mullan, *Plagues and Politics,* 191.

47. Quoted in Webster, *Government and Health Care,* 677.

48. Quoted in Kunitz, "Explanations and Ideologies of Mortality Patterns," 386–94; Mullan, *Plagues and Politics,* 187–91; Webster, *Government and Health Care,* 676–77.

49. N. Pearce, "Traditional Epidemiology, Modern Epidemiology, and Public Health," *American Journal of Public Health* 86(5) (1996): 680.

50. Ibid., 680–82.

51. Duffy, *The Sanitarians,* 283–84; M.G. Marmot and J.F. Mustard, "Coronary Heart Disease from a Population Perspective," in *Why Are Some People Healthy and Others Not? The Determinants of Health of Populations,* eds. R.G. Evans, M.L. Barer and T.R. Marmor (New York: Aldine De Gruyter, 1994), 194–95.

52. R. Taylor, M. Lewis and J. Powles, "The Australian Mortality Decline: Cause-Specific Mortality 1907–1990," *Australian and New Zealand Journal of Public Health* 22(1) (1998): 41–42.

53. Marmot and Mustard, "Coronary Heart Disease from a Population Perspective," 189–200.

54. Quoted in K. Garrety, "Actor-Networks, Social Worlds and Controversy: The Case of Cholesterol, Dietary Fat and Heart Disease," unpublished paper, School of Science and Technology Studies, University of New South Wales, 1996, 8.

55. Ibid., 1–19.

56. R. Reader, *The National Heart Foundation of Australia and Heart Disease in Australia: An Account of the Foundation's First Twenty Years* (Gundaroo: Brolga Press for National Heart Foundation, 1996), 5–12.

57. "The National Heart Foundation of Australia," *Medical Journal of Australia* 1 (1969): 461; "The National Heart Foundation of Australia," *Medical Journal of Australia* 1 (1961): 941; Reader, *The National Heart Foundation of Australia and Heart Disease in Australia,* 117, 143.

58. Reader, *The National Heart Foundation of Australia and Heart Disease in Australia,* 140–41, 167–71.

59. R. Walker and D. Roberts, *From Scarcity to Surfeit: A History of Food and Nutrition in New South Wales* (Kensington: NSW University Press, 1988), 121–23, 126–28, 146–48; Reader, *The National Heart Foundation of Australia and Heart Disease in Australia,* 223.

60. P. Magnus, "The Cardiovascular State of Australia: Good or Bad News?" *Medical Journal of Australia* 164 (1996): 517–18.

61. Taylor, Lewis and Powles, "The Australian Mortality Decline," 42; National Health and Medical Research Council, *Promoting the Health of Australians: Case Studies of Achievements in Improving the Health of the Population, December 1996* (Canberra: AGPS, 1997), 2.

62. J. Goodman, *Tobacco in History: The Cultures of Dependence* (London: Routledge, 1993), 90–107; Wilson, "The Historical Decline of Tuberculosis in Europe and America," 367; R. Walker, *Under Fire: A History of Tobacco Smoking in Australia* (Carlton: Melbourne University Press, 1984), 34, 54, 84; National Health and Medical Research Council, *Promoting the Health of Australians,* 1.

63. I. Tyrrell, "The Anti-Tobacco Reform and the Temperance Movement in Australia: Connections and Differences," *Journal of Royal Australian Historical Society* 84 (1) (1998): 10–22; "Cancer and Tobacco Smoking," *Medical Journal of Australia* 2 (1950): 523.

64. M. Susser, "Epidemiology in the United States after World War II: The Evolution of Technique," *Epidemiologic Reviews* 7 (1985): 162–63; "Carcinoma of the Lung," *Medical Journal of Australia* 2 (1960): 265; Goodman, *Tobacco in History,* 124–25.

65. Quoted in "Carcinoma of the Lung," 266.

66. Goodman, *Tobacco in History,* 10–11, 126–27.

67. D. Collingridge and C. Reeve, *Science Speaks to Power: The Role of Experts in Policy Making* (London: Frances Pinter, 1986), 123–41; Webster, *Government and Health Care,* 133–35, 242–45, 424–26, 665–69.

68. Quoted in Mullan, *Plagues and Politics,* 149.

69. Quoted in A.M. Brandt, "The Cigarette, Risk, and American Culture," *Daedalus* 119(4) (1990): 164.

70. Ibid., 163–72; Mullan, *Plagues and Politics,* 149–50.

71. "Medical Matters in Parliament: Cigarette Smoking," *Medical Journal of Australia* 1 (1964): 776; "Smoking and Health," *Medical Journal of Australia* 2 (1965): 338–39; Walker, *Under Fire,* 34, 87–88.

72. "Cigarette Advertising and Television," *Medical Journal of Australia* 1 (1967): 398.

73. Ibid., 397–98; Walker, *Under Fire,* 87–92.

74. Walker, *Under Fire,* 97–110; National Health and Medical Research Council, *Promoting the Health of Australians,* 4–5.

75. Walker, *Under Fire,* 110–12; National Health and Medical Research Council, *Promoting the Health of Australians,* 1, 6–9.

76. Beaglehole and Bonita, *Public Health at the Crossroads,* 72–73; "Prophylaxis against Road Accidents," *Medical Journal of Australia* 2 (1965): 795–96; A. Johnson, "Some Social and General Aspects of Traffic Accidents," *Medical Journal of Australia* 2 (1966): 161–63; see M. Lewis, *A Rum State: Alcohol and State Policy in Australia* (Canberra: AGPS, 1992), 17.

77. J. McGeorge, "Driving under the Influence," *Medical Journal of Australia* 1 (1942): 105–8; N.M. Gutteridge, "Driving under the Influence," *Medical Journal of Australia* 1 (1942): 271–72.

78. F.S. Hansman, "Driving under the Influence of Intoxicating Drink," *Medical Journal of Australia* 2 (1953): 388–90; A.J. McMichael and A.J. McLean, "Alcohol and Road Accidents in Australia: Corroborative Population-Based Evidence," *Community Health Studies* (3) (1980): 281–84.

79. *Commonwealth Parliamentary Debates,* H. of R. 60 (20 August 1968): 299; H. of R. 130 (14 December 1982): 3400; H. of R. 118 (1–2 May 1980): 2591–93.

80. R. Room, "The Dialectic of Drinking in Australian Life: From the Rum Corps to the Wine Column," *Australian Drug and Alcohol Review* 7 (1988): 430; Report of Royal Commission into Sale, Supply, Disposal or Consumption of Liquor in State of Victoria, *Victoria Parliamentary Papers*, 2, 1964–65, 949–94.

81. National Health and Medical Research Council, *Promoting the Health of Australians*, 15–21; A. Woodward, "Epidemiology and Public Health in South Australia," in *Health for All: The South Australian Experience*, ed. F. Baum (Kent Town: Wakefield Press, 1995), 130–33; *National Alcohol Strategy: A Plan for Action 2001 to 2003–04* (Canberra: Commonwealth Department of Health and Aged Care, 2001), 45.

82. Lewis, *A Rum State*, 6–10.

83. A.W. Martin, "Drink and Deviance in Sydney: Investigating Intemperance, 1854–55," *Historical Studies* 17 (1977): 342; A.J.C. Mayne, *Fever, Squalor and Vice: Sanitation and Social Policy in Victorian Sydney* (St. Lucia: University of Queensland Press, 1982), 134; W. Phillips, "'Six O'Clock Swill': The Introduction of Early Closing of Hotel Bars in Australia," *Historical Studies* 19 (1980): 250–66.

84. W.F. Bynum, "Chronic Alcoholism in the First Half of the 19th Century," *Bulletin of History of Medicine* 42 (1968): 160–85; R.M. MacLeod, "The Edge of Hope: Social Policy and Chronic Alcoholism, 1870–1900," *Journal of History of Medicine and Allied Sciences* 22 (1967): 215–45; C. McCarthy, *Inebriate Retreats: Their Origin, Utility, Necessity, and Management* (Melbourne: Stillwell, 1888), 9–12; S. Garton, "Bad or Mad? Developments in Incarceration in New South Wales, 1880–1920," in *What Rough Beast? The State and Social Order in Australian History*, ed. Sydney Labour History Group (Sydney: Allen and Unwin, 1982), 98; S. Garton, "'Once a Drunkard Always a Drunkard': Social Reform and the Problem of 'Habitual Drunkenness' in Australia, 1880–1914," *Historical Studies* 53 (1987), 43–44; "The Treatment of Inebriates," *Australasian Medical Gazette* 25 (1906): 481; J. Bostock, "Alcoholism and Its Treatment," *Medical Journal of Australia* 1 (1939): 137–38; Lewis, *A Rum State*, 111–18.

85. P. Healy, *Patterns of Drug Use in Australia 1970–1977* (Sydney: Health Commission of NSW, 1978), 18; J.B. Bungey and C.J. Winter, "Alcohol Consumption Patterns in South Australia, 1983," *Medical Journal of Australia* 144 (1986): 6; "Alcoholism," *Medical Journal of Australia* 1 (1961): 55; *South Australia Parliamentary Debates* 2 (26 October 1961): 1582–83; *Queensland Parliamentary Debates* 248 (21 March 1968): 2488–91; *Victoria Parliamentary Debates* 291 (22 October 1968): 1097–101; *Western Australia Parliamentary Debates* 205 (8 October 1974): 2084–86; *New South Wales Parliamentary Debates* 153 (25 March 1980): 5811–15; E. Single and T. Rohl, *The National Drug Strategy: Mapping the Future: An Evaluation of the National Drug Strategy 1993–1997* (Canberra: AGPS, 1997), 31.

86. S.J. Minogue, "Alcoholics Anonymous," *Medical Journal of Australia* 1 (1948): 586–87; A.V. McKinnon, *Castle of Shadows* (Sydney: Devonshire Press, n.d.), 9, 15–23, 38–42, 76–78; P. Stolz, "The Australian Foundation on Alcoholism and Drug Dependence: A National Perspective," in *Alcohol in Australia: Problems and Programmes*, eds. A.P. Diehm, R.F. Seaborn and G.C. Wilson (Sydney: McGraw-Hill, 1978), 227–43.

87. "The Alcoholism Treatment Package," *Lancet* 2 (1977): 489.

88. Report of (Honorary) Royal Commission to Inquire into Treatment of Alcohol and Drug Dependents in Western Australia, *Western Australia Votes and Proceedings,* 6, 1973, 52.

89. M. Sargent, *Drinking and Alcoholism in Australia: A Power Relations Theory* (Melbourne: Longman Cheshire,1979), 167; *Alcohol Policies in the United Kingdom: Report by Central Policy Review Staff,* 1979, VIII, 9, 70, 77.

90. Quoted in R. Room, "The World Health Organization and Alcohol Control," *British Journal of Addiction* 79 (1984): 86–88.

91. A. Paton, "The Politics of Alcohol," *British Medical Journal* 290 (1985): 1.

92. K. Bruun, *Dilemmas in Drug Control Policy* (Melbourne: Alcoholism Foundation of Victoria, 1972), 4–10; R.E. Kendell, "Alcoholism: A Medical or a Political Problem?" *British Medical Journal* 1 (1979): 367–71; Paton, "The Politics of Alcohol," 1–2; J. Cavanagh and F. Clairmonte, "Alcoholic Beverages: Dimensions of Corporate Power," in *The World Alcohol Industry with Special Reference to Australia, New Zealand and the Pacific Islands,* ed. J. Cavanagh, F. Clairmonte and R. Room (Sydney: Transnational Corporations Research Project, University of Sydney, 1985): 1–9; A. Wodak, "Australian Alcohol Consumption," *Medical Journal of Australia* 144 (1986): 1–2.

93. Quoted in D. Manderson, *From Mr Sin to Mr Big: A History of Australian Drug Laws* (Melbourne: Oxford University Press, 1993), 40.

94. Quoted in ibid., 44.

95. Ibid., 9, 40–42, 54–55, 61–64, 71, 95–97, 105–25.

96. Ibid., 117, 123, 126–30, 143–47, 159.

97. "Research into Alcoholism and Drug Dependence," *Medical Journal of Australia* 2 (1972): 518–19; Senate Select Committee on Drug Trafficking and Drug Abuse Report, *Commonwealth Parliamentary Papers,* 8, 1971, 9, 84.

98. K.M. Roger, "Strategy for Drug Abuse Prevention: The National Drug Education Program," in *Drug Trade and Drug Use,* ed. G. Wardlaw (Canberra: Australian Foundation on Alcoholism and Drug Dependence for Australian National University, 1982), 29–35; Manderson, *From Mr Sin to Mr Big,* 152; *Commonwealth Parliamentary Debates,* H. of R. 80 (12 September 1972): 1243.

99. P. Baume, "Opening Address," in *Drug Trade and Drug Use,* ed. Wardlaw, 1–2.

100. *Drug Problems in Australia: An Intoxicated Society? Senate Standing Committee on Social Welfare Report* (Canberra: AGPS, 1977), 12.

101. Manderson, *From Mr Sin to Mr Big,* 170–72; *Commonwealth Parliamentary Debates,* S 84 (19 March 1980): 795–800.

102. Quoted in Room, "The Dialectic of Drinking in Australian Life," 432.

103. D. McDonald, H. Brown, M. Hamilton, M. Miller and E. Stephenson, "Australian Drug Policies 1988 and Beyond: A Drug Campaign Evaluation," *Australian Drug and Alcohol Review* 7 (1988): 500–504; Room, "The Dialectic of Drinking in Australian Life," 432; Manderson, *From Mr Sin to Mr Big,* 188–90.

104. *Draft National Health Policy on Alcohol in Australia. Presented to Ministerial Council on Drug Strategy,* 6 November 1987, 5; *Commentary on National Health Policy on Alcohol in Australia: Presented to Ministerial Council on Drug Strategy, 6 November 1987,* 2–11; *Advertiser,* 23 April 1988, 5 January 1989; *Age,* 25 March 1989; D. Hawks, "The Watering Down of Australia's Health Policy on Alcohol,"

Keynote Address to Winter School in the Sun: Lifestyles, Culture and Drugs Conference, Brisbane, 1989, 7.

105. Hawks, "The Watering Down of Australia's Health Policy on Alcohol," 9–16; *National Health Policy on Alcohol in Australia: Presented to Ministerial Council on Drug Strategy: Adopted 23 March 1989,* 6–8.

106. Quoted in Single and Rohl, *The National Drug Strategy,* 59.

107. Ibid., vii–viii, 3–66; *National Alcohol Strategy,* 5.

Chapter 3

The Concept of Community Health

After twenty-three years of Liberal-National Party governments in Canberra, the country returned a Labor government, headed by Gough Whitlam, in December 1972. An energetic, reforming government strongly committed to the pursuit of social justice, the Whitlam administration was not short on policy objectives, especially in the health and social welfare areas. It was sometimes less clear about the detailed means by which the objectives were to be reached. The Community Health Program tended to suffer from such lack of coherence, a defect that was made worse by the speed with which reforms were introduced—in the belief that Labor, not being the "natural" government, might well not have much time to promote its plans to advance social justice. Where conservatives had tried to restrict state intervention, relying on economic growth to furnish the wherewithal by which individuals would provide for themselves, and seeing social welfare only as a safety net for those whom the market and family failed, the Whitlam government saw state intervention as a means by which to advance the welfare of all citizens. It sought to advance, not restrict, state intervention in education, housing and urban development, as well as health.

While the return of Labor to power saw the resurrection of major federal initiatives in prevention through the Community Health Program, it is well to remember that prevention was a minor theme in health policy compared with concern for equitable access to curative and rehabilitative services through a universal health insurance scheme, Medibank, and a hospital cost-sharing scheme. Where federal support for health since 1949, under conservative governments, had taken the form of subsidizing of private expenditures, it now involved expansion of the public sector, through direct provision of personal services. An important reason for Labor's concern with adequacy of health care services was the fact that Whitlam, himself the member for a disadvantaged Sydney electorate, was acutely aware of the service deficiencies in the quickly growing outer suburbs of Sydney and Melbourne. Indeed, shortcomings in these areas of Sydney had been highlighted by New South Wales health authorities, who were already planning regionalization of administration and development of community-oriented services under a new Health Commission.[1]

THE CONCEPT OF THE COMMUNITY HEALTH CENTER IN THE UNITED STATES AND BRITAIN

The health center movement in the United States has roots in the 1890s, in attempts to alleviate the lot of immigrants in the slums of Chicago and New York. The work of the local dispensary, the key source of medical assistance for the urban working class, was being modified by voluntary social workers like Lillian D. Wald and Mary Brewster at New York's Henry Street Settlement and Jane Addams at Chicago's Hull House. Prevention and social assistance were provided, as well as rudimentary health care. Inspired by Wilbur C. Phillips's idea that infant milk stations could also provide health education in their neighborhoods, the Milwaukee City Health Department established a health center providing infant and maternal health care in a Polish neighborhood in 1911. The mothers themselves were involved in the running of the center. When Phillips went back to New York City, he organized a group to encourage creation of democratic neighborhood facilities. A neighborhood project was set up by Phillips and his wife in Cincinnati in 1918, but the city government withdrew its backing in 1920 in the face of criticism from local doctors and charges of support for "socialism." Projects in Pittsburgh and Philadelphia also failed to take root, but New York, Boston and Buffalo proved more receptive ground. Dr. Sigismund Goldwater, health commissioner for New York City, created in 1914 a health district of thirty-five thousand people on the Lower East Side of Manhattan. A medical inspector and three nurses served the district. It carried out home visiting and health education, as well as inspection of infants and schoolchildren.

The health center movement grew when the poor health of recruits in World War I sharpened consciousness of health matters. There were in 1920 seventy-two health centers in forty-nine cities but ten years later 1,500, about 50 percent of which received municipal funding. Although some specialized in child health or ear, nose and throat conditions, they all pursued prevention. In New York in the 1920s, municipal health centers were closed by a hostile city government, but in 1934 Mayor Fiorello La Guardia reestablished city support. Federal funding permitted the building of new health centers. By 1936 New York was split up into twenty-two health districts. To create a greater presence for the health districts in the central health administration, a new Bureau of District Health Administration (into which the child and school hygiene bureaus were dissolved) was set up. At the same time, the community was kept involved through the establishment of two committees for each district, one representing its doctors and its other, religious and social groups. The 1940s saw the recession of the health center movement in the United States as immigration declined, per capita incomes increased and the medical profession resisted challenges to private provision of primary care services.[2]

The medical profession had reacted strongly to the growth of public provision of primary care services in the late nineteenth and early twentieth centuries. It charged that free-standing and hospital dispensaries—about a hundred throughout the country by 1900—were treating some patients able to pay for the services of private practitioners. In fact, however, New York State law of 1899 punished patients who understated their incomes, and dispensaries seem to have catered mainly to poor families. A 1911 survey of Manhattan dispensaries showed that 90 percent of patients could not afford private care. To avoid the stigma of charity medicine, some working-class families used doctors employed by fraternal societies under contract, on a salaried or capitation basis. As in Australia, the organized profession disliked contract practice because of the poor remuneration and because it took patients away from the fee-for-service system. The American Medical Association in 1913 had agreed to accept contract practice only where there was an income limit for members. By 1920 or so, contract practice had become insignificant. In the 1920s and 1930s, the AMA went on to fight group practice and prepaid care, using as a primary argument the proposition that they were a step toward socialized medicine.

As specialization increased in the 1940s and 1950s, the number of general practitioners declined, especially in inner, urban areas, where the poor were concentrated. General practitioners accounted for 80 percent of doctors in 1931 but only 28 percent in 1963. Those who could afford private care attended different specialists for different conditions. In the 1960s, in the large cities, the hospital outpatient department and the emergency room were the sources of primary care for the poor. The neighborhood health center concept revived in this situation of inadequate distribution of primary health care.

Liberal critics of federal health policy, like Milton Roemer, pointed in the 1950s to excessive bias toward hospital construction and called for comprehensive, community-based services. State psychiatric hospitals were already in the 1950s declining in population as the use of tranquilizers enabled patients to be seen on an outpatient basis and as federal funding for nursing homes allowed a transfer of aged people with senility problems to these facilities. Professional enthusiasts for community psychiatry advanced persuasive therapeutic arguments, in any case, against institutionalization and in favor of treatment in the community. The John F. Kennedy administration, advocating a new approach to psychiatric illness and intellectual disability, in 1963 persuaded Congress to support construction of community mental health centers. Later, funds for staffing were provided. These programs established a direct connection between the federal government and local communities. However, because it was intended as a demonstration program, the concept was not permanently funded. Moreover, like the neighborhood health centers program, it was always comparatively marginal in health care.

Kennedy's advisers had begun to develop an antipoverty program, but it was Lyndon Johnson's "War on Poverty" that finally committed the federal government to redistributive reform and heavy involvement in health care support. The Office of Economic Opportunity (OEO) had become involved with local community action groups in health care, and a decision was taken to support demonstration health centers offering comprehensive care. The first was established in Boston, a second in rural Mississippi, and others followed. After Congress authorized funds for such services in 1967, the OEO over four years supported establishment of around a hundred neighborhood health centers and similar projects.

The Department of Health, Education and Welfare (HEW) assisted with establishment of fifty other centers. The centers were to provide a wide range of health care for poor communities and at the same time employ local people and involve community members in their operation. As elements of a national demonstration program, the centers functioned outside the established health bureaucracies. But Medicaid, the federal health care program for the poor, did not cover many of the services provided by the centers. In the late 1960s another long-term source of income was severely restricted when it was mandated that only 20 percent of center registrants could be paying patients. This removed the centers as serious competitors for private practitioners. Now essentially dependent on government funds, the centers were highly vulnerable to any adverse change in federal policy. HEW planned in the later 1960s to have a thousand centers, serving a population of twenty-five million, in place by 1973 and to use the center program rather than Medicaid to provide health care for poor areas. But such extensive plans were not implemented. It was Medicaid that received the bulk of funds, even when evidence existed that the centers promoted community health and cut demand for hospital services through prevention and early treatment. The reason was that Medicaid was reconcilable with major, established health interests. Medicaid ensured that the bad debts of hospitals did not accumulate, and it presented no threat to private practice. The centers would survive the conservative Richard Nixon and Ronald Reagan administrations, carrying on into the 1980s.

President Nixon's "New Federalism" of 1969 aimed to get rid of much of the categorical grant programs structure introduced by the Kennedy and Johnson administrations, to make state and localities responsible for such matters, and in general to reduce substantially federal subsidization of health activities. But Nixon faced a liberal Democratic Congress ready to defend many of the programs associated with the War on Poverty. The health center program was strongly supported by senior officials of the Department of Health, Education and Welfare (renamed the Department of Health and Human Services in 1980) for the life of the Carter administration. Reagan began his presidency with a Republican Senate and a House having only a small Democratic majority. Even so, Congress rejected a number of times President Reagan's proposal to submerge the center program in a block grant to the states for health services, although it accepted that the states should be more involved in the running of the program.

The center program never grew into a serious challenge to mainstream private medicine, and it never fulfilled the hopes of early supporters of the centers in the OEO and HEW that it would serve populations other than the poor and thus help transform the national health care system, as a cost-effective means of providing primary care and preventive services. The centers remained peripheral to the national health care system precisely because they were limited to serving the poor, a residual population that neither hospitals nor private practitioners were interested in serving.[3]

In Britain, the Dawson Report of 1920, which (as noted in *The People's Health*, volume 1) reviewed the future of medical services in the United Kingdom, proposed establishment of primary health centers integrating preventive and curative services and run by general practitioners. Not only did it include the (rather vague) notion of health maintenance as opposed to cure of disease, but its collectivism challenged the deep-rooted individualism of general practitioners. Thus the report was shelved. However, the concept of the health center, housing a range of health personnel, did not disappear from the world of health planning. In the 1930s, the Labor Party, the Socialist Medical Association and the Medical Practitioners Union gave a prominent place in policy to the concept. The center concept was prominent in early wartime versions of the NHS, but doctors became hostile because they linked it with salaried service under local authorities.

As the NHS was in process of establishment, the centers appeared about to become significant parts of the new organization. Even the British Medical Association (BMA) saw them as acceptable experiments that might well develop into the basis of general practice and the focus of neighborhood preventive, curative and social services. But this key feature of the NHS did not become established, for a number of reasons. First was the failure of the two dozen existing clinics, run by local authorities and mutual aid societies and allowed to continue as health centers, to thrive. Second was that in the Labor government's negotiations with the BMA in 1948, it became clear that the BMA would accept only modification of the established panel system as the basis of general practice. But the restriction of the health center concept to new practice locations, like housing projects, itself ran into insuperable problems: virtually no funds were available for capital development, and in Birmingham and Sheffield the support of local practitioners was lost. The result was cautious progress involving development where no viable alternative was possible. Even this way forward was blocked when preference in policy was given to group practice over center development. Only eight centers were built by 1956, with a further two built by 1960. A small number of others were opened through cooperative arrangements between local health authorities and organizations like the Nuffield Provincial Hospitals Trust. Many local authorities sought government support to open new centers, but in the main they failed to get approval. Many centers became caught up in the competition among general practitioners for patients. Local doctors often saw patients on center premises in order to forestall other doctors from capturing them. Cooperation in centers between doctors and local authorities was often poor. Overall, patients received no great advantage from attending centers.[4]

While the centers had been seen, at the beginning of the life of the NHS, as a way of integrating the three branches of the service, general practitioner wariness and government unwillingness to spend for capital development resulted, as we have seen, in little center growth. A survey by the Medical Practitioners Union published in 1960 found as few as fourteen centers—of which four were in Scotland—providing for fewer than 250,000 people and representing only seven hundred thousand pounds in capital expenditure.

In the second half of the 1960s, various developments improved the situation of general practitioners. Following work by the College of General Practitioners (from 1967, the Royal College), the Royal Commission on Medical Education proposed reforms that lifted the status of general practitioners to that of the hospital-based specialists—reforms concerning undergraduate and postgraduate education and the general practitioner role in medical schools. Moreover, the BMA's 1965 Family Doctors Charter led to a new contract for general practitioners that meant better financial conditions, with contributions to the cost of ancillary staff and to rents and rates on practice premises. The contract encouraged more positive attitudes among practitioners. These developments and the government's fiscal interest in transferring resources from expensive hospital medicine to cheaper and more prevention-oriented community services pushed the growth of health centers.

By 1974, there existed 566 centers in England, twenty-nine in Wales, and fifty-nine in Scotland. By 1978, there were 815 in England, and they housed 20 percent of practitioners. But while primary health care was doing well in the family practitioner services area, it was subject to spending constraints in the hospital and community health services sector. Indeed, both the Harding and the Acheson Reports in the 1980s expressed concern about the future of primary care teams. Earlier, the Royal Commission on the National Health Services of the late 1970s had said cautiously that primary care teamwork was at an early state of development. In the late 1980s, expert commentators were still critical of the adequacy of primary care in rural and inner-city locations, especially inner London, noting that some doctors still saw themselves as having no role other than "responding to episodes of illness."[5]

THE COMMUNITY HEALTH CENTER CONCEPT IN AUSTRALIA

Although the concept flowered most brilliantly in the 1970s in Australia, it was not new. Indeed, if we break down the idea into its significant component parts, some may be discerned in earlier examples of community-based health services. These significant parts include highlighting of the role of the "community"—an often vague term, but usually implying some sort of local, social network and often carrying egalitarian and democratic overtones that might be expressed as nonprofessional, nonbureaucratic, local citizen participation in the management of the health facility; prevention and support rather than cure as the basis of organization, resulting in prominence for health education; geographical, social and economic accessibility of services for all citizens; provision of services on a regional basis; serious attention to social and psychological factors in the causation of illness and in its treatment; and greater recognition of the role of nonmedical health professionals in service delivery and policy discourse. Douglas Gordon, a distinguished public health figure and longtime professor of social and preventive medicine at Queensland University, saw the essence of community health in 1979 even more simply, as a focus on health in communities or social groups, with emphasis on prevention rather than cure. Prevention would include early diagnosis and support for the disabled, as well as the aged. Focus on the group entailed prevention, because the study of health in groups "often shows us how to prevent disease." Unlike traditional public health, however, community health tried to involve the general practitioner very extensively in preventive work.[6]

Of course, as I observed in *The People's Health,* volume 1, community-based (as opposed to hospital or domiciliary) prevention-oriented services catering to infant and, in a more limited way, maternal health needs were set up in Australia in the early twentieth century. But these were doctor dominated in relation to organization, and authoritarian and directive in relation to patients. They were influenced by a background ideology of "national efficiency" and "race" improvement, and by a strong pronatalism. By the 1970s, community health was informed by the more egalitarian and democratic culture of the times and by considerations of social justice rather than "national efficiency." I also observed that J.H.L. Cumpston, a leading national hygienist and the preeminent public health figure of the first half of the twentieth century, recommended to the federal Royal Commission on Health of 1925 that the country be split up into health districts. Each district was to have a health center supervised by a salaried public health doctor, who would coordinate preventive work and the activities of non-medical public health workers. Clinical work would be carried out by local private practitioners, who would be paid fees for service. The royal commission recommended a national public health scheme of this type, but the recommendation was never implemented. Earlier, the reforming NSW Labor minister of public health, Frederic Flowers, who had sought to make public hospitals available to all citizens as a matter of right, not just to those too poor to afford private care, had envisaged community-based dispensaries as the source of ambulatory care for tuberculosis sufferers. In 1912 he had persuaded some friendly societies to allow use of their dispensaries for this purpose, only to find progress blocked by opposition from private medical practitioners and pharmacists. Nonetheless, a government-subsidized dispensary was opened in inner Sydney by the National Association for Prevention and Cure of Consumption.

In 1941, Cumpston and Raphael Cilento, with Harold Dew and J. Newman Morris, drew up as a committee of the NHMRC a report, *An Outline of a Possible Scheme for a Salaried Medical Service,* which the full NHMRC endorsed as a basis for discussion with the medical profession. The NHMRC saw three particular strengths in the proposal: it united preventive and curative services; it ensured that remote areas would obtain adequate medical services; and it would create socially equitable access to medical services. As in Cumpston's 1925 scheme, the country would be split up into health districts, and the district health officer, employed by the national health authority, would supervise the normal range of public health and preventive activities. Local general practitioners, paid part-time salaries, would provide primary care in district centers and would refer serious cases to the local public hospitals.[7] The Chifley federal Labor government's National Service Act of 1948–49 did in fact divide the country into health areas supervised by district health officers. It also provided for regional clinics, where preventive work would be done by local doctors employed on a sessional basis. The bulk of curative work would continue to be done by private practitioners under government-subsidized, fee-for-service arrangements, whereby half the scheduled fee was paid by the patient and half by the federal government. Labor lost power in late 1949 before this national health service could be set up.

As noted earlier, psychiatry was much influenced by the idea of community-based services in the 1960s. Indeed, reformers among psychiatrists hailed community psychiatry as the "third psychiatric revolution." Gerald Caplan, a well-known American exponent, saw them as having a regional focus and as providing early treatment that would prevent hospitalization. They would also support patients discharged from hospital and promote mental health education as a means of primary prevention. However, the movement of public policy to the right and economy in welfare expenditure in the 1970s put brakes on the growth of community psychiatry. The community centers themselves ran into difficulties. In the large cities, the absence of strong natural communities meant that genuine participation was often difficult to build. Moreover, the desirable degree of community participation became a point of conflict. Some centers opted for more limited participation through advisory boards, while others chose total community control. Disputes also existed about the emphasis to be placed on social reform as opposed to purely clinical matters. Overestimation of the capacity of preventive work to reduce the prevalence of chronic psychiatric illness, as well as of the effectiveness of crisis intervention, led to some discrediting of the community mode of practice.

Reviewing community psychiatry in Australia in the mid-1970s, the *Medical Journal of Australia* pointed out that ever since psychiatric hospitals had begun placing patients in the community, professionals had disagreed on whether they were gaining independence or were being callously neglected.[8] In fact, focus on community psychiatric work had begun in the late 1950s in Australia. In 1958, the NSW Mental Health Act modernized mental health legislation. It repealed the 1898 Lunacy Act, abolishing certification and committal on the sole ground of psychiatric illness. It provided for the first time for community workers—mental welfare officers—to visit patients on leave at home. The following year, regional planning of psychiatric services began, with North Ryde Psychiatric Centre—the first new psychiatric facility in the state since 1924—acting as a model. It provided a regional service on a basis of only 0.4 beds per thousand population. In 1961 the Health Advisory Council issued an *Interim Report on Preventive Psychiatry.* This document stressed prevention, decentralization and community orientation. In Australia, as in the United States and Britain, the availability of new psychotropic drugs in the 1950s enabled acute symptoms of significant conditions to be alleviated to the extent that reintegration of many hospital patients into the community was feasible. However, the drug revolution reinforced, rather than initiated, the movement toward community-based services.

A more cost-effective solution to psychiatric hospital overcrowding seemed to be to deal with the problems in the community. The weekly cost per patient in NSW increased from $17.39 in 1959–60 to $111.85 in 1972–73. Even if an inflation rate of 5 to 8 percent is allowed for this period, the rising cost of psychiatric hospitals is clear. The impact of the community psychiatry movement can be seen in the decline of the NSW hospital patient population, which went down from an average of 12,505 in 1961 to 8,250 in 1972, despite the fact that admissions increased from 12,660 to 20,987 in this period. In Queensland, the director of psychiatric services, Basil Stafford, was impressed by the emphasis placed in the English Mental Health Act of 1959 on open hospitals and community psychiatry. Queensland legislation in 1962, like the 1958 NSW act, sought to modernize the basis of psychiatric treatment. From the 1960s onward, mental health professionals were educated in community principles. Some acted as consultants to voluntary community agencies, which in turn applied preventive crisis intervention, in the belief that it would reduce demand for professional services. Victoria, which began the process of modernization earlier than any other state, created a Mental Hygiene Authority in the early 1950s. This body developed plans for regionalization of services and community-oriented psychiatric units. By 1961, two units were operating in relation to psychiatric hospitals at Ballarat, a major provincial town, and at Larundel, Melbourne, while a third was coming into operation in the heavily populated Latrobe Valley. By 1970 there were ten clinics in Melbourne itself.

In South Australia, W.E. Mickleburgh, a senior psychiatrist, having been influenced by developments in the United Kingdom, helped initiate in the mid-1960s community-based facilities. The first day-hospital and first aftercare hostels were established, and the first mental health visitors were trained. A community mental health center was opened in Adelaide in 1967, and three years later a second center was established. Starting in 1959, discharges from Claremont Hospital in Western Australia increased. The institution began to empty, as a parallel decline in the readmission rate took place. A day hospital was opened at Shenton Park, and more aftercare hostels were set up. Also, from 1959 on mental health officers worked in the community with patients and their families.

Tasmania modernized its mental health legislation in 1963 with the passing of a new Mental Health Act similar to Queensland's. This act promoted the growth of informal admissions; by 1965, informal patients constituted 75 percent of the patient population. In 1967, new legislation intended to integrate the professional, academic, administrative and community aspects of mental health was passed.[9] Reflecting on the advance of community psychiatry at the end of the 1960s, the NSW director of psychiatric services, W.A. Barclay, wrote: "There has been a considerable growth of community services during the past year. . . . [R]eduction of resident patients in psychiatric hospitals in the face of a substantial increase in the number of patients . . . can only be effected with humanity and safety if there is a corresponding growth in community mental health services."[10]

The push toward community-based services was also affecting other areas of health services, especially in NSW. Dr. Sidney Sax, a South African–trained doctor who had been much influenced by Dr. Sidney Kark's experiments with community health services in South Africa (Kark's ideas were expressed in *The Practice of Community Oriented Primary Health Care* [1981]), was made chairman of a Consultative Committee on the Care of the Aged set up by the NSW health minister in the Askin Liberal-Country Party government, A.H. Jago, in mid-1964. Sax, NSW director of geriatric services and later director of research and planning, reported to the health minister in August 1965, proposing development of community services at two levels—at the local level, personal services like home aides; and at regional level, general practitioner and allied health services, domiciliary nursing, and specialized geriatric units in general hospitals. The community services would prevent the aged from being prematurely hospitalized and would assist in the postdischarge period if they were.

From the mid-1960s various inquiries had examined the question of a structure enabling integrated development of NSW health services. In 1965, Health Minister Jago proposed to the chairman of the Public Service Board that an inquiry into health services organization be instituted. G.C. Eglington presented a report on the matter at the beginning of 1968. The report recommended, inter alia, unification of all health services under one administrative authority (the idea of a single health commission); decentralization and regionalization of services; at the local level, integrated, community services able to do all preventive work, treat all illness but the most complex, and carry out all investigations; and representation of consumer interests. A committee chaired by Sir Kenneth Starr submitted a report on community health services to the minister in November 1969, recommending a health commission to replace the Health Department, the Hospitals Commission and the Ambulance Transport Service Board; significant regionalization and decentralization of services; redefinition of the role of boards of public hospitals; and ongoing use of the advice of health professional and community groups in administration of services. Thus, it emphasized decentralization and accessibility of services, plus responsiveness to community wishes. In 1971, the premier, Robin (later Sir Robert) Askin, publicly stated the intention of the government to create a health commission of the type recommended by the Starr report. The following year Jago introduced legislation to the state parliament constituting a health commission, to function as a corporate body under the minister. He noted that in NSW, as in some other parts of the world, the indivisibility of the health of the person would now be reflected in the integrated nature of health administration. In April 1973 the Health Department became the Health Commission, when the department and the Hospitals Commission were incorporated into the new body.[11]

In November 1971, the first community health center providing a comprehensive range of services for a defined local community was officially opened. Queenscliff Health Centre, originally a diagnostic center for children from remote country areas visiting Sydney through the Royal Far West Children's Home, now offered facilities in child health, mental health, dental health and health education for the people of the Manly-Warringah area, on the northeastern side of Sydney Harbor. In May 1972, the second center, the Blacktown Health Centre, located in a socially disadvantaged, outer western suburb of Sydney, was opened. Offering a comprehensive range of services, it was established in the grounds of Blacktown District Hospital.

At the end of 1972, a community center was opened to provide services for an inner-city, socially disadvantaged population. The Glebe Community Care Centre, serving the suburbs of Glebe, Forest Lodge, Annandale, Ultimo and Pyrmont, worked closely with hospitals, general practitioners and nursing homes in its catchment area. By mid-1974, the staff was seeing ninety-eight people a day, of whom fifty-seven were seen at home. A small research team was part of the center, and the center functioned in close association with the Community Care Teaching Unit of Royal Prince Alfred Hospital (RPAH), one of the teaching hospitals of the University of Sydney Medical School.

Indeed, the center's origins lay in the teaching unit. Dr. Sidney Sax had been asked in 1970 by the hospital's project planning team to write a brief on the RPAH's involvement in community and geriatric medicine in its immediate community. The hospital authorities accepted Sax's proposals. A community medicine committee (having representatives of the hospital, the university, local municipal councils, the AMA, the Royal Australian College of General Practitioners and local general practitioners) of the planning team obtained in 1971 funds from the Ramaciotti Foundation, a Sydney-based private funder of medical research, to create a Community Care Teaching Unit. Dr. Andrew Harper became the founding director of research and training at the unit; his first task was the setting up of the Glebe Community Care Centre. From April 1975, community services in the rest of the hospital's defined community were provided through the Newtown Community Care Centre, which because of the federal government's establishment of the Hospitals and Health Services Commission in 1973 could be supported by federal funds. Thirty percent of the population served by the center were recent immigrants from Yugoslavia, Turkey or South America.[12]

The Queenscliff, Blacktown and Glebe community health centers in NSW predate the national community health center program introduced by the federal Labor government in 1973. Other community-based centers also predate the national program. In July 1971, about two hundred members of Sydney's Aboriginal community set up the Aboriginal Medical Service (AMS) as an incorporated body in Redfern, an inner-city, low-income suburb. Its staff was initially volunteer. The aim was that the center be staffed and administered as much as possible by Aborigines. Within a short time the Federal Health Department funded the posts of a doctor, nurse and some ancillary staff. By 1978, the federal Department of Aboriginal Affairs was funding twenty-six full-time posts. Offering primary care services, the AMS targeted key health needs of the Aboriginal community: nutrition, immunization, child health and alcohol abuse.[13] Because the AMS was recognized by the major hospitals as having the trust of the community, it could play an important part in liaison between the two.[14]

A NATIONAL COMMUNITY HEALTH CENTER PROGRAM

Before the Whitlam Labor government took office at the federal level in late 1972, conservative coalition governments had provided some money for such community-based services as domiciliary nursing and home care for the aged. But the states argued that proper reform required far more federal funding. Dr. Brian Shea, South Australian director general of medical services, observed in 1970, "The inescapable fact is that all state treasuries are rapidly running out of financial resources to maintain health and hospital standards at optimal levels."[15]

Only a short time before the McMahon Liberal-Country Party government lost office in October 1972, the National Congress of the Australian Hospitals Association was addressed by representatives of the major parties on health policy. The Liberal minister for health, Sir Kenneth Anderson, indicated that the government was essentially satisfied with the status quo as established by the 1970 update of the health insurance system. The Labor shadow minister for health and social welfare, Bill Hayden, on the other hand, declared that Labor would substantially increase federal funding, recognizing that as the federal government enjoyed an 85 percent share of public revenue, it had to become more involved if the states were to develop comprehensive services. He identified nine specific policy initiatives to be pursued: first, a Hospital and Health Services Commission (HHSC) to work with the states to develop regionalized health services, improve public health services, encourage growth of district general hospitals, and establish community health care centers; second, enlargement of the general practitioner's role by education of medical students in community medicine, funding of training for family practice and provision of community health staff to support the work of the general practitioner; third, introduction of universal health insurance; fourth, development of domiciliary and nursing home services; fifth, introduction of a national school dental health program; sixth, initiation of a national Aboriginal health program; seventh, preventive and occupational health and rehabilitation services, to be significant aspects of the new health program; eighth, assistance to the states to develop community mental health services as a priority and to provide psychiatric inpatient services in general hospitals; and ninth, ongoing evaluation of the various programs.

Soon after the Whitlam government assumed office, two new bodies were established to carry out Labor's health policy: the Health Insurance Commission, which had the job of introducing the universal health insurance scheme, Medibank; and the HHSC, more of a policy-making organization, charged with increasing the supply of health services. As Sidney Sax, who became chairman of an interim committee pending enactment of legislation to create the HHSC, recorded, there was a marked feeling of urgency among government ministers. The minister for health, Dr. Douglas Everingham, said to Sax at their first meeting, "Bear in mind that we are elected for a term of three years only!"[16] The Department of Health lost responsibility for the health insurance scheme to the Department of Social Security, which came under Bill Hayden's control as minister for social security, while the HHSC remained with the Department of Health. Dr. Sax later suggested that this division of responsibilities rendered coordination of health policy less effective, and the speed with which implementation took place increased the distance between various planning and policy groups. He further suggested, however, that because the HHSC consciously sought to work closely with the Health Department, even though it enjoyed direct access to the minister, the HHSC and department successfully coordinated policy development and management.

Prime Minister Whitlam had, when announcing the intention to establish the HHSC, predicted a significant role for prevention and community health services: "Health is a community affair. Communities must look beyond the person who is sick in bed or who needs medical attention. . . . The Commission will be concerned with more than just hospital services. Its concern and financial support will extend to the development of community-based health services and the sponsoring of preventative health programs."[17] Yet the Whitlam government's support for health advancement and community services was a minor theme in health policy compared with its concern with universal health insurance through Medibank. Medibank not only underwrote "sickness" care but perpetuated the predominant fee-for-service system, giving private practitioners direct access to federal funding. Thus, as with its successor, Medicare, all patients became "private," in the sense that they might see a general practitioner, knowing that most of the fee would be covered by federal funds.[18] One well-informed commentator has suggested that the community health policy began as a "political surrogate for a national health service" to win the support of Labor's left wing for national health insurance. As we shall see, the community health program was to be sidelined by the conservative Fraser Coalition government in the later 1970s, and it would slip farther from view when specific funding was replaced by a share of general, tax-sharing grants to the states.[19]

The interim committee of the HHSC began work in early April 1973 and by late May had tendered its report on the Community Health Program (CHP) to the Whitlam government. The CHP was to provide, in a coordinated way, facilities for prevention, treatment, rehabilitation and related welfare needs. The aim was "to encourage the provision of high quality, readily accessible, reasonably comprehensive, coordinated and efficient health and welfare services at local, regional, state and national levels." The community to be served would be consulted about development of services and would, "where appropriate," be involved in that development.[20] The following services were to be available in defined regions or localities:

1. Information and counseling services to improve habits, conditions and environments that dispose to health disorders
2. Preventive action such as immunization
3. Detection procedures to reveal preclinical phases of disease

4. Motivation of individuals to seek care as soon as departures from normal health are perceived
5. Diagnostic and treatment services during illness
6. Rehabilitation and supportive services for people with continuing disabilities
7. Assistance for people with chronic disability in adapting to sheltered living or working conditions.

Following consultation with state health authorities, the HHSC proposed federal funding be of two types: block grants to the states to cover capital and operating costs of facilities; and specific grants to the states or nonprofit organizations for individually approved projects that could be progressively included in a regional system. Funds would also be provided for a few national projects like the Family Medicine Program, a scheme run by the College of General Practitioners to train doctors in general practice. The report believed that community centers would offer coordinated primary care from teams of health professionals; those with chronic diseases or disabilities would have a choice between institutional and community care. Members of the community would cooperate with health professionals to solve the local community's health and related problems. The report's authors also believed that such centers would generate great opportunities for professional education and research, and that in the shift from hospital inpatient care to community services they would provide the means to reduce the considerable rate of increase in health service spending. For 1973–74, the CHP received ten million dollars. Under the Mental Health and Related Services Assistance Act, 1973, federal funds were provided for capital and maintenance costs of community-based mental health and alcohol and other drug services, and $7.5 million was made available for 1973–74. Initially constituting a separate program, the community mental health services were later integrated into the CHP.

The CHP was certainly an advance on the traditional health services in terms of meeting the health needs of the population. But with the luxury of hindsight, we can see that the HHSC report was conceptually unclear and intellectually limited in its analysis of how to advance the health status of the Australian people. Although reference was made to the effect of the social environment on health, the focus of the program was on individuals. The analysis of the causes of ill health also was rather shallow. The HHSC appears to have intended to use mainly individualistic means to promote secondary prevention. In any case, the CHP functioned in a virtual policy vacuum.[21] The social bases of ill health may have been acknowledged, but the practice was "to help individuals cope through their personal choices, however limited their options may be, with the larger ongoing causes of illness related to income and job inequities or agricultural and marketing policies and practices."[22]

The conceptual ambiguities of the CHP left it open to narrow interpretations by certain state health officials who, focusing on an individualistic approach to prevention, saw the problem as one of unhealthy lifestyle choices by ignorant or misinformed people. They thus supported individual counseling or mass media health education to persuade individuals to change faulty habits or not to take them up, and also to attend screening programs. A study of eight Queensland centers revealed that their activities were very different from the aims strongly endorsed in state policy documents and supported by center staff. Thus, 50 percent of staff gave high priority to primary prevention, but only 7 percent of their time was actually given to this area; in any case, they did not believe that the primary aim was being achieved. Community work received very little attention. The overwhelming emphasis was on work with individual clients or the therapeutic (secondary prevention) use of small-group work. Most center resources went to day-to-day client demands and to established interventions known to professional staff.

Organizationally, the community health services failed to link up with public health efforts in a way that would have allowed primary and secondary prevention to function as complementary aspects of a fully health-promoting policy. Primary care is concerned with high-risk and sick persons; it functions on an interpersonal basis. Public health policy is concerned with well persons and total populations, and it focuses on long-term health interests. While primary care promotes primary prevention for some acute health problems, it mainly focuses on secondary prevention, reducing risk and containing the severity of sickness. It benefits people, particularly the very young and elderly, in the short and medium term. Public health policy, however, offers primary prevention of risks, influencing common, underlying causes of major health problems so it benefits people, particularly through the middle-adult years, in the medium to long term. Community health centers have in principle the capacity to bridge individual and collective approaches at the local level. While offering individual services for secondary prevention (and a limited degree of primary prevention), they may support or even initiate collective attempts to change community living conditions—for example, by increasing people's awareness of the larger economic, policy and environmental factors adversely influencing health and how to act to change them; or by initiating efforts to advance new health policies.[23]

In 1972, at the beginning of the experiment with community health centers, Charles Kerr, professor of preventive and social medicine at the University of Sydney, warned that if the health center concept did not extend beyond the primary medical care model and the general practitioner's existing arrangements with other health professionals and agencies, it would be no advance over the established situation. First, the center had to be under a single management and related to the administration of the health region in which it was located; otherwise, it would reproduce the fragmentation of health services—private practitioners, public hospitals, health department components, medical school interests and voluntary agencies—already existing. Second, it had to provide a real team approach if it were to deal adequately with the range of health conditions in the community. The key team member would be the doctor. But unfortunately, the conservatism of medical educators had resulted in a generation of doctors not well qualified for community practice, because understanding of chronic disease and preventive medicine had not been adequately imparted to them.[24]

In 1974, Andrew Harper, director of research and training of the Community Care Teaching Unit, Royal Prince Alfred Hospital, Sydney, was publicly critical of official failure to use Australian and overseas data on organization, planning, management and evaluation as the CHP was being implemented. He was concerned that the lag of overall planning behind center development might lead to even more fragmentation of health services. He was also critical of the medical profession's conservatism and its suspicions that the CHP foreshadowed socialization of health and medical services: "While on the one hand the medical profession is growing more and more fragmented through specialization, the need is for more and more integration of professional services."[25]

The CHP was formally reviewed by the HHSC in 1976, near the close of the first triennium of funding. The HHSC, in presenting an overview of the program, observed that it had "attempted to place a different emphasis on health care, in that it has fostered an approach of prevention through education and outreach programs, and encouraged the development of community based diagnostic, therapeutic and rehabilitation services."[26] It had funded more than seven hundred projects; over three hundred more were ready but had been deferred because of lack of funds. It had sponsored initiatives in addition to community health services, in health education, community geriatric services, community mental health services, alcohol and drug treatment, community rehabilitation services, domiciliary nursing, women's health, youth services, rural health and staff training programs. It had made "some smaller inroads" into such special-needs as immigrant health, Aboriginal health, health transport, family planning services and occupational health. The projects operated at national, state, regional and local levels. While most were run by the state health authorities, a significant proportion was run by nongovernment organizations under the supervision of the states. Moreover, the breadth and flexibility of the program were evidenced by the way the various states emphasized the different aspects of the community health services.

By the close of 1975, with over 2,200 employees, the community heath projects offered at least some improvement for around half of those people residing in areas of service scarcity. An estimated 15 to 20 percent of the population was in areas seriously deficient in services. More than three hundred projects were funded in rural areas; 40 percent of the program's funds underwrote projects having considerable rehabilitation emphasis; and some effort went into health education. But community health centers were the prime focus. Some women's health centers were set up to evaluate their effectiveness in providing for women, while refuges were provided for women and dependent children who were homeless or in danger of abuse. These housed in 1977–80 an estimated twelve thousand women and fifteen thousand children. The "serious uncertainty" among the states concerning the continued funding of the program—it was funded by annual parliamentary appropriation—had, however, inhibited development of services and coordinated regional planning.

The program's efforts to counter service fragmentation were later negated, according to Dr. Sax, by "the lack of enthusiasm shown by administrators of special purpose grants when their absorption into broader schemes was proposed [by the HHSC in its 1976 review] with a view to promoting flexibility in administration."[27] Rigidity of attitudes on the part of health professionals, especially doctors, proved another serious obstacle for the CHP. In its 1976 review the HHSC deplored the fact that many health professionals narrowly viewed the CHP as "a health-center building program," merely enabling premises and records to be shared. Doctors too often equated centers with salaried medical practice and saw them as threats.

The Australian Medical Association (AMA) had in 1972 published its own report on health centers, *Health Centres in Australia,* which gave the centers a supporting role in relation to the general practitioner, who retained primary responsibility for the patient. The AMA was opposed to salaried medical practice in centers but endorsed practice on a fee-for-service basis. The HHSC, however, noted in the 1976 review that the Royal Australasian College of Physicians and the AMA strongly supported "team medicine." It also noted that the federal AMA in a 1974 submission to the National Inquiry into Poverty had accepted salaried practice in some health centers in areas deficient in medical services, as well as the need to develop centers in localities other than underprivileged areas, so that they would not become exclusively identified with poverty and low socioeconomic status. Of other medical associations, the socially progressive Doctors' Reform Society warmly supported the CHP, whereas the conservative General Practitioners Society, which rejected state involvement in health care, totally opposed it. The HHSC's 1976 review proposed further education of doctors as the answer to medical suspicions.[28]

COMMUNITY MEDICINE AND COMMUNITY NURSING

In May 1971, the University of Sydney Faculty of Medicine had accepted its curriculum committee's report proposing a reconstructed five-year (instead of six-year) medical course. A working party chaired by Professor Charles Kerr devised guidelines for a new course in behavioral and social sciences that would focus on social and behavioral factors in medicine and community practice. Half the course would involve work in the community to promote experience of team work with other health professionals. The committee's proposals, incorporating those of the working party, were substantially accepted by the faculty in August 1972, and the new medical course began in 1974. Changes were also being proposed at the federal level. In July 1972, the minister for education and science in the McMahon Liberal-Country Party government, Malcolm Fraser, established a committee chaired by economist Professor Peter Karmel to advise the Universities Commission on the future of medical education. One year later, the committee's report, *Expansion of Medical Education,* was published. To meet projected needs to 1991 (one doctor per 543 people), the committee proposed that new medical schools be set up at the University of Newcastle and the James Cook University of North Queensland (each now has a medical school). This major proposal was matched by one for establishment of departments of community medicine in existing medical schools.

The new Whitlam Labor government, after the Universities Commission had endorsed the Karmel committee's recommendations, offered funding for departments of community practice in December 1973, with the proviso that they operate in cooperation with the new community health centers. The minister for health, Dr. Douglas Everingham, had appointed a committee on health personnel and training under the chairmanship of Sidney Sax in July 1973. Among the Sax committee's recommendations was one that the HHSC draw up guidelines for training, especially in the light of the important changes to practice demanded by the CHP. The committee noted the need to promote a community perspective in medical education. It called for chairs and departments of community practice devoted to "the principles and practice of promoting health and the delivery of primary health care in situations outside hospitals."[29] The 1973 report of the Interim Committee of the HHSC, also chaired by Sidney Sax, had called for courses in community practice, urging federal funding for projects involving use of community health facilities for such courses.

The professional bodies, for their part, were developing community-oriented training programs. In the 1960s, the Medical Education Committee of the Royal Australasian College of General Practitioners (RACGP) had introduced the Vocational Training Program, the forerunner of the Family Medicine Program (FMP). In this way the committee saw general practice developing as a specialty in its own right. In 1973–74, the FMP received a $1.1 million grant through the CHP. The project was the largest single undertaking funded by the program. By mid-1974, 238 graduates were enrolled in the FMP, which the RACGP developed in cooperation with the Federal Health Department to raise the standards of general practice and to relieve the chronic shortage of general practitioners in rural and outer metropolitan areas. In January 1976, Ian Webster was appointed founding professor of community medicine at the University of New South Wales Medical School. Professor Webster, in an early statement of his credo, argued that the division of medicine into preventive, curative and rehabilitative arms was harmful and that this defect had been reinforced in Australia by the nature of the National Health Service as created by the 1953 federal legislation, because it excluded preventive medicine. While Medibank was less discriminatory against the aged and invalid pensioner, it too penalized the general practitioner who wished to do preventive work. Both were illness oriented. Community and personal values about health had to change. Medical practice had to be reoriented toward prevention if prevention was to become viable.

Webster noted that community medicine had existed under different names in medical practice for some time, whether as public health, social medicine or preventive medicine. But it had been separated from mainstream medicine, which awarded high status to specialists in specific disease processes in individuals. This individualistic orientation reflected, in fact, the historical influence of private enterprise in medicine—that is, medical practice as small business. He hoped the current development of general practice and primary medical care heralded a closer relationship between community and mainstream medicine.[30]

In 1975, Charles Bridges-Webb, a Victorian general practitioner, had been appointed as the first holder of the chair of community medicine at the University of Sydney Medical School. His department was focused on the education of general practitioners and on person-to-person dimensions of health care. For Bridges-Webb, the most important aspect of community medicine was provision of personal health care for individuals, although another dimension related to "aspects of environment," health education and prevention plus assessment and planning based on social medicine and epidemiology—public health disciplines concerned with health and disease in whole populations.

Public health nursing has a history going back to the beginnings of infant welfare work in Australia round 1900, but it was better established in the nursing educational and practice systems in other Western countries. In Australia, nursing education and practice were dominated by the demands of hospitals, which followed the medical treatment model, and by the reparative paradigm of hospital nursing. In the decades following World War II, slow change occurred in this situation as new Colleges of Nursing and new postgraduate courses, influenced by nurses exposed to public or community health nursing overseas, came into being. Public health nursing itself shifted from a social administration to a primary health care and community development model. The state began to support change in the 1970s in new plans for tertiary education for nurses and the introduction of the community health programs.

The Royal Victorian College of Nursing (RVCN) had unsuccessfully urged Melbourne University in 1946 to set up postgraduate courses for nurses. In early 1949 the NSW College of Nursing (NSWCN) had been formed. Soon after the College of Nursing, Australia (CNA) had been established in Melbourne, with the aim of promoting postgraduate education. The intention was to establish branches in each state. With the creation of Colleges, state-based special interest groups (SIGs) for nursing specialties were established. Infant welfare and industry nurses formed vocal SIGs, acting as advocates for the public health perspective. But the dominance of hospital practice meant that progress toward better education in community nursing practice was slow. Thus, in Victoria in the 1950s refresher courses for infant welfare nurses, lasting up to three weeks, were offered on an annual basis by the Health Department. Yet funding could not be obtained to offer training to enable sisters to deal with emotional and social problems of children not covered in basic or midwifery training. Even in the early 1960s, when in practice the traditional emphasis on feeding problems in infant work gave way to more stress on emotional and social development, training lagged behind. Individual nurses pioneered new practice in infant welfare work. The same was the case in public health nursing with Aborigines in the 1950s and '60s.

In Western Australia, Sister Pat McPherson (who worked for the AIM), combining communication skills and public health skills in immunization and nutrition and health assessment, pioneered preventive work in the oppressive conditions faced by Aboriginal communities. As importantly, she raised awareness in official circles of the need to promote such work. The Western Australia Department of Public Health proceeded to adopt her methods, appointing the first public health nurse. The AIM realized that it was not dealing merely with health problems but with the larger issue of social change and reform. In the Northern Territory, nurses carried out surveillance and immunization work in the 1950s, although they generally lacked specialist training. Traveling by air or four-wheel-drive vehicles, they carried out surveys of child health, leprosy case finding, Mantoux testing and BCG vaccinations; they also provided treatment. The first survey sister was appointed in 1954, two more were appointed in 1959, and five more appointed in 1965. Sister Kettle, the senior survey nurse, well understood the cooperative nature of modern health promotion, writing in 1969: "To date the health service has been essentially one of 'care.' The role needs to . . . become one of promotion of self-help among Aborigines. . . . Health cannot be imposed upon people. It must be won in partnership with them. . . . The key personnel in the field programme will be public health nurses . . . who require public health training to prepare them for their role in promoting better health practices through self-help."[31]

Employers continued to provide courses. Doris Bardsley, superintendent of maternal and child welfare in Queensland, developed in the early 1950s a new child welfare nurse's certificate that upgraded the existing infant welfare course. The colleges of nursing also were active. The NSW college offered a sister tutor course that included work on nutrition, public health, preventive medicine, bacteriology, educational psychology and the practice of education. From 1949 the colleges and the School of Public Health and Tropical Medicine at Sydney University offered a joint certificate of industrial nursing, available to unmatriculated students. The CNA offered a diploma in public health nursing from 1959. The first two students graduated in 1961, but student numbers remained small. Distance and cost barred interstate nurses from attending the Melbourne-based national course; most students were from Victoria. The CNA from the mid-1960s offered post-certificate courses in maternal and child welfare and in tuberculosis nursing. The RVCN at the same time developed courses in occupational health/industrial nursing, as well as a generic public health nursing course. Lack of state financial support for postgraduate education severely restricted demand for courses. The Victorian health minister in 1964, in reply to a request by the Victorian state committee of the CNA for scholarships for a postgraduate public health course, wrote that adequate, specialized courses already existed in infant welfare, school nursing and in tuberculosis community nursing. By the early 1970s a few scholarships were available through the CNA and the NSWCN for public health–style courses.[32]

In 1968, Rae Chittick, an emeritus professor at the McGill University School for Graduate Nurses in Canada who had originally been a public health nurse, presented a damning report on the narrowness and inadequacy of hospital-based nurse education in Australia. She advocated university programs for nurses, arguing that their absence had blocked the growth of public health nursing. She also noted the "great indifference" that many nurses remembered of the medical profession to their long-term hopes and aspirations. Patricia Chomley, founding director of the College of Nursing in Australia, 1949–64, similarly wanted development of generic public health nursing posts in Australia, seeing as a great disadvantage the fragmentation of public health nursing into maternal and child welfare, tuberculosis, industry, and school health.

By the late 1960s, courses in public health nursing were developing. The Tasmania Health Department improved on the traditional infant welfare certificates by offering a six-month course in child health including pediatrics, nutrition, child development, public health and social services, principles of health education and study of the preschool child. The NSWCN offered an occupational health nursing course full-time over three months, and the Occupational Health Division of the NSW Health Department provided a free lecture course for nurses working in industry. We have seen how Sister Pat McPherson pioneered public health nursing in outback Aboriginal communities in Western Australia and how her work inspired creation of public health nursing posts in that state. The Northern Territory and Queensland by the early 1970s were establishing generic public health nursing positions as part of their health services. Such posts typically required general, midwifery and child health certificates plus such qualifications as a health visitor's certificate. Often the candidate was required to earn the diploma of public health.

Pilot nursing education programs in tertiary institutions were introduced in 1974. In a massive transfer, all education programs had been shifted to the tertiary sector by the 1990s. A variety of postgraduate courses, including community health and maternal and child health, came to be offered along with preregistration general courses. Advocates of change thus did not directly challenge the preeminence of the medical profession or of the medical model of health care. The advent of the Whitlam Labor government, with its redistributive social and health policies, reinforced the trend away from the hospital-based model of nursing education and practice—first, by making tertiary education, including nurse education, more accessible, by meeting the full costs of higher education; and second, by introducing the CHP, which required speedy development of formal courses in community health (public health nursing was now called "community health nursing") and continuing education in the area.

Community nursing sought to promote health, not simply to deal with illness, and to work in teams with other health professionals, as agents of social change. In addition to health assessments, immunizations and referrals, nurses in the community setting sought to promote better social and emotional environments for their patients. As one infant welfare nurse recorded in the mid-1970s,

> "We obtain food orders for the hungry, clothing for the cold in the winter. . . . We read government letters to migrants, ring up employment agencies to find jobs for the jobless[;] . . . contact voluntary agencies to pay for a family to get the gas put back on[;] . . . contact police for protection for beaten wives[;] . . . encourage families to seek medical assessment of retarded children, go with them for moral support, listen to, support and advise agitated mothers[;] . . . find a private corner where a woman or man can cry without the waiting room looking on."[33]

The CHP brought with it the generalist community nurse, devoted to prevention of illness, health counseling and promotion and therapeutic and rehabilitation work. "Infant welfare sisters" became "community health nurses." Where the infant welfare nurses of the early twentieth century had been involved in social control as well as health advancement, the community nurse of the mid-1970s sought to provide social support as well as health promotion.[34] Indeed, the CHP stimulated evaluation of nurse education nationally in the face of changing modes of health care delivery and of demand for personnel from the quickly growing community health services.

A diploma in community health nursing developed by the NSWCN was the first such qualification in Australia. The first students began studies in

January 1974 at the New South Wales College of Paramedical Studies (which became the Cumberland College of Health Sciences in 1975 and is now the Faculty of Health Sciences of the University of Sydney). The course aimed to provide for the growing autonomy of nurses in areas like design and implementation of health-promotion and education programs, preliminary screening and assessment of patients, and family counseling. It covered health promotion, health maintenance, environmental and social factors influencing health, family health, and electives like maternity care; it aimed to prepare nurses to work with families, at-risk groups like the aged, and minorities like immigrants.[35]

The CHP affected the School of Public Health and Tropical Medicine at the University of Sydney. The federal health minister, Dr. Everingham, asked a committee of the HHSC chaired by Sidney Sax to review the activities of the school and make recommendations about its future in the light of national needs in health education, teacher education for health profession educators, health services research, epidemiology and environmental health and related concerns. The committee's report proposed establishment of a National Institute of Health, which would have both educational and research responsibilities and would also draw up national priorities for the improvement of health. Consultations with the university, the Federal Health Department and others followed. The cabinet then asked the Tertiary Education Commission to report on the matter. The commission recommended that the school be renamed the Commonwealth Institute of Health to reflect better its new concerns; that funding continue to be provided by the Federal Health Department and that the university continue to be responsible for academic standards and supervision of research programs; and finally that research and evaluation functions remain primary but that teaching activities gradually expand. On the fiftieth anniversary of the school, 3 March 1980, the Commonwealth Institute of Health replaced the school. The growth of community health centers in creating an expanding demand for staff had helped change the school's orientation. Its concerns now included health administration, health education and promotion and health services research, as well as its long-established concerns with tropical medicine, parasitology and epidemiology.[36]

The introduction of the CHP in 1973 gave rise to another new category of health professional—the community physician. By 1976, there were in New South Wales alone fifty posts for community physicians. There were problems of role and functional identity. Moreover, communication between the physicians carrying out this new role was inadequate. In June 1981, a group of community physicians met in the Department of Community Medicine, Royal Prince Alfred Hospital, Sydney, to consider a number of issues—confusion over the definition of community medicine; role problems, such as generalist versus specialist community physicians (for example, child health or geriatrics); lack of training opportunities; lack of professional credibility; uncertainty as to whether the community physicians should affiliate with the Royal Australasian College of Physicians or form a new body; difficulties of recruiting young physicians; the validity of the continuing separation of traditional public health and community health; and the need for a body to try to influence public policy and its likely overlap with groups like the Doctors' Reform Society. The meeting decided that a new society could play a valuable role in three areas: ongoing training, definition of skills and knowledge required by community physicians, and professional support. Doctors J. Ward, S. Morey, P. Niall, G. Goldstein and D. Krol were nominated to draw up proposals for a further meeting.[37]

Four and a half years later, in February 1986, the inaugural annual general meeting of a national body of community physicians, chaired by Dr. Sue Morey of NSW, an early appointee at the pioneering Glebe Community Health Centre and a key figure in the organization of the national body, took place in Sydney. The first Council of the Australian Association of Community Physicians included, in addition to Dr. Morey, Professor S. Leeder (NSW) and Doctors J. Best (NSW), P. Brown (NSW), R. Clark (NSW), L. Forster (NSW), J. Powles (Victoria), J. Harrison (Victoria), E. Maynard (South Australia) and W. Beresford (Western Australia). Present at the meeting were physicians from New South Wales: A. Adams, N. Andersen, M. Azmi, H. Beange, J. Best, P. Brennan, P. Brown, G. Carreon, C. Cullen, S. de Burgh, J. Dewdney, E. Endacott, C. Ewan, L. Forster, G. Goldstein, R. Hall, P. Havlacek, J. Hohnen, M. Hohnen, S. Irvine, M. James, D. Jeffs, M. Kearney, D. Lange, S. Leeder, R. Leitner, J. Lennane, A. Lloyd, E. May, P. Moffitt, S. Morey, P. Mowbray, C. Mukerjee, J. Pereira, P. Prabhu, R. Resnik, P. Shea, J. Stanhope and P. Tait; from Victoria, J. Cooper, N. Crofts, J. Harrison, L. Knight, A. Morsy, B. Monheit, J. Powles, R. Webster and P. Zimmet; from Queensland, K. Burns and R. Waugh; from South Australia, A. Radford; from Tasmania, J. Curran, T. Dwyer and V. Younger; and from the Northern Territory, F. McConnel.[38]

The new association established that 761 medical practitioners nationally had qualifications relevant to community medicine. From the outset the association was involved in training and qualifications issues. The Hawke Labor government had commissioned an eminent American public health expert, Professor Kerr White, to report on national public health education and research support; the president, Dr. Morey, and the treasurer, Dr. Jack Best, had talks in mid-1986 with the federal health minister, Dr. Neal Blewett, and the federal minister for community services, Senator Don Grimes, about White's proposal for training fellowships in public health. The association was not happy with his proposal that the NHMRC solely administer the fellowships, suggesting instead that the association do so, alone or jointly. It also offered to provide the ministers with a statement of the core skills, knowledge and attitudes required by a doctor practicing public health and community medicine.[39] The association, however, was unable to wrestle control of the fellowships from the NHMRC.

Still seeking a more secure professional future, the association explored the possibility of becoming a faculty of the Royal Australian College of Medical Administrators (RACMA), but the college was cautious, and basic differences existed. While the community physicians were focused upon population medicine and epidemiology, the administrators were concerned with financial management in institutional, especially hospital, environments. In August 1987, discussions were held with the Royal Australasian College of Physicians (RACP) about forming a Faculty of Community Medicine. Three association members, Professors Stephen Leeder and Richard Heller (University of Newcastle) and Morey, were to develop plans for a training program within the college framework—although discussions continued with the RACMA. The majority of community physicians in Australia having been trained in the United Kingdom, consultation with British community physicians seemed appropriate. Morey talked with the president of the Faculty of Community Medicine of the Royal Colleges of Physicians of the United Kingdom, Dr. Rosemary Rue, and others about the development of the British faculty. They found that the role of community physicians in the United Kingdom was under review by a committee chaired by the chief medical officer, Sir Donald Acheson. Professor Walter Holland, a distinguished public health physician and the teacher of a number of senior Australian public health doctors, such as Stephen Leeder, visited Australia and told the annual conference of the association in 1988 that the Acheson report had recommended that the specialty of community medicine revert to the traditional name, "public health" and also that, in a further revival of the public health function, district health authorities within the National Health Service appoint directors of public health as consultants in public health medicine—at a notional rate of 15.8 consultants per million population. Professor Holland also talked to the Secretary of the RACP, David Teller, about the formation of the United Kingdom Faculty of Community Medicine and its relationship with the Royal Colleges of Physicians in Britain.[40] The association ultimately found a permanent home as the Faculty of Public Health Physicians of the RACP.

THE STATES AND THE COMMUNITY HEALTH PROGRAM

New South Wales led the way in the reform of health services in the 1960s. After a long time as the opposition, the new Liberal state government was keen to promote its image and to unify control of health services, which was then shared between the Hospitals Commission (a statutory authority responsible for administration of the Public Hospitals Act of 1929, which required it to inspect and determine the subsidies paid to hospitals), and the

Health Department. Within the department, public health and mental health services operated independently. Pressure was coming from people within the department and from academics for comprehensive care of the individual and family within their community environment, as was being done in Britain and Scandinavia. Wary of his public service advisers, who had served Labor governments for almost two and a half decades, the new health minister, A.H. Jago, employed G.C. Eglington to inquire into organization of health services. His interim report on Community Health Services and the Public Hospitals Act—no final one was presented—became the basis for a formal inquiry. Eglington recommended that the government be responsible for all services (including those provided by voluntary organizations); that the central health authority be the central planning and policy agency; and that regionalized services center on the hospital as the primary community agency, as in New Zealand. A committee was formed under the chairmanship of Kenneth Starr, medical director of the NSW State Cancer Council; its other members were Sir Edward Ford, former director of the School of Public Health and Tropical Medicine, the University of Sydney; Dr. R.L. Harris, honorary physician, Royal Prince Alfred Hospital; Dr. N. Larkins, medical secretary, NSW Branch, AMA; J.H.D. Marks, chairman of the Development and Finance Corporation; N. Oakes, assistant under secretary, State Treasury; J.D. Rimes, permanent head, NSW Health Department; H. Selle, chairman of the Hospitals Commission; and D. Smith, chairman of the Riverina Region Hospitals Advisory Council. It recommended the following in November 1969: establishment of a Health Commission to replace the Health Department, the Hospitals Commission and the Ambulance Transport Service Board; significant regionalization and decentralization of administration; and a mechanism by which the views of professional and community groups would influence how health services were delivered.

In a policy speech in January 1971, the premier made clear that the government intended to create a Health Commission. A consultative document put out by the health minister in April 1972 looked forward to a "stage one," which would put a Health Commission in place by 1973; and a "stage two," in which the commission's role would be laid down along the lines of the Starr committee's proposals, if accepted, to remove the executive independence of the general hospitals and make the commission the employer of hospital staff, under the Industrial Arbitration Act. The Health Commission Act of 1972 provided for a commission comprising a chairman and deputy (one of whom was to be a doctor) plus four members. The commission would have divisions of personal health services, environmental and special health services, manpower and management services and finance and physical resources. Stage one elicited no opposition, but stage two called forth a storm of protests from groups like the Catholic hospitals and the medical profession, which feared their autonomy would suffer. Retreating, the government did not proceed with stage two.

The commission came into being in April 1973, with Dr. R. McEwin as chairman, G. Slough as commissioner for manpower and management services, Dr. D. Storey as commissioner for environmental and special health services, Dr. W. Barclay as commissioner for personal health services, and K. Boylan as commissioner for finance and physical resources. The Ambulance Transport Board did not come under the commission until 1976. Under the act, the commission's function was that of "promoting, protecting, developing, maintaining and improving the health and well-being of the people of New South Wales to the maximum extent possible."[41] The one-to-one relationship between a commissioner and the bureau responsible for his area of concern caused various problems. The commission operated more like four different empires than a unified whole. Objective appraisal of bureau activities by the commission as a whole and each successive commissioner was limited by the close relationship of commissioner to bureau.[42]

In 1976 a task force inquiry into management proposed that the secretary to the commission assume the functions of the Manpower and Finance Bureaus and that the latter be abolished. Then, the post of "Director of Medical and Allied Services" was created, having responsibilities in health services paralleling those of the secretary (now director of administration) in administration. The Bureaus of Personal Health Services and Environmental and Special Health Services were dismantled, and a number of new health-related divisions established, along with separate divisions of planning and research.

The Wran Labor government, first elected in 1976, was reelected in 1981. L.J. Brereton, who replaced K.J. Stewart as health minister, immediately appointed a task force to reduce the commission's staff of Central Office employees. Minister Brereton, responding to the task force report, indicated that the commission would be replaced by a department. A department was set up in December 1982, with Bernie Mackay, former chairman of the South Australian Health Commission, as the secretary.

While much had been made at the time of the commission's creation of making the organization of health services conform to a holistic approach to health promotion, a significant political reason for creating a statutory authority organization had been to "depoliticize" the Hospital Commission's recommendations concerning resource allocations. This was no longer important. Moreover, Premier Wran had a number of times overruled decisions about health services by Minister Stewart and his commission staff in what was an electorally sensitive area. The decision to disband the commission was taken also because of budget constraints forced by reductions in federal grants to the states. One of the key features of the commission's organization was to have been regionalization; however, because of ambivalence about the idea at the highest levels of the commission, the originally intended degree of devolution of administration was never achieved. Even so, the 1976 task force pointed to gains from regionalization, such as additional specialist services and implementation of the community health program.[43]

With the regionalization (essentially decentralization) of administration that had followed creation of the Health Commission in 1973, New South Wales was well placed to accept the commonwealth's proposal to fund community health centers. Victoria in 1978 and South Australia in 1981 also established health commissions, with the aim of integrating health services but in a way that would allow individual institutions greater independence from government than a centralized department would permit. Victoria and South Australia also regionalized administration. Having greater concentration of population than NSW, they pursued delegation of administration rather than geographical decentralization. Queensland, which traditionally had a very centralized administration, was to implement regionalization in 1991.

The responses of the states to the CHP were influenced by such factors as the party political color of the government, the policy of the organized medical profession, the extent of community involvement in services and the state of development of services. The Liberal government of NSW was suspicious of the Whitlam Labor government's health policy. Yet it allowed the Health Commission to work cooperatively with the CHP. A major constraint was the government's understanding with the AMA in NSW that no general practitioner services would be provided by health centers under the control of the commission, in order to ensure that the centers' salaried doctors did not compete with private practitioners. Even family planning and vaccination services were "outlawed." The centers were not supposed to promote themselves or charge for services. Little funding flowed to projects organized by community groups, although a small number of feminist-inspired women's health centers were set up. These did offer primary medical care, as did Mount Druitt Polyclinic and Peakhurst Health Centre, because when established they served areas where general practitioners were scarce. Moreover, in some extrametropolitan areas doctors charging fee-for-service shared buildings with centers.[44]

The Victorian conservative government, locked in political battle with the Whitlam government, would not allow state centers to open. Commonwealth funds were directed to community groups; such arrangements on occasion were organized by federal Labor politicians. Most voluntary group centers included general practitioner services, usually on a fee-for-service basis. Later, the Victorian government assumed responsibility for the CHP, providing its share of funding, although the earlier centers remained to a large extent outside its control.

In its 1976 review of the CHP, the HHSC observed that in Victoria the development of prevention and health education programs, like the growth of a team approach, had been slow to emerge. The conservative Queensland coalition government willingly accepted commonwealth funding, using it mainly to develop existing health services. Major projects included the extension of care at Brisbane's Central Assessment Clinic for the intellectually handicapped; comprehensive health resource centers in places like Rockhampton and Redcliffe; and a regional center in Townsville. A large, purpose-built health center was established at Inala, a working-class Brisbane suburb in great need of primary health services. The HHSC 1976 review noted that centers in Queensland cooperated well with surrounding private practices.

The conservative government in Western Australia evinced a broadly similar response. The majority of early projects were sponsored by the mental health authority. Large, purpose-built community health centers were also built. These offered primary medical care on a fee-for-service basis, as well as a wide range of allied services. Health education was part of all projects, while community nurses were widely employed in counseling people requiring specialized care.

In South Australia and Tasmania, where Labor governments were in power, a range of programs, including centers employing salaried doctors, was set up. Local medical associations in Tasmania mustered considerable opposition to such centers. Progress with the CHP was slower in this state than elsewhere, because of the need to integrate community and mental health services, limited resources, and the existence of a district medical service, which was already an effective community health provider. Domiciliary nursing, the reach of which was expanded in 1976, brought great benefit to the aged and psychiatrically ill, reducing the demand for hospital beds. Similarly, in South Australia, domiciliary care programs greatly reduced demand for institutional care. In this state, three types of projects flourished under the CHP: large, purpose-built community health centers offering primary medical care on a fee-for-service basis; training courses for allied health professionals, especially those establishing new roles, like that of the community nurse; and projects offering domiciliary and rehabilitation services for the aged and disabled. The CHP here was marked by considerable community participation in decision making about services.[45]

In the Australian Capital Territory, a London firm of health planners—Llewelyn-Davies, Weeks, Forestier-Walker and Bor—had been commissioned by the National Capital Development Commission in 1968 to advise on Canberra's future health needs. Reporting in 1970, the planners proposed a health commission to coordinate ACT health services (in mid-1975 the Capital Territory Health Commission was born). The firm also proposed multidisciplinary and easily accessible community health centers. In early 1971, the ACT branch of the AMA held a special meeting to consider policy on community health centers. Medical opinion was divided, with concerns being expressed about staffing, confidentiality of records and the independence of private practitioners working in centers.

Dr. Ron Wells, director of ACT Health Services, had in January 1971 received ministerial approval for two pilot centers. The accession of the Whitlam government in 1972 reinforced his position. Wells and his deputy, Bernie Mackay, easily persuaded the federal health minister, Everingham, that they should proceed quickly with pilot centers at Melba (where salaried general practitioners worked) and Scullin (where there were private practitioners) in the fast-growing Belconnen area of Canberra. Public meetings and extensive media coverage helped counteract misinformation about the new centers. By mid-1976, seven complete community health centers and Evatt, a "mini" one, were operating; twenty-six salaried doctors were on staff. Three years later six more centers were open. Kippax community health center had opened in May 1975 with both salaried and private practitioners, a mixture for which the local community had shown preference in a 1974 survey. Although personal relations were good between the salaried doctor and the three private practitioners in the center, there was not much professional contact; the latter did not join the salaried health professionals and office staff in the common room. However, while local community committees were initially attached to centers, none survived very long. Wells believed even the salaried staff did not want to share the administration with community representatives. Moreover, determined leadership was not forthcoming from the committees.[46]

The Northern Territory, like the ACT administered by the commonwealth, established several community health centers in rural areas and provided accommodation for community nurses in remote areas. A training program for Aboriginal health aides was introduced, and local Aboriginal communities were encouraged to propose people for training. Staffing of health centers was a continuing problem in the 1970s.[47]

By the beginning of the 1980s, at least seventy-five centers across Australia (excluding the ACT) offered primary medical care part or full-time. Of these, nineteen centers had salaried or sessional doctors—in full-time-equivalent terms, fifty-nine doctors—while about two hundred doctors practiced under fee-for-service arrangements (see table 3.1).[48]

The conservative Fraser Liberal-National Party government came to power in the mid-1970s, at time when the national economy was in a serious recession. Holding a monetarist economic philosophy, it aimed, in Treasurer Phillip Lynch's words, "to lessen public intervention in the private sector" and ensure "there are reductions in government spending, a reduction of the deficit and a cutback in excess liquidity."[49] Although the Fraser government promised in November 1975 to preserve the CHP, with its 350 health centers of various types, it effectively ended federal funding for it by mid-1981 through a series of fiscal policy changes—health block grants, cutbacks, and then absorption of funding into general tax-sharing grants to the states without conditions or monitoring.

Table 3.1
Primary Medical Care in Centers Funded under the Community Health Program, 1980–81

ξ	Fee for Service	Salaried or Sessional	Total
NSW	3	6	9
Victoria	26	6	32
South Australia	13	1	14
Western Australia	8	3	11
Queensland	0	1	1
Tasmania	5	2	7
Northern Territory	2	*	2+

ξ The ACT had a separate financial appropriation and had four centers with salaried doctors, two with private practitioners and three with a mix of salaried and private practitioners.
*In the Northern Territory, the federal government funded only a small part of community health services. A number of centers had salaried doctors.

Source: *Report to Health Commission by Standing Committee on Community Health, November 1981* (Sydney: NSW Health Commission, 1981), 28.

In 1974–75, the Whitlam Labor government had provided 90 percent of CHP operating costs and 75 percent of capital costs. In 1977–78, the Fraser government contributed 75 and 50 percent, respectively. From 1978 to 1979, it provided 50 percent of each cost component. Total federal funding, which had been forty-seven million dollars in 1975, fell to below thirty-nine million in 1978 in constant (1975) dollars. Per person in constant (1975) dollars, it fell from $3.39 in 1975 to $1.75 in 1982, a 48.5 percent decline. The community health centers offering primary care suffered the greatest losses. In 1976–77 to 1980–81, most states reduced sharply rates of increase in expenditure on centers. Compared with other states, South Australia did not reduce the rate of increase so much. Tasmania, in the beginning the lowest-spending state, kept up increases through 1980–81.

In the two years after the Fraser government introduced the tax-sharing regime in 1981, the three states reduced real CHP spending on average 17.1 percent per person per year; the range was 14.1 percent in NSW to 19.9 percent in Tasmania. But it was less the tax sharing and the real cuts in support for the CHP than the greater financial responsibility placed on the states for hospital support that led to a real decline in community health services, especially in the CHP.[50] National (state and federal) spending on community health declined between 1979 and 1982 as a percentage of total health spending (see table 3.2).

In September 1978, the NSW Public Service Board told the Health Commission that it would have to eliminate 1,062 positions. The commission chose to shed fifty laboratory posts, 612 posts in mainly psychiatric hospitals, and four hundred from community health. But no general hospital posts

Table 3.2
Government Spending on Community Health, 1979–82

Year	Hospital	Medical	Community Health
1979–80	46.9%	17.6%	2.41%
1980–81	47.0	17.0	2.45
1981–82	46.6	17.1	2.37

Source: *Review of the Community Health Program* (Strawberry Hills: Australian Community Health Association, 1986), 27.

were in danger. The board and the Treasury thought there would be no backlash, because community health lacked media support, and even federal Labor seldom criticized the Fraser government. However, a grassroots protest, later called the "Save Community Health Campaign," applied political pressure to the Wran state government, distributing press releases and urging voters to write to their members of Parliament. The Doctors' Reform Society accused the government in the press of favoring general hospitals over community health services. Soon after, the *Sydney Morning Herald* ran feature articles on the extravagant expenditure on hospitals. In mid-1979, when it became likely that the imminent federal budget would include a further 5 percent cut in funding, an interstate campaign led by a group of health centers and community groups from the more vigorous Victorian community-run centers was mounted. When the federal government restored five million dollars to the community health finances, the campaign leaders believed they had achieved a victory.

In New South Wales, community health campaigners, who were largely drawn from CHP staff, formed themselves in 1980 into the Community Health Association of NSW. The new body advocated annual expansion of the program, representative area health boards, assignment of 15 percent of hospital savings to centers, growth of primary prevention, local and national health promotion, and social and environmental programs linked with center activities. The association tried to influence public opinion through press releases and organization of forums.

After the election of the Hawke Labor government in 1983, the federal health minister, Dr. Blewett, offered funding for a national community health association. In early 1984, the NSW body met with sister associations in Victoria and South Australia that had been formed about the same time as the NSW association. They established the Australian Community Health Association (ACHA), in order to develop a national movement and lobby the federal government more effectively. ACHA was very active over the next decade and a half, coordinating state association activities, running national community health conferences, lobbying governments, reviewing the CHP, and sponsoring innovations like the Community Health Accreditation and

Standards Program (a comprehensive, national management device) and the Healthy Cities Australia project. But the 1980s and 1990s saw in Australia, as in other liberal democratic states, a convergence of the policies of left and right-wing parties. The Hawke and Keating Labor governments, 1983–96, pursued aspects of the neoconservative economic policy of market reliance to allocate resources but softened the impact by a commitment to social justice and state intervention in social policy. From 1996 onward, the Howard Liberal-National Party coalition government, like the Reagan administration in the United States and the Thatcher government in the United Kingdom, pursued an uncompromising, radical-right policy of reducing and privatizing public services, deregulating economic activity and cutting welfare support. It reduced state intervention and the size of government to a greater extent than any Australian government in the previous fifty years. In general terms, such an ideological climate is uncongenial to public health, which critically depends on state regulation and intervention. More particularly, it is unconducive to the growth of community health services. Indeed, funding cuts for community health centers, especially in Victoria and South Australia, where historically they have been strongest, marked the 1990s. In 1997, ACHA was forced to close down its Sydney secretariat when its modest federal funding was withdrawn.[51]

EVALUATION OF THE COMMUNITY HEALTH PROGRAM

In 1989–90, of total Australian health expenditure—federal, state and local government and private—51.6 percent went to hospital and other institutional services, 18.3 percent went to medical services, and only 4.4 percent to community and public health services, although a very small amount of hospital spending was also allocated to community services. The very small size of funds directed to community health clearly made it difficult to achieve the ambitious aims laid down for the CHP in the 1973 Sax report: to provide improved community health services in areas of significant unmet need; to promote aspects of health care, prevention, health maintenance and rehabilitation that had been neglected; and to offer an alternative to more costly institutional care.

In his 1979 report on health promotion in Australia, Professor Lindsay Davidson, principal of the School of Public Health and Tropical Medicine, University of Sydney, noted that of an estimated federal expenditure on health and drug education of $2.040 million in 1977–78, just over half was spending on specific health education projects under the CHP. The rest was spending on the National Drug Education Program ($750,000) and by the Federal Health Department directly on health and drug education ($254,000). CHP projects specially directed to prevention or health education numbered twenty-four in Victoria, nineteen in NSW, four in Western Australia, three in Queensland and one in Tasmania, as well as nine national projects. While the CHP was the largest source of health-promotion manpower in Australia, some community health centers were underused by their communities. This appeared to be especially the case in NSW. Moreover, they were used largely to fulfill previously unmet needs for curative services. While emphasis on prevention was supposed to be built into the work of the two hundred centers, this "has been slow to evolve, and preventive services still play a relatively minor role in the overall functioning of most community health centers, whether this is judged from client utilization rates or from staff job descriptions," said Professor Davidson.[52] Research on community need for health promotion and preventive services, he concluded, was urgently required.[53]

Writing five years later, in 1984, Nick Crofts, president of the Victorian branch of the Doctors' Reform Society and a doctor (then at the Collingwood Community Health Centre but with long experience in health centers), saw the basic variation among centers to be their relative emphasis on prevention and treatment. The problem was communities themselves sometimes demanded treatment rather than preventive services; health professionals could be more radical in their conception of health priorities than the citizens they served. At Collingwood Community Health Centre (located in an inner Melbourne working-class area), the staff found "it insurmountably difficult to . . . redirect our efforts to prevention, because the community knows it needs primary care." In the scramble for primary care, national planning priorities disappeared. Crofts concluded that generally the "much-touted" shift to prevention had not developed properly and that basically the centers had become vehicles for the alternative delivery of medical services. He proposed that the main reason why centers had failed to be effective sources of preventive work was that they continued to look upon prevention as simply another service to be delivered: "The linking of health . . . with the power to make the important decisions in one's own life, to control one's own destiny, has made only the vaguest of inroads into CHC practice."[54]

Writing a year later, Crofts said that movement toward prevention-oriented activities required individual health professionals to change their mind-set from one of problem solving to one of "seeing life in terms of . . . actualisation." The difference between treatment and prevention is one of timing; treatment, he argued, is a delayed preventive program—and a costly one, in terms of resources and human suffering. Health improvement requires social-structural change empowering the powerless to exercise true choice. In this social health perspective, the community health center of the future would need to employ experts in social-structural change—sociologists, lawyers, public relations experts, economists, and political lobbyists—whose work would be complemented by that of epidemiologists, public health practitioners and community physicians. Those involved in the CHP, Crofts declared, had to decide whether to act as social-change agents in cooperation with local citizens or to continue as agents of social control, supporting social institutions that produced ill health.[55]

In late 1986, the report of a review of the CHP carried out under the auspices of the Australian Community Health Association was presented to the Federal Health Department. The review made two major observations about the program. First, despite the commonwealth's absence (except for a few nationally funded projects) from the program after 1981, community health services had become established firmly as part of health services in all states and territories. Also, these services exhibited a "surprising degree" of similarity of approach across states. But this apparent progress had been bought at the price of changing the health center program's priorities, to the extent of largely surrendering its original objective—to make community-based health promotion and prevention the primary goal of the health care system. The reviewers' second observation was that community health had thereby become reduced to an "illness-focused, residual service providing mainly tertiary and some secondary prevention"—that is, care of those with chronic illnesses and early detection and treatment of disease. It was in that sense that the original objective of the program—changing priorities from expensive, specialist, curative services to community-focused, primary-care services emphasizing primary prevention and community participation—had to a large extent been lost to sight. Given the smallness of the program relative to the overall health system, the program's failure to attain this objective was understandable. But the result was that primary health care, the gateway to the health system and a major determinant of health costs, still lay in the private sphere, largely outside public control. On grounds of cost containment and health advancement, the reviewers argued, the domination of the health system by costly institutional and specialist curative services had to be ended. A national primary care program, of which publicly funded community health services would be the core, needed to be developed if primary health care was to serve people in their communities through quality treatment, early intervention and, above all, prevention of illness and promotion of positive health.[56] On figures for 1983–84, 86 percent of CHP funds were spent on management and relief of illness, only 11 percent on primary prevention. Thus, the pattern was that of traditional care, similar to the emphasis in community outreach programs of hospitals.

The other major area of innovation (besides orientation of services toward primary prevention) envisaged originally for the CHP had been community participation in the functioning of centers. We have noted earlier how this flourished early in the ACT and then died out. The 1976 HHSC review of the CHP had called for more community involvement, seeing the best model as one of staff and community representation on the management committees of centers. The states varied in the degree to which communities were involved in administration. No formal involvement existed in Queensland, although informal participation may have occurred in some programs. In

Tasmania, as in Queensland, the structures and ideology of hospital-based domiciliary nursing dominated community health. Because of this, community involvement was not strong. There were exceptions—the Royal Hobart Hospital had established in the 1980s an advisory council for centers under its aegis, and the Kingsmeadows center had a local management committee, although it did not control the budget.

Western Australia had little community health structure and no community participation in administration. A health advisory network that allowed for community involvement was developed in the mid-1980s, but advisory committees, when set up, had failed. Northern Territory Health had a separate division for Aboriginal and Community Health. While for Aboriginal communities local participation was viewed as desirable, the matter was ignored in relation to European communities. Nurses from the Rural Health Service in Alice Springs (in the central part of the territory) were expected to involve themselves in community affairs. In Darwin, Aboriginal health workers ran some services, and Aboriginal control was a long-term official objective.

In South Australia, the CHP benefited from a general government commitment through the 1970s and 1980s to social reform. The Dunstan Labor government (1970–79) was receptive to the concept of community health, and the Tonkin Liberal government (1979–82) provided reasonably secure funding. In Dr. John Cornwall—minister of health from 1982 to 1985 and minister of health and community welfare, 1985–88, in the Bannon Labor government—the community health movement had an energetic supporter who paid serious attention to the idea of community involvement and provided a sense of direction to community health in South Australia. In the mid-1980s, organized community involvement was initiated via a "sector advisory committee" structure in the metropolitan, or central, health sector. The southern sector introduced a community health advisory committee, and the western sector had a steering committee and project officer. In 1985, Health Minister Cornwall introduced statewide consultation procedures to identify what the community saw as the objectives of the health system and to set up machinery allowing community participation in policy development and service planning.

Victoria enjoyed a history of community involvement stronger than that of any other jurisdiction in Australia. The early years of the CHP had seen community groups threaten to use direct federal funding from the Whitlam government as a way of persuading a reluctant Liberal state government to provide funds through the Hospitals and Charities Commission. The community-based management boards of community health centers continued to give the CHP in Victoria a strong local focus. The Labor health minister, Tom Roper, set up a committee in mid-1983 to review community health services and establish a plan for effective development, in order to avoid the "scramble" of the 1970s. Among the recommendations of the committee, which reported in mid-1985, was that District Health Councils, introduced under regionalization arrangements and based on an average population of a hundred thousand people, be open to input from the community and not dominated by health care organizations. Because District Health Councils would be rather distant from local communities, the committee proposed creation of local health groups in order to form a link between consumers of health services and the councils. The groups would be based on local government areas and composed of representatives of local government, health providers, consumer groups and individuals. Community participation was not only built into the Victorian community health centers but was part of the superior levels of health service organization. In the event, regionalization was a slower process than originally envisaged. Forty-three District Health Councils throughout the state were planned, but by the end of the 1980s only sixteen had been funded.[57]

In New South Wales, the Health Commission's 1977 detailed policy of goals and progress measures for community health disappeared in the face of the withdrawal of federal funding. The division of community health of the central health authority was abolished when the health bureaucracy began to be reorganized in 1982. As central policy direction in the health system declined, the eleven health regions approached community health in various ways, according to local conditions. There was a widespread tendency in the NSW health system, as in other states, to see community health as only domiciliary care. Staff posts formerly funded by federal money were not filled when they fell vacant. Unlike the situation in South Australia and Victoria, the new Area Health Boards enjoyed little community input, although the legislation of 1986 on which they were based gave them responsibility not only for financial management but promotion of community representation. The Health Department continued to run community health centers with minimal community participation.

The consumer-rights movement helped to promote community participation in health services, although the movement historically enjoyed mixed success in NSW. After American consumer advocate Ralph Nader's famous victory in automobile safety over General Motors in the 1960s, the consumer movement spread throughout the Western world. In 1973, the Medical Consumers Association (MCA) was established in Victoria and soon after in New South Wales. Compared with the role given consumers in health services planning and management in the United Kingdom, the New South Wales organization's function was limited—essentially, helping patients with complaints and making submissions to official inquiries into health matters. However, in 1978–79 the Wran government made funds available for a consumers' representative body in the outer Western Sydney Western Health Involvement program. While in Victoria the first concern of the MCA was the debate about national health insurance—Medibank—one of its projects was a discussion program for consumer and community representatives on community health center management committees. The discussion program, Health Feedback, was funded through the CHP in 1973–74. In the 1980s a number of discussion programs were employed in the District Health Councils program.

In the later 1970s, the Australian Consumers Association (ACA) began to focus on health questions. With the return of Labor to power at the federal level in 1983, a more positive approach to consumer participation in federal health policy and planning became possible. In May 1985, eight consumer and community groups got together to petition the federal health minister, Dr. Blewett, to create machinery for community participation in the work of the Federal Department of Health, citing the WHO strategy of "Health for All by the Year 2000" (HFA), which emphasized the need for governments to set up such mechanisms. The Doctors' Reform Society, the Australian Consumers' Association and the Australian Federation of Consumer Organisations, among others, supported the petition. Blewett set up a review committee, which sought the views of consumer and community groups but did not seek involvement by traditional health interests like professional and industry groups. At the close of 1986, sixteen consumer and community interests came together to form the Consumers' Health Forum of Australia, an independent, incorporated body funded by the Federal Health Department.

The minister instructed his department to consult the forum on major health policy matters, explaining that it would "increase access by community, consumer and user groups to decision making within the department, including policy, research priorities, budget allocation and regulatory and legislative change."[58] It was to be a counterbalance to the influence of established professional and industry groups. The AMA expressed concern that "the medical model for prevention/treatment of illness should be discarded in favor of a wider, social welfare approach." Moreover, it was anxious about "advocacy in some quarters of abandonment of scientific principles in health care and their replacement by humanistic ones."[59] In the early 1990s, the consumer movement sought greater government recognition of the consumer voice in health matters. The final background paper put out under the federal Labor government's National Health Strategy in 1993 asserted that greater participation would arise from a statement of consumer rights, a position strongly supported nationally by consumer and community groups and influenced by the example of the Patients' Charter in the United Kingdom. States and territories under the Medicare Agreements, 1993–98, agreed to draw up a Public Patients' Hospital Charter that would contain rights like access to public hospital on the basis of clinical need (not possession of health insurance) and provision of information on public hospital services that were available to public patients.[60]

New South Wales lagged behind states like Victoria and South Australia in setting up machinery to advance consumer and community representation.

However, it pioneered in the field of machinery to process complaints about health care, establishing an independent Complaints Unit as early as 1984. Queensland and Victoria subsequently created complaints commissions. In contrast to NSW, which prosecuted health providers, these commissions pursued conciliation. The trend was toward establishment of complaints units in other jurisdictions, a trend encouraged by the spirit of the 1993–98 Medicare Agreements between the states and commonwealth.[61]

THE LEGACY OF THE COMMUNITY HEALTH PROGRAM

The historical legacy of the CHP has been mixed. There seems little doubt that in the formative years of the CHP, 1973–75, the federal Labor government did not clearly identify what the primary objective of the program was—whether to constrain health expenditure by treating patients in the community so they would not have to be hospitalized, or to pursue prevention. In the event, as we have seen, a disproportionate amount of CHP funding and effort was devoted to treatment and care, not to prevention. It was also left unclear whether the emphasis in prevention should be on individuals and small-group interaction or on community-level attempts to change attitudes and behavior or address structural inequities.

There was, moreover, an inherent problem in the provision of primary medical care. Many private practitioners opposed the team-based, multidisciplinary concept of the community health center, especially where salaried doctors were employed, because it offered an attractive alternative to established general practice and could be seen as a threat to the long-term viability of private practice itself. Certainly, the 1976 review of the CHP and a 1985 federal discussion paper played down the importance of personal medical care in centers, apparently to soothe the anxieties of private medical practitioners. But in a larger perspective—even in the period of the Whitlam government, before the decline in federal support with the Fraser government—the CHP received very limited funding in absolute terms or relative to Medibank, the universal health insurance scheme. Medibank itself not only supported "sickness" care rather than health promotion but underwrote the private, fee-for-service system. Medicare, when introduced in early 1984 by the Hawke Labor government as a virtual reincarnation of Medibank, continued the underwriting of private, fee-for-service medicine.

Yet the CHP arguably achieved a number of significant things. The program created a body of health professionals, mostly employees of the program, who brought (and still bring) commitment to community health ideals into policy and practice. It helped to reduce, at least to some extent, the influence of the dominant biomedical culture on professional practice and consumer expectations. The needs of disadvantaged groups were served to an extent inconceivable without the program. However great the failure to advance prevention, health education and health promotion received unprecedented recognition, and the ground was better prepared for the coming of the "new public health" than might otherwise have been the case.[62]

NOTES

1. S. Sax, *A Strife of Interests: Politics and Policies in Australian Health Services* (Sydney: George Allen and Unwin, 1984), 101–2; J. Raftery, "The Social and Historical Context," in *Health for All: The South Australian Experience,* ed. F. Baum (Kent Town: Wakefield Press, 1995), 19–20.

2. J. Duffy, *The Sanitarians: A History of American Public Health* (Urbana: University of Illinois, 1990), 214–16.

3. A. Sardell, *The U.S. Experiment in Social Medicine: The Community Health Center Program, 1965–1986* (Pittsburgh: University of Pittsburgh Press, 1988), 23–28, 34–38, 44–46, 77–78, 164–66, 193–94, 225–26; P. Starr, *The Social Transformation of American Medicine* (New York: Basic Books, 1982), 364–72.

4. C. Webster, *The Health Services since the War,* vol. 1, *Problems of Health Care: The National Health Service before 1957* (London: Her Majesty's Stationery Office, 1988), 380–87.

5. Quoted in C. Webster, *The National Health Service: A Political History* (Oxford: Oxford University Press, 1998), 131–32; J. Kinnaird, "The British National Health Service: Retrospect and Prospect," *Journal of Public Health Policy* 2 (1981): 390–91.

6. D. Gordon, "The Future of Community Health," in *Community Health in Australia,* ed. R. Walpole (Ringwood: Penguin Books Australia, 1979), 129–30; M. Crouch and C. Coulton, *The Course of Community Health in New South Wales: 1958–1982* (Kensington: School of Sociology, University of New South Wales, 1983), iv–v.

7. See M.J. Lewis, "Editor's Introduction," in J.H.L. Cumpston, *Health and Disease in Australia: A History,* ed. M.J. Lewis (Canberra: Australian Government Publishing Service [hereafter AGPS], 1989), 18.

8. M. Lewis, *Managing Madness: Psychiatry and Society in Australia 1788–1980* (Canberra: AGPS Press, 1988), 88–89; "The Psychiatric Patient in the Community," *Medical Journal of Australia* 1 (1975): 797.

9. Lewis, *Managing Madness,* 80–89; Crouch and Coulton, *The Course of Community Health in New South Wales,* 5.

10. Quoted in Lewis, *Managing Madness,* 88.

11. Crouch and Coulton, *The Course of Community Health in New South Wales,* 7–16; Standing Committee on Community Health Services, Health Commission of NSW, 1979, *Writings and Decisions of Health Commission of New South Wales Which Relate to Community Health* ([Sydney]: [NSW Health Commission], [1979]), 23–24, 30–31; Lewis, *Managing Madness,* 94.

12. Crouch and Coulton, *The Course of Community Health in New South Wales,* 17–20; S. Morey, "The Newtown Community Centre: Integrated Health Care for the Local Community," *R.P.A. Magazine* 73 (1975): 20–21; S. Sax, "Community Medicine and Geriatric Medicine at Royal Prince Alfred Hospital," October 1970, 1–2, Papers of Dr. S. Morey, Sydney; Report of Meeting of Darlington Committee, 16 December 1971, Royal Prince Alfred Hospital, Camperdown, NSW, 1, Papers of Dr. S. Morey, Sydney.

13. Crouch and Coulton, *The Course of Community Health in New South Wales,* 17.

14. T. Fagan, "The Aboriginal Medical Service," *New Doctor* 34 (1984): 20.

15. Quoted in G. Gray, *Federalism and Health Policy: The Development of Health Systems in Canada and Australia* (Toronto: University of Toronto Press, 1991), 172.

16. Quoted in Sax, *A Strife of Interests,* 103.

17. Quoted in E.G. Whitlam, "Health Politics and Programs from Lyons to Keating," *New Doctor* 61 (1993): 29.

18. Sax, *A Strife of Interests,* 101–3; Whitlam, "Health Politics and Programs from Lyons to Keating," 29–30; M. Cohen, "Unintended Consequences of Medicine," *New Doctor* 43 (1987): 11.

19. N. Milio, *Making Policy: A Mosaic of Australian Community Health Policy Development* (Canberra: Department of Community Services and Health, 1988), 16.

20. Quoted in Raftery, "The Social and Historical Context," 21.

21. Sax, *A Strife of Interests,* 103–7; Raftery, "The Social and Historical Context," 22–23.

22. Milio, *Making Policy,* 22.

23. Ibid., 22–31.

24. C. Kerr, "Self-Help Via Community Health Centres," *Medical Journal of Australia* 2 (1972): 1133–34.

25. "Like 'Rediscovering the Wheel'?" *AMA Gazette* (2 May 1974): 17.

26. *Review of the Community Health Program: Report from Hospitals and Health Services Commission, March 1976* (Canberra: AGPS, 1976), 29.

27. Sax, *A Strife of Interests,* 216.

28. *Review of the Community Health Program,* 29–45; Crouch and Coulton, *The Course of Community Health in New South Wales,* 21, 32; Sax, *A Strife of Interests,* 141–42.

29. Quoted in Crouch and Coulton, *The Course of Community Health in New South Wales,* 38.

30. Ibid., 11, 20, 36, 38, 40, 43, 49; *Review of the Community Health Program,* 7–8; I.W. Webster, "Where Healing Starts," in *Community Health in Australia,* ed. Walpole, 38–40.

31. Quoted in H.M. Keleher, "Australian Nursing: For the Health of Medicine or the Health of the Public?" (Ph.D. dissertation, La Trobe University, Bundoora, 1999), 225.

32. Crouch and Coulton, *The Course of Community Health in New South Wales,* 49; C. Bridges-Webb, "Community Medicine: Little Sister or Big Brother?" in *Community Health in Australia,* ed. Walpole, 65; H.M. Keleher, "Australian Nursing," 207–42.

33. Quoted in Keleher, "Australian Nursing," 247.

34. Ibid., 243–48.

35. Crouch and Coulton, *The Course of Community Health in New South Wales,* 35.

36. D. Lee, *School of Public Health and Tropical Medicine* (Sydney: School of Public Health and Tropical Medicine, 1980), 40–42; Crouch and Coulton, *The Course of Community Health in New South Wales,* 40–41.

37. Minutes of Meeting of Community Physicians, 3 June 1981, Royal Prince

Alfred Hospital Department of Community Medicine, 1–2, Papers of Dr. S. Morey, Sydney.

38. Australian Association of Community Physicians, Minutes of First Annual General Meeting, King's Cross, 28 February 1986, 1–4, Papers of Dr. S. Morey, Sydney.

39. *Snow's Field: The Voice of the Community Physicians* 1(1) (1985): 1; 1(3) (1986): 1–2.

40. Ibid., 2(3) (1987): 1–2; 2(4) (1987): 2; 3(1) (1987): 2–3; 3(2) (1988): 1–2.

41. Quoted in C.J. Cummins, *A History of Medical Administration in New South Wales 1788–1973* (Sydney: Health Commission of NSW, 1979), 158.

42. Ibid., 152–59; S.J. Duckett, "State of the Health Service: Structural Change in New South Wales Health Administration—or Sisyphus Revisited," *Community Health Studies* 8(2) (1983): 193–95.

43. Duckett, "State of the Health Service," 195–98.

44. New South Wales Correspondent, "The State of the Health Service: New South Wales," *Community Health Studies* 3(1) (1979): 42; G.R. Palmer and S.D. Short, *Health Care and Public Policy: An Australian Analysis* (South Melbourne: Macmillan Education Australia, 1994), 120.

45. *Review of the Community Health Program,* 30–35; Palmer and Short, *Health Care and Public Policy,* 120–21.

46. K. Powell, *Canberra's Health, 1950–1994: A Stormy Growth* (Gundaroo: Brolga Press, 1999), 254–60.

47. *Review of the Community Health Program,* 37.

48. *Report to Health Commission by Standing Committee on Community Health, November 1981* ([Sydney]: [NSW Health Commission], [1981]), 27–28.

49. Quoted in F.K. Crowley, *Tough Times: Australia in the Seventies* (Richmond: Heinemann Australia, 1986), 311–12.

50. N. Milio, "The Community Health Program under Federal Fiscal Austerity," *New Doctor* 29 (1983): 37–41.

51. New South Wales Correspondent, "The State of the Health Service," 43–44; Milio, *Making Policy,* 295–97; D. Broderick and P. Laris, "The South Australian Community Health Association," 233–36; F. Baum, *The New Public Health: An Australian Experience* (Melbourne: Oxford University Press, 1998), 44–48.

52. L. Davidson, S. Chapman and C. Hull, *Health Promotion in Australia 1978–79* (Canberra: AGPS, 1979), 101.

53. Ibid., 93–96, 100–102; Palmer and Short, *Health Care and Public Policy,* 13–14, 123–24; Sax, *A Strife of Interests,* 101–2; Raftery, "The Social and Historical Context," 19–20.

54. N. Crofts, "Community Health Centres: A Personal Experience," *New Doctor* 41–42 (1986): 51–53.

55. N. Crofts, "Community Health: Where Do We Go From Here? Preventive Interventions," *New Doctor* 37 (1985): 9–11.

56. *Review of the Community Health Program—1986* (Strawberry Hills: Australian Community Health Association, 1986), summary, n.p.

57. Ibid., 16, 31–62, 78; Raftery, "The Social and Historical Context," 28–29; *Report of Ministerial Review of Community Health Services, May 1985* (Melbourne:

Government Printer, 1985), i–iv, 43–44, 83–84; P. Broadhead, S. Duckett and G. Lavender, "Developing a Mandate for Change: Planning as a Political Process," *Community Health Studies* 13(3) (1989): 246–47.

58. Quoted in L. Sylvan and D. Legge, "Community Participation in Health," in *Health Promotion: The Community Health Approach,* ed. M. Miller and R. Walker (Bondi Junction: Australian Community Health Association, 1989), 65.

59. Quoted in ibid., 66.

60. *Review of the Community Health Program—1986,* 65–70, 79; Sylvan and Legge, "Community Participation in Health," 64–66; E.M. Bates, *Health Systems and Public Scrutiny: Australia, Britain and the United States* (London: Croom Helm, 1983), 78, 174; Palmer and Short, *Health Care and Public Policy,* 321; T. Pentes and A. Owen, "Community Participation in NSW Area Health Boards," in *Health Promotion,* ed. Miller and Walker, 270–71.

61. Palmer and Short, *Health Care and Public Policy,* 321.

62. Ibid., 124–26; Raftery, "The Social and Historical Context," 30–34; Cohen, "Unintended Consequences of Medicine," 11.

Chapter 4

The New Public Health: Promise and Performance

Throughout its history, public health in Australia has been quick to embrace compelling ideas from overseas. The sanitary idea, which launched the "old public health," with its focus on improvement of the physical environment (and from about 1900, the health of population groups with special needs), was eagerly imported from Britain. The idea of community health services emphasizing primary health care and prevention that flourished in the 1960s and 1970s was shared with a number of Western countries, as we have seen. The policy of "Health for All by the Year 2000" (HFA), again emphasizing primary health care, was taken up in Australia in the 1980s. It lies at the heart of the "new public health."

The Hawke Labor government had committed itself to support for the Community Health Program (CHP) in its 1983 election campaign. After winning the election, it provided eighteen million dollars for community health under its Medicare Agreement with the states. But the federal government did not offer leadership in community health policy; it focused on implementation of Medicare, the national health insurance program. The CHP did not become the mechanism by which the commonwealth advanced health promotion and disease prevention in the 1980s and '90s. Yet, the longer-term importance of the CHP and the community health movement that grew out of it should not be underestimated. Ideologically, the community health movement facilitated the reception of new public health ideas in Australia. As we have noted previously, the CHP brought into being a body of committed health professionals and administrators who were to continue to exercise an influence on policy.[1]

THE INTERNATIONAL CONTEXT

The community health movement was an important domestic factor in the rise of the new public health in Australia. But the international arena was also the source of policy ideas. As early as 1948, the World Health Organization had supported a definition of health that substituted a social and holistic perspective for a strictly biomedical one. WHO defined health as "a state of complete physical, mental and social well-being, not merely the absence of disease or infirmity." This perspective was not absolutely new. Certainly, the international sanitary conferences held from 1851 to 1903 and the Office International d'Hygiène Publique (from 1907) had limited their interests to quarantine control of communicable diseases, especially cholera, plague and yellow fever. After World War I, the League of Nations Health Organization had likewise been concerned with international control of particular communicable diseases, broadening its interests to major problems such as malaria, syphilis, tuberculosis and leprosy. But the League had in the 1930s begun to be concerned with what later became known as "horizontal" public health issues—general primary health care issues like nutrition, housing, hygiene and physical fitness—as opposed to "vertical" policy, focused on particular diseases. This broader, social approach prepared the way for the new conceptualization of health expressed in the 1948 WHO definition, although WHO's priorities in its early years reflected in practice the vertical, or one-problem/one-solution, strategy.

There were good reasons for the vertical approach. Malaria, tuberculosis and venereal diseases were very prevalent in economically developing countries. As discussed earlier, the scientific achievements of the Second World War, in particular the coming of the "magic bullet" penicillin, and DDT, seemed to endorse a monocausal approach. In any case, the science of the day was more at home with specifics than generalities. The approach was reinforced by the availability in the 1960s of new insecticides to attack the vectors of diseases like onchocerciasis, or "river blindness," prevalent in Africa. The approach was legitimated also by the success of the campaign to eradicate smallpox, the ancient scourge, from the world in the 1970s. It was further supported by the success of international child-immunization campaigns against diphtheria, tetanus, whooping cough, measles, poliomyelitis and, with BCG vaccine, tuberculosis. The vertical approach suited the economic development theory of the time, which envisaged that "trickle-down," effects of economic growth would raise the living standards of even the poor and ultimately produce better health (as Thomas McKeown in large part argued it had in the West). The approach did not require diversion of domestic investment and foreign aid resources from productive economic development to health service expansion in less developed countries.

However, both epidemiological and development theory began to change in the 1960s. The ecological approach, classically illustrated in the work of Scrimshaw, Taylor and Gordon on the interaction—synergy—of nutritional status and (some) infections, showed that the condition of the host as well as the virulence of the parasite determined the relationship between host and parasite. Disease had multiple causes.

The new view was supported by epidemiological experience in developing countries, where the pneumonia-diarrhoea complex was a major cause of illness and death. This situation resulted from a variety of pathogens and reflected the host's nutritional status. Moreover, development theory itself was changing. The human-capital approach to economic development, which encouraged investment in health and education to raise productivity, was compatible with the ecological view, because health services had to deal with various major causes of disease. Horizontal rather than vertical, disease-oriented programs were now advocated by development experts. In any case, a number of poorer countries, eschewing foreign aid for ideological reasons, were achieving through social and primary health care programs remarkable reductions in infant and child mortality rates, as well as increases in life expectancy. China, Sri Lanka, the Indian state of Kerala, and Costa Rica pursued horizontal social programs with such features as mass education, equitable distribution of public health measures and primary health care, adequate caloric intake across the population, and substantial political and social commitment to implementation.

At the same time, the WHO-supported malaria-eradication campaign was foundering. The incapacity of medical "generals" to roll back permanently the malaria enemy with biological "weapons" alone was manifest. The assistance of experts on social and economic organization—anthropologists, sociologists, economists and geographers—had to be sought. While the demise of the malaria-eradication campaign and the withdrawal of funding by America, the major funder, was the primary reason for the death of the vertical concept, political and organizational changes were rendering it impractical in any case. In the postcolonial era, the entry of a large number of new nations into WHO made coordination in vertical programs a prescription for organizational disaster. The health infrastructures of many newly independent countries were inadequate for effective participation in vertical campaigns, which require a capacity to follow an eradication timetable in step with other countries.[2] Thus, where in its first decades WHO was to a large extent disease oriented in policy and dominated by medical professionalism, by the 1970s the organization was becoming politicized and conflict ridden.

In the 1950s and 1960s, WHO, like UN agencies generally, had pursued Western-based technical approaches, but the next decade saw developing nations pushing for broader programs. The annual World Health Assembly ceased to be concerned essentially with exchange of information and became marked by lobbying over specific policy issues. Although they lacked the West's financial capacity to affect budgets, Third World countries had power in formal voting, because of their numbers. They used it in the 1970s to challenge established policy in international agencies; one such challenge was represented by the HFA program of WHO. Halfdan Mahler, WHO director-general from 1974 to 1986, himself supported this radical review of health policy. In 1975, he initiated the push for HFA, with its emphasis on international equity in health and on primary health care as the means to its goal.

The 1960s and 1970s were also a period of radical critiques of modern biomedicine's contribution to health advancement. Ivan Illich sought to show modern technology-driven medicine was itself a source of illness. In Britain, Peter Townsend and Tudor Hart pointed to the failure of medicine to end social inequalities in health status. Thomas McKeown's historical study of mortality decline, a work that was becoming widely quoted, seemed to point up the limitations of biomedicine. In his Rock Carling lecture of 1976 McKeown put in order of importance as contributions to historical health improvement in England and Wales "limitations of family size (a behavioral change), increase in food supplies and a healthier physical environment (environmental influences) and specific preventive and therapeutic measures."[3] Five years earlier, in the Rock Carling lecture of 1971, Archie Cochrane had raised the question of effectiveness and efficiency in health care in proposing what two decades later would become the basis for the international, scientific movement of evidence-based medicine. Even in affluent Western countries, the escalating cost of health care was beginning to concern governments. In any case, curative medicine was producing a diminishing health gain for a steeply rising level of investment. A 1974 Canadian report, *A New Perspective on the Health of Canadians*—which came to be known as the Lalonde report, after the Canadian health minister, Marc Lalonde—saw health care as only one of four "health fields." The other three were human biology (genetics), the environment and individual lifestyle. If the developed Western countries were more cautious about HFA and the primary health care approach than Third World countries, which warmly embraced them, the advent of HFA did encourage, as we shall see, the introduction of national health goals and targets in Europe and in Australia.[4]

In September 1978, WHO and the United Nations Children's Fund (UNICEF) jointly sponsored an international conference on primary health care in Alma Ata, in the Soviet Union. The conference produced the Declaration of Alma Ata, which called upon all governments and health and development workers to pursue the principles of HFA. While primary health care was to be the vehicle for achieving health for all, community participation and intersectoral action were seen as vital. More specifically, the declaration saw health as a fundamental right; gross inequalities in health status between developed and developing countries, and within countries, as unacceptable; and community participation in health care planning and implementation as a right and duty of citizens. It envisaged primary health care as providing promotive, preventive, curative and rehabilitative services; as involving health education, promotion of proper nutrition, safe water and basic sanitation, maternal and child care (including family planning), immunization against major infections, prevention of endemic diseases, appropriate treatment of common conditions and provision of essential drugs; and as requiring coordinated efforts by all sectors related to development, not simply the health sector. It called upon all governments to formulate national policies to promote primary health care.[5]

On the larger social stage, beyond health and medicine, the postwar era saw the proliferation of social-change movements in the Western world—such as feminism, consumerism, environmentalism, black rights, and lesbian and gay rights and the peace movement. These activists created an ideological climate in which the values of the new public health flourished more easily. While pursuing different political agendas, the movements nevertheless shared a common commitment to challenging injury, injustice and oppression by dominant social groups and value systems. They all used the language of social justice: equity, human rights, participation and empowerment. The focus on rights shifted from concern with civil and political to social and economic rights. Community advocates and commentators debated the social rights of citizenship, evincing renewed interest in ways to advance participatory democracy.

Disillusioned with the hierarchical structures and bureaucratization of traditional political parties and trade unions, the new social movements tried to build alternative forms of democracy. Egalitarianism in interpersonal relationships and democratic decision making were valued as ends in themselves. Members of movements demonstrated in practice the social changes they desired. Unlike political parties, they did not pursue state power but typically made demands upon the state—for land rights, equal pay and affirmative action legislation, homosexual law reform, demilitarization and disarmament and government measures to protect the biosphere. Many supporters were from the "new middle class." Because of greater access to advanced education, they could understand political, social and economic affairs from theoretical perspectives. The new social movements promoted a rights-based rhetoric and worldview in which egalitarianism, democratic decision making and the sovereignty of the community were key elements. They called for attention to the needs of individuals. But they strongly valued the benefits of community, especially nonhierarchical, cooperative relationships.

The period after World War II also saw great changes in the nature of the state in Australia and other Western countries. In approximate chronological order, the transformations were the welfare state, the bureaucratic state, the corporatist state and the managerialist state. Moved by social deprivation, the prescriptions of Keynesian economic theory for full employment and pressure from the labor movement, governments established statutory benefits and support programs. The welfare state created greater employment opportunities for social work and allied "human service" professionals. From the 1960s and 1970s on these professionals were influenced by the values of the social change movements. They began to advocate philosophies of empowerment and community development to assist both individuals and communities to gain access to benefits or, more radically, to change the system. But as the welfare state developed so did bureaucratization, with the executive gaining in power relative to the legislative function. Bureaucracy, rules based and process oriented, sought standardized outcomes. Legislation providing social benefits or enabling market regulation often did not create rights so much as grant bureaucrats wide discretionary powers.

More recently, the state has taken on a corporatist character, whereby administrators have mediated between interest groups, which have to possess considerable material and intellectual resources to advocate their cases effectively. One commentator on the evolution of corporatism in the United States has noted that interest-group intermediation has meant "underrepresentation of poor and diffused interests."[6] In Australia, community and consumer groups have in some instances formed peak bodies like the Consumers' Health Forum, the Australian Council of Social Service, and the Australian Council on the Ageing. These bodies use professional staffs, in order to increase their capacity to contribute to national policy debate and decision making.

In the last decade or so, further changes to the nature of the state have occurred as managerialism has replaced regulation and bureaucratic process with the allocative mechanism of the market, thereby turning citizens into customers of the state. The Westminster parliamentary model of government has, in one rather extreme assessment of the Australian situation, been replaced by the "competitive franchise model of government."[7] Administrators are managers of franchises; requiring no particular expertise in their areas of work, they pursue a net-benefit-maximization approach and apply cost/benefit analysis. Like corporatism, this approach shuts out poorer interests, which cannot command the expertise necessary to meaningful participation. A number of commentators argue that the future growth of participatory democracy is seriously at risk because managerialist practices like competitive tendering and contracting-out of services basically undermine the pursuit of community development.[8]

The HFA, with its commitment to community participation and intersectoral action, implied a new view of health promotion. But because of its emphasis on primary health care, the HFA strategy seemed more immediately applicable to developing countries than to the high-technology medical and health care systems of developed countries. However, the European region of WHO sought in 1985 to make HFA meaningful for European countries by developing targets for improved health status reflecting HFA principles. WHO Europe sponsored meetings aimed at developing the concept of health promotion. These culminated in an international conference on health promotion in developed countries held at Ottawa in November 1986.

The conference produced the Ottawa Charter, which captured the imagination of the health promotion community in Western countries.[9] The charter restated significant HFA principles, stressing that health was critically dependent on political, economic and social conditions. It identified five main action areas for health promotion: building healthy public policy, creating supportive environments, strengthening community action, developing personal skills, and reorienting health services from illness reduction toward health promotion. It envisaged three processes by which citizens might start to control their own health—mediation, enablement and advocacy. The international movement advocating health promotion progressed farther with the second international conference, in Adelaide, Australia, in April 1988. That conference focused on the issue of healthy public policy, identifying equity and accountability as its key aspects. Areas of action identified as having priority were women's health, nutrition, alcohol and tobacco, and the natural environment. In June 1991, the third international conference was held in Sundsvall, Sweden. The focus there was on creating physical, social and economic environments that promoted health but were reconcilable with sustainable economic development.[10]

Macdonald and Bunton suggest that viewed internationally, health promotion, as both a term and a concept, was first introduced to the Western world in the Canadian Lalonde Report. This, as we noted earlier, saw four "causes" of disease and death—inadequate health care services, lifestyle (behavioral) factors, environmental pollution, and human biology. Thus positive individual (behavioral) and environmental (structural) change would advance the health status of the population. The development of health promotion as a specific public health activity, or body of expertise, and the emergence of the new public health movement became intertwined. As we have seen, the 1986 Ottawa conference grew out of the HFA strategy of WHO. The Ottawa Charter became a definitive reference point for health promotion action. In turn, health promotion as a professional activity, drawing on the concepts of the social and behavioral sciences, became an integral part of the new public health. Health promotion grew out of health education. Yet it sought to remedy traditional health education's neglect of structural factors. In Britain, health education in a formal sense may be dated from the setting up of the Central Council for Health Education in 1927. But the activity, as part of public health practice, dates back to the movement of public health in Britain, and elsewhere in the Western world, from a focus on environmental sanitation to concern with the lifestyle of individuals in the last years of the nineteenth and the early years of the twentieth century—the education of mothers in infant care, of schoolchildren in personal hygiene, and of the population at large about control of infectious disease, both epidemic and chronic (like TB and syphilis).[11]

Health education has usually meant education about diet, exercise and body functioning, although it has also been about how to gain access to health services. A fundamental failing of the focus on individual lifestyle has been the assumption that rationality in decision making prevails. Another has been blindness to the way economic, social and political factors contextualize and constrain individual choice. Disadvantaged people lack the material and, indeed, cultural resources to pursue healthier lifestyles.

In the 1970s, social psychology advanced a number of theories through which behaviorally oriented health education sought to produce changes in individual behavior. "Social learning theory," commonly associated with the name of A. Bandura, looks particularly at the individual's belief in his or her capacity to alter his or her behavior, and at the social influences on learning about behavior. Change is produced by motivating, by providing skills for behavior change, by developing support networks to maintain change, and by reinforcing change. The "health belief" model, put forward by M.H. Becker, sees individuals carrying out cost-benefit analysis as a result of which change will occur, or will not. They do this in terms of likely susceptibility to illness or injury, and the severity thereof, and the likely efficacy and personal benefit. In the 1980s and '90s, other models were introduced. The theory of "reasoned action" as advanced by Atzen and Fishbein (1980) has it that behavior follows from "intention" to behave in a particular manner. Intention results from a combination of the individual's belief about the behavior and his or her perception of how significant persons might judge or evaluate that behavior. The "stages of change" theory associated with J.O. Prochaska and C.C. DiClemente (1984) suggests that individuals go through five stages when changing behavior. They often do not advance smoothly through the stages—as yet no intention to change, contemplating change, preparing for change, behavior change for a brief period, and maintaining change over a long period. In the "health action" model, intention to act results from the interaction of beliefs, motivation and normative factors. In contrast to other theories based on social psychology, it allows for the influence of environmental factors on action. Significant in the model is the individual's self-esteem. This is strongly influenced by the individual's beliefs about his or her competence and control of the situation.

One common application of social-psychological knowledge has been social marketing, particularly popular in the United States. Promotion through mass media campaigns to reach target audiences is common. Australia has a history of using mass media campaigns to promote behavioral change at the population level. Both federal and state governments have been willing to fund mass campaigns in relation to health problems like smoking, road accidents and heart disease. Health promotion foundations in three states—Victoria, South Australia and Western Australia—have used funds from tobacco taxes for social marketing.

Like the social-psychological models, however, social marketing fails to allow for structural constraints on individual behavior. Indeed it may encourage blaming of the victims while promoting unrealistic expectations of individual responsibility among disadvantaged groups. Another weakness of the behavioral approach is the assumption that better health is a prime concern of everybody—that people, given adequate information, will choose rationally the path to better health. Even when the individual enjoys good social and economic conditions, health is only one of various considerations bearing upon everyday decision making. Finally, individual behavior-change programs have not enjoyed great success. In the Multiple Risk Factor Intervention Trial (MRFIT) in the United States, after six years of exposure to efforts to change their eating and smoking behavior, men at high risk of coronary heart disease had made little change in behavior. Moreover, even if the program is successful, new candidates for the high-risk group in the population will be recruited, because the structural factors influencing the behavior have not changed. Health-related behavior takes place in social contexts. Thus low-income, single mothers in the United Kingdom continued to smoke, because it provided one of the few sources of pleasure available to them. It offered brief respite from the demands of child care in a social context that did not otherwise provide relief.[12]

THE UNITED KINGDOM EXPERIENCE

As already noted, health education by local authorities and voluntary bodies goes back to the 1890s when personal health services began to develop, at first to save infant lives but later to reach schoolchildren and tuberculosis and VD sufferers. Health education work expanded into new territory as public VD clinics were set up in the wake of the 1913–16 Royal Commission on VD, maternity and child welfare clinics were established from 1918, and the tuberculosis sanatoria proliferated in the 1920s. The proposition that maternal efficiency in infant care was more important than poverty in prevention of infant disease and death heightened the role of health education. Financial retrenchment in the 1920s made it even more attractive to the Health Ministry.

Ministry officials, supported by the former health minister, Christopher Addison, wanted in the early 1920s a central organization under the ministry to replace local authorities in the field of health education. But financial restraint prevented realization of such ambitions. The ministry encouraged the Society of Medical Officers of Health to pursue the work. In September 1927, a Central Council for Health Education came into being. In an introduction to a 1928 health education handbook for schoolteachers, Sir George Newman clearly related self-responsibility for health behavior to citizenship and morality, and health advancement to "national efficiency." The handbook stated that "the first duty of a citizen . . . is to make himself a strong, long-lived, capable citizen, able to work and produce, the guardian and maintainer of a home[,] . . . loyal, patriotic, 'a friend and helper of mankind.'"[13]

Through the 1930s, the Central Council supplied to local authorities for a small fee posters and copies of its monthly journal, *Better Health.* It assisted with organization of health weeks and exhibitions. It took advantage of the burgeoning documentary film industry and produced films on TB, diphtheria, housing, infant health and other public health concerns of the time. *Better Health* enjoyed sales of 57,500 in its first year; by 1929, sales of two hundred thousand were claimed. In its pages, women were depicted as the natural protectors of family health. While much material was directed at them, little on their own health problems appeared. The journal, like the Central Council itself, did not concern itself with the connection between poverty and ill health, even in the economically depressed 1930s. A few radical doctors and social scientists, like G.C.M. M'Gonigle and Richard Titmuss, pointed to poverty, not ignorance, as the cause of undernutrition and related ill health, but they had limited impact. Where in the 1920s Newman, as chief medical officer, had identified cooking lessons as the answer to poor nutrition, his successor, Sir Arthur MacNalty, went as far as to admit that "poverty and lack of proper implements prevent many girls from attempting to apply in their homes the lessons which they are given at school."[14]

Advice on "economical cookery" and "wise spending on food supplies" was commonly offered by the journal. Thus in December 1930 it suggested that cheap fish like skate, catfish and bream might be included in the family diet; "Gardening for Health" was a long-running feature. Not only was the journal likely to have little appeal for working-class citizens, because of its parish-magazine style, but the often exaggerated claims in its advertising for foods and beverages were at odds with the sober nutritional material in articles. This contradiction reflected the wider contrast between the very limited health education efforts and the growth of commercial advertising in the interwar period, despite the international economic depression. By 1937, a hundred million pounds was being spent on commercial advertising.[15]

When the National Health Service began, it seemed that health education might enjoy considerable prominence, but this hope soon faded. Health education by the early 1950s lacked direction, except for the traditional concern of local health authorities with maternal and child welfare. Cost concerns about health care and the influence of the ideas of critics like McKeown raised the issue of a greater role for prevention.[16] The Central Council for Health Education and the Scottish Council for Health Education had continued to assist local authorities with education after the NHS came into being. But their role shrank as the status of the medical officer of health declined, as did the role of local government in health. In the course of the 1950s, as important new health education issues, like smoking and health, began to emerge and more established issues, like sex education and family planning, took on new aspects, it became clear that the two central councils lacked both resources and direction. The Health Ministry decided to set up an inquiry. When the Scottish Health Department expressed interest, the inquiry embraced both councils, with Lord Cohen of Birkenhead as chairman. The committee was asked to look not only at "fresh fields" for health education but to advise on what methods were likely to be effective in the future. It commenced its labors in July 1960. Officials became concerned that members were failing to come to grips with their brief, but in May 1964 a report was finally published.

The report failed to deliver answers concerning new areas of endeavor for health education. Its proposals concerning centralized organization of health education and the creation of a new profession of "health educator" were widely discussed, but the committee, in effect, left the matter of organization to the central health authorities. Official opinion was split between those who believed effective education was possible only if health departments took direct responsibility and those who wanted a semi-independent authority to continue. The latter view prevailed. The Scots decided to keep their existing council for purposes of training, while having the central authorities assume responsibility for all other health education functions. The Treasury was not happy about funding a new central health education authority, and conflict between it and the Health Ministry delayed progress. Ministerial intervention ended the logjam. In 1968 a new Health Education Council (HEC), a registered charity, was set up. In the same year, the Scottish Home and Health Department established a Health Education Unit to prosecute health education work. The unit came to be seen as successful in an era when health education in the United Kingdom was not an especially vigorous field. The new HEC quickly became caught up in important promotional work when the Labor secretary of state for social services, Richard Crossman, requested the council to mount antismoking campaigns as a matter of priority.

By the 1970s, pressure from the preventive medicine lobby for a more coherent policy on prevention was matched by strong public opinion in favor of government action. Politicians were sensitive to the pressure. The Social Services and Employment Sub-Committee of the Commons Expenditure Committee, chaired by Labor's Renée Short, carried out a major review of prevention. It wanted more action on alcohol and tobacco control, diet, family planning, screening for cancer and promotion of sport, and as well stronger support for health education, especially mass media campaigns. The director of the HEC had told the inquiry that the Department of Health and Social Security (DHSS) and the Department of Education and Science had been hostile to the HEC's efforts.

The central health authorities, seeking to regain the initiative, speedily put together a consultative document, *Prevention and Health: Everybody's Business,* which appeared under the names of the four secretaries of state for the respective parts of the United Kingdom in March 1976. The document's concern with individual responsibility for health was heartening for the Treasury, which was eager to see financial restraint applied by the DHSS.

Although the government pointed to key areas for action like tobacco, alcohol and other drugs and sensible diets and fluoridation to prevent dental caries, it did not commit itself unequivocally to action. Subsequently promises were made to publish papers on specific preventive topics. *Prevention and Health* became the central pillar of the DHSS argument that health departments had fundamentally altered policy toward prevention.

To illustrate its conversion to prevention, the Labour government issued in December 1977 a white paper, also titled "Prevention and Health," which put health education at the forefront of preventive strategies. The Scottish Health Education Unit, while formally part of the health department, was considered more effective than the more autonomous HEC, which covered the remainder of Britain. The new initiative in prevention policy improved the lot of the HEC both in terms of material resources and freedom of action. Its 1978 "Better Health: Look after Yourself" campaign came to be regarded as indicating a real advance in the HEC's effectiveness. But its relationships with the DHSS and with ministers remained at times difficult. TheHEC's life was made unstable by the turnover of chairmen—six in 1968–79. Moreover, while health education funding increased more than 100 percent in 1977–79, the expenditure of health education agencies was a tiny fraction of the total NHS budget in 1979—a mere 4.7 million pounds, or around 0.05 percent of the budget.[17] In November 1986 the secretary of state for social services announced that the HEC would be replaced by the Health Education Authority within the NHS from April 1987.[18]

The Thatcher Conservative government, elected in May 1979, quickly set out to reduce public spending, including that on the NHS. It was also intent on introducing structural and management reforms to promote the efficiency of the NHS and on encouraging alternative health care provision through private and voluntary channels. It was the beginning of a more ideological approach to health policy. It signaled the end of the consensus that had existed since the NHS was set up. Plans for reorganization were made public in a consultative document, *Patients First,* published in December 1979. The key reform was abandonment of the area level of administration and the creation in April 1982 of 192 District Health Authorities (which became Statutory Health Authorities) and delegation of power to units of management. Scotland and Wales, having more simple structures, were little affected by the reforms. While small savings were made on management costs, the administrative loss was that health authorities and local authorities were no longer overlapping or coterminous. Family Practitioner Committees became authorities, able to hire in their own right and directly responsible to the DHSS; Special Health Authorities were created to administer the London postgraduate teaching hospitals.

Facing in 1988 widespread dissatisfaction with paediatric intensive care, essentially a funding issue, the Thatcher government conducted a review of services. The health professions were excluded from this review. As a result, an internal "market" was introduced to the NHS in 1990, with competition replacing planning as the mode of allocating resources. The market was created by dividing the NHS into "purchasers" and "providers." The hospitals were providers, which sold services to health authorities, the purchasers. General practitioners were encouraged to become fundholders, funded by monies diverted from health authorities. They too became purchasers of hospital services.

The new system caused much controversy and was criticized by most organizations that represented health workers. Not only were equity and the public service ethic lost and commercial attitudes and methods inappropriately imposed in health care, but the economic efficiencies won by the market mechanism were dubious. The additional cost of the bureaucracy was 1.7 billion pounds a year. The NHS's long-established low level of administrative costs (around 6 percent) was doubled. The Labour opposition made abolition of the internal market a major part of its election platform in 1997, and it was elected to government with a massive majority in Parliament in May. The Blair Labour government indicated its intended changes in a white paper of December 1997: reducing bureaucracy (purchasing bodies to be cut from 3,600 to five hundred); the emphasis to be on quality, not quantity (for example, a health authority would devise a health improvement program for its area—a strategy to meet health needs); equity (fundholding to be replaced by primary care groups); openness to the public (hospital trust board and health authority board meetings to be open); and a central role for primary care (a primary care group within the parameters of the health improvement program would commission hospital services for patients, drawn from its population of about a hundred thousand people).[19]

In a retreat from the community medicine concept, by the mid-1980s "public health" was being employed again to describe population-level health concerns. The chief medical officer, Sir Donald Acheson, in 1986 chaired an inquiry into "the future development of the public health function . . . following the introduction of general management into the Hospital and Community Health Services."[20] In his 1988 report, Acheson concluded that five key problems existed: the need for information about population health nationally and locally to support the policy-making process, the need to advance health promotion and disease prevention activities, the need to clarify the role of public health doctors, the need to establish the locus of responsibility for communicable diseases, and the need to improve health authorities's capacity to evaluate health service outcomes. Of the inquiry's thirty-nine recommendations, the first was that henceforth the medical specialty of community medicine be called the specialty of "public health medicine."

Along with this resurrection of policy interest in public health, including health promotion, came a considerable growth of concern about social inequalities in health in Britain. *Inequalities in Health,* known as the Black report, was presented in April 1980 to the Conservative secretary of state, who gave it a cool reception. In 1987, the Health Education Council published *The Health Divide: Inequalities in Health in the 1980s,* which reviewed evidence on inequalities since the Black Report. (The question of health inequalities in Britain and elsewhere will be discussed at length in the following chapter.)

The Acheson Report, among other things led to growth in the number of training positions in all regions for public health physicians. Funding was reserved for an additional fifty trainees a year for four years. However, the training and career development of nonmedical public health professionals was not provided for. As concern about costs of management grew in the 1990s, career opportunities for public health physicians narrowed. Capacity to recruit new trainees diminished. Further, nonmedical professionals like nurses and social scientists, whose salaries were smaller, carried out public health functions.

From the 1960s, epidemiology gradually became part of undergraduate medical courses. Postgraduate courses likewise developed. Modern, properly structured, postgraduate courses in public health were available at the London School of Hygiene and Tropical Health from 1970, and other centers quickly offered the same. The conditions of specialist training in public health from 1974 were akin to those of other specialties—part or full-time training with academic fees paid by the employing authority. The salaries of public health physicians employed by local authorities were in the interwar period comparable to those of most general practitioners or consultants. But with the coming of the NHS, public health salaries ceased to be as good as those of clinicians. Given the other attractions of clinical medicine in the 1950s and '60s, the quality and number of recruits to public health medicine fell away. The NHS reforms of 1974, however, made the salary levels of public health doctors the same as those of hospital doctors. In 1972, the three Royal Colleges of Physicians of the United Kingdom formed the joint Faculty of Community Medicine (later the Faculty of Public Health Medicine), which meant that the specialty of public health medicine now had a professional body able to "bring together all the interests, academic and service" and to "undertake all the assessment needed during and at the end of general professional training," as the Todd Report on medical education had envisaged in 1968.[21]

THE AMERICAN EXPERIENCE

The origins of health education in the United States were caught up in the health center movement that began in Chicago and New York in the 1890s. I have already looked at the development of health centers, but it needs to be repeated that education of the individual and of families in the community was seen in the United States too as an important means of promoting infant and child health and of controlling tuberculosis and VD. While neighbourhood center projects faltered in Pittsburgh, Philadelphia and Cincinnati, they took root in New York, Boston and Buffalo. The New York City Health Department was the first municipal body formally to establish health education facilities, setting up a Bureau of Health Education in 1914. To ensure that health education work was community-based, the department in the same year set up the first district office on the Lower East Side of Manhattan. Nurses carried out education work in homes, and health inspectors encouraged voluntary acceptance of sanitary codes through health education. By the late nineteenth century, municipal health departments were producing regular health publications for the general public as well as for doctors and teachers. They cooperated with school boards to promote health education classes.[22]

The 1920s were a period of expansion of health departments as states and municipalities supported the growth of new divisions, one of which was health education. The growing number of public health nurses was well placed to carry out health education work. One reason for the growth of health education in the conservative 1920s was that its focus on individual behavior change threatened no powerful economic or political interests. Unlike child health clinics or school medical services, it did not evoke the private medical profession's fears of competition for patients; unlike housing reform and occupational health, it did not threaten the incomes of landlords and employers.[23] Leading public health figure, Charles-Edward Winslow, noted in 1923 the great potential of health education: "The dominant motive in the present-day public health campaign is the education of the individual in the practices of personal hygiene. The discovery of popular education as an instrument in preventive medicine, made by the pioneers in the tuberculosis movement, has proved almost as far-reaching as the discovery of the germ theory of disease thirty years before."[24]

The first decade and half to two decades after World War II was the golden age of curative medicine and federal investment in biomedical infrastructure—hospitals and research facilities. The 1960s were a time when the "New Frontier," "Great Society" and "War on Poverty" programs of John Kennedy and Lyndon Johnson attempted to redistribute health resources to the poor and the elderly through the mechanism of neighbourhood health centers, Medicare and Medicaid. At this time the aim of health education was to encourage use of health services—early attendance for care, participation in screening and immunization programs and use of child and family planning clinics. The 1970s, however, saw the economies of the Western world caught between inflation and rising unemployment. Governments responded by trying to contain steeply rising health costs, which in the United States were increasing at about 20 percent per annum, substantially in advance of the general inflation rate.

In 1971 President Nixon publicly discussed the "health maintenance organization" (HMO) as a means by which to contain costs. The HMO Act of 1973 introduced incentives for the practice of preventive medicine. While the government later abandoned its requirement that HMOs wanting federal certification had to provide health education, HMOs continued with programs like weight control and smoking cessation. The U.S. Public Health Service offered grants and loans to encourage development of HMOs. The President's Committee on Health Education, 1973, proposed that citizens be educated for self-care and restraint in their use of health services (something of a reversal of the approach in the 1960s). It also proposed that health education be increased in schools and at workplaces.

The National Health Planning and Resource Development Act of 1974 identified health education as a planning priority. In the same year, a Bureau of Health Education was established within the Centers for Disease Control. While government cost containment and the need to induce behavioral change to deal with chronic diseases was one force pushing the advance of health education, another was the blossoming of a popular self-help health movement. This produced a boom in commercial products like dietary and other health books, health courses and packaged "wellness" programs for employers. Voluntary health bodies and philanthropic organizations contributed to the growth of health education. The American Heart Association sponsored an early meeting of health educators and behavioral scientists to discuss means of lowering the prevalence of cardiovascular illness. For the ten years beginning in 1977, the W.K. Kellogg Foundation provided funding for demonstration projects in health promotion in schools, hospitals, universities, workplaces and community settings. In 1985, the Henry J. Kaiser Family Foundation committed itself to ten years of funding for a national health promotion program. Two years later, the Robert Wood Johnson Foundation announced it would provide twenty-seven million dollars for community-oriented preventive programs in the area of drug abuse. In 1976, the Office of Health Information and Health Promotion, later the Office of Disease Prevention and Health Promotion, was established within the U.S. Public Health Service. J. Michael McGinnis, who became head of the office, was soon to create a national policy basis for health promotion in the United States. Moreover, at the same time a body of new research, underwritten by the National Institutes of Health and the National Center for Health Services Research, was emerging. This research showed that health promotion was effective.[25]

Soon after Joseph A. Califano assumed office as secretary of health, education and welfare in the Jimmy Carter administration in 1977, he asked the surgeon general, paediatrician Dr. Julius Richmond, to prepare a report on disease prevention. Dr. McGinnis took direct responsibility for the task. *Healthy People: The Surgeon General's Report on Health Promotion and Disease Prevention, 1979* became the guiding light for health promotion in the

United States. Secretary Califano stated in his foreword, "You, the individual, can do more for your own health and well-being than any doctor, any hospital, any drug, any exotic medical device." The report strongly emphasized individual responsibility, although it also referred to "harmful social conditions" like poverty, hunger and ignorance.[26] It mentioned the mushrooming national expenditure on health care—from twenty-seven billion dollars in 1960 to $192 billion in 1978—but pointed out even this great increase in spending had not delivered marked improvements in health. Prevention was an idea whose time had come.

The innovative aspect of the report was its setting of national health goals related to five major life stages to be achieved by 1990: to reduce infant mortality by at least 35 percent, to below nine per thousand births; to reduce deaths of children (one to fourteen years) by at least 20 percent, to below thirty-four per thousand population; to reduce mortality in fifteen- to twenty-four-year-olds by at least 20 percent, to fewer than ninety-three per thousand; to reduce deaths among twenty-five- to sixty-four-year-olds by at least 25 percent, to fewer than four hundred per thousand; and to reduce the average number of days per year of restricted activity from acute or chronic conditions by 20 percent, to fewer than thirty days, for people sixty-five years and older.[27]

The Public Health Service then developed specific targets or objectives relating to these broad goals, which appeared in 1980 in the report *Promoting Health/Preventing Disease: Objectives for the Nation*. These objectives were laid down for fifteen priority areas: high-blood-pressure control, family planning, pregnancy and infant health, immunization, sexually transmitted diseases, toxic agent control, occupational health and safety, accident prevention and injury control, fluoridation and dental health, surveillance and control of infectious diseases, smoking and health, alcohol and other drug misuse, physical fitness and exercise, and control of stress and violent behavior. The Public Health Service had spent a year consulting with five hundred expert individuals and organizations. Also, public comment was invited on draft proposals.

The report was intended to be a sort of manual for use by key figures in the private and public sectors. It would serve as well to help future assessors track the nation's success in prevention. The objectives were intended for well people, and few dealt with secondary prevention (detecting disease conditions at an early stage, such as screening for breast cancer). As a national prevention strategy, the objectives required the federal government to provide leadership and strategic support, but state and local authorities were expected to provide "local roots" for the strategy. The report briefly acknowledged the potential for controversy about the causes of ill health and their remedy. There would be controversy over "the appropriate role of government in fostering personal behavior change," "the philosophy and psychology of throwing responsibility for serious health problems back to the victim," and "the role of business and industrial processes in health and disease."[28]

A "mid-course review" by the Office of Disease Prevention and Health Promotion in 1985 found that just under half of the objectives had been achieved. It called for action to reduce social inequalities in health status. By the later 1980s, some considerable reductions in aggregate death rates from leading causes of death had been achieved. In 1970–87, the age-adjusted mortality from heart disease declined by 33 percent, from cerebrovascular disease by 55 percent, from accidents by 35 percent, and from chronic liver disease and cirrhosis by 40 percent. The result was that the overall death rate declined by 25 percent.

The United States was the first country to develop health goals and targets in a comprehensive national strategy to advance health status. In the late 1980s and 1990s, as we shall see, Australia and the United Kingdom likewise tried to develop systematic approaches to setting and pursuing health goals and targets.[29]

PUBLIC HEALTH RENAISSANCE IN AUSTRALIA

On taking office in 1983, the Hawke federal Labor government preoccupied itself in the health area with implementation of Medicare, the universal, tax-funded health insurance scheme it initiated in February 1984. Medicare differed from Medibank in that a specific levy of 1 percent on taxable income was imposed to help pay for the scheme. Free care in public hospitals was reintroduced, but private health insurance funds could provide insurance for private patients in private or public hospitals. The medical profession had "philosophical" objections to Medicare. However, it did not demonstrate the hostility it had shown to Medibank in the mid-1970s, although some concessions concerning payments of medical benefits for services in hospitals were made following a dispute between some sections of the profession and the New South Wales and federal Labor governments in 1984. The new scheme's basic components were similar to those of Medibank: universal coverage for a large part of the cost of medical services, free public hospital care, and the income tax as the source of funding of the scheme.[30]

While the new federal government was heavily focused on health insurance at first, it later turned its attention to implementation of the HFA strategy in Australia. When WHO adopted HFA by the Year 2000 as a global strategy in 1981, Australia, by endorsing the strategy, committed itself to the articulation of goals and targets to improve the health of the population and remove health inequities. Adoption of the strategy also meant a commitment to reorient the health system away from its traditional focus on treatment of illness and toward promotion and protection of health. While the development of national health policy in the second half of the 1980s accorded with this reorientation, it is important to recognize that resource allocation remained very much in favor of treatment and care, as tables 4.1 and 4.2 show.

As these tables indicate, the percentage of total recurrent health expenditure in Australia spent on community and public health services between 1983 and 1995 remained very small. From a low of 3 percent in 1982–83, it rose to a high of 5 percent in 1991–92 and remained at that level in 1994–95. This may be compared to spending on treatment services—spending on hospital services of well over 40 percent and on medical services of 17 to 18 percent in the same period.

The Background: Health Education in Australia

The companion volume to this book shows how infant mortality, especially from diarrheal and associated conditions, was a massive urban health problem, particularly for the poorer classes, in nineteenth-century Australia, as it was in Britain and the United States. This and other problems of infant rearing in Antipodean conditions gave rise to an indigenous health education literature on infant care. These manuals were often written by doctors but sometimes by nonmedical authors like Mrs. Annie Elliss of Sydney, who published *The Australian Baby* in 1902. The Australian Health Society sponsored publication in Melbourne of Dr. C.D. Hunter's *What Kills Our Babies* in 1878 and Dr. James Jamieson's *Diseases Which Should Be Prevented* in 1882. P.E. Muskett, a Sydney doctor who published works on infant and child health in the 1880s and 1890s, brought out a manual of general health education, *The Illustrated Australian Medical Guide,* in Sydney in 1903.[31]

In the early twentieth century, public health authorities initiated organized infant welfare work, and the state carried out health education. Dr. W.G. Armstrong, the pioneer of such work in Australia, described infant health education in inner Sydney in the early 1900s:

> A daily list of all births . . . is obtained . . . ; within a few days after registration, the home of each child born in a poor neighbourhood is visited by a woman inspector of the municipal council, who interviews the mother, talks to her confidentially on the management of the child . . . and earnestly inculcates cleanliness, leaving, also, at each house a copy of a brief . . . leaflet setting forth the dangers of infantile diarrhoea, and giving instructions on the feeding of infants.[32]

The New South Wales Department of Public Health produced a pamphlet on infant care in 1909 (reprinted in 1911 and 1913) *How to Take Care of Babies during the Summer Months.* Nonofficial manuals like Nurse Edith Aitken's *Australian Mother's Own Book* (Sydney, 1912) continued to appear. Dr. Margaret Harper, a prominent figure in the infant welfare movement and

Table 4.1
Total Recurrent Health Expenditure (Public* and Private‡), Australia, 1982/83–1988/89

	1982–83		1983–84		1984–85		1985–86		1986–87		1987–88		1988–89	
	A$m	%	A$m	%	A$m	%	A$m	%	A$m	%	A$m	%	A$m	%
1) *Institutional*														
(a)Total Hospitals	5,758	46.4	6,253	45.1	6,789	44.7	7,372	42.9	8,483	43.4	9,306	43.1	10,326	42.5
(b) Other	1,323	10.7	1,532	11.1	1,654	11.0	1,849	10.8	2,106	10.8	2,273	10.6	2,487	10.2
2) *Non-InstitutionalServices*														
(a) Medical	2,174	17.5	2,469	17.8	2,685	17.7	3,091	18.0	3,471	17.8	3,887	18.0	4,359	17.9
(b) Dental	560	4.5	660	4.8	725	4.8	879	5.1	996	5.1	1,107	5.1	1,253	5.2
(c) Other Professional	342	2.8	420	3.0	532	3.5	572	3.3	663	3.4	763	3.5	961	4.0
(d) Community Health Services	297	2.4	342	2.5	417	2.8	† 689	4.0	† 725	3.7	† 825	3.8	† 957	3.9
(e) Other	1,238	10.0	1,395	10.0	1,516	10.0	1,921	11.2	2,186	11.2	2,400	11.1	2,766	11.3
3) *Health Promotion and Prevention*	72	0.6	89	0.6	121	0.8	† –	–	† –	–	† –	–	† –	–
4) *Research*	165	1.3	171	1.2	194	1.3	234	1.4	287	1.5	313	1.5	337	1.4
5)*Administration*	485	3.9	534	3.8	538	3.5	565	3.3	611	3.1	695	3.2	856	3.5
Total Recurrent Expenditure	12,414	100.0	13,865	100.0	15,171	100.0	17,172	100.0	19,528	100.0	21,569	100.0	24,302	100.0

*Federal, state and local government
‡Health insurance funds and other private sources
†Includes the old categories of community health services, and health promotion and illness prevention, of which the second category accounted for 22 percent of the combined figure in 1985–86, 26 percent in 1986–87, 27 percent in 1987–88, and 28 percent in 1988–89.

Source: *Information Bulletin 2: Australian Health Expenditure 1982–83 to 1984–85* (Acton: Australian Institute of Health, 1987), 4–6. *Health Expenditure Bulletin 10* (Canberra: Australian Institute of Health and Welfare, 1994), 12–19.

Table 4.2

Total Recurrent Health Expenditure (Public* and Private‡), Australia, 1989/90 and 1991/92–1994/95

	1989–90		1991–92		1992–93		1993–94		1994–95	
	A$m	%	A$m	%	A$m	%	A$m	%	A$m	%
1) *Institutional*										
(a) Total hospitals	11,059	41.4	12,149	38.9	12,464	38.0	12,675	37.1	13,536	37.0
(b) Other	2,720	10.2	3,136	10.04	3,191	9.8	3,252	9.5	3,393	9.3
2) *Non-Institutional Services*										
(a) Medical	4,878	18.3	5,928	19.0	6,422	19.6	6,884	20.2	7,371	20.1
(b) Dental	2,442	9.1	1,652	5.3	1,709	5.2	1,831	5.4	1,943	5.3
(c) Other professional			1,291	4.1	1,397	4.3	1,244	3.6	1,443	3.9
(d) Community and public health†	1,165	4.4	1,555	5.0	1,651	5.0	1,701	5.0	1,823	5.0
(e) Other	4,443	16.6	3,923	12.6	4,312	13.2	4,921	14.4	5,037	13.8
3) *Research*			464	1.5	500	1.5	534	1.6	627	1.7
4) *Administration*			1,125	3.6	1,113	3.4	1,099	3.2	1,418	3.9
Total Recurrent Expenditure	26,707	100.0	31,223	100.0	32,759	100.0	34,141	100.0	36,591	100.0

*Federal, state and local government

‡Nongovernment sector: private health insurance funds, individuals, and spending by workers' compensation and compulsory motor vehicle third-party insurance providers on health services.

†This includes the old categories of community health services, and health promotion and illness prevention.

Source: G.R. Palmer and S.D. Short, *Health Care and Public Policy: An Australian Analysis* (South Melbourne: Macmillan Education Australia, 1994), 14. *Health Expenditure Bulletin 12* (Canberra: Australian Institute of Health and Welfare, 1996), 27–29. *Health Expenditure Bulletin 13* (Canberra: Australian Institute of Health and Welfare, 1997), 14.

early paediatrician, brought out *The Parents' Book* in Sydney in 1926. This had run to nineteen editions by 1945.[33]

The achievements in preventive medicine of Australian military forces during World War I and the important role of war propaganda inspired innovation in health education when peace returned. Dr. Harvey Sutton (principal medical officer with the NSW Education Department and later founding principal of the School of Public Health and Tropical Medicine at Sydney University), Dr. J.S. Purdy (health officer of the Sydney City Council), and Dr. Richard Arthur (eugenicist and later NSW minister for health) founded Sydney's annual "Health Week" in 1921, during which public lectures were supplemented by an exhibition in Sydney Town Hall. The idea soon after inspired similar efforts in Brisbane, Melbourne, Adelaide and Newcastle. Health Week, which continued until 1950, was well supported by the press and, as radio became more popular, by radio stations. In 1939, broadcasts were made over eight Sydney stations.[34]

On the other side of the continent, new approaches to health education were also tried in the interwar years. In the early 1930s, the Western Australia Public Health Department ran a health section at the annual Royal (Agricultural) Show in Perth. By 1939, the correspondence section of the infant health service of the Public Health Department was using radio talks as well as newspaper articles to reach mothers. The Health Education Council in Queensland, with representatives from the Health and Education Departments and various voluntary and other agencies influential in the community, had a regular newspaper column and bought radio time; it also produced a standard reference book on health for schools. It obtained much access to the mass media gratis because of professional contacts. The more conventional media of pamphlets and posters were also exploited. But by the early 1950s, apart from Health Week in New South Wales and the work in Queensland, health education was languishing in Australia.

In 1955, the Federal Health Department organized in cooperation with WHO a national seminar on health education at the Australian National University in Canberra. Each state and territory was invited to send two representatives. Western Australia's representatives then visited Brisbane to learn about the work of the Queensland Health Education Council. They strongly recommended that a similar body be created in their state. In 1956 the council, composed of representatives of the Health and Education Departments, the Parents and Citizens Federation, Country Women's Association, Red Cross Society, Employers' Federation, Trades Hall, the Local Government Association, the Australian Broadcasting Commission, commercial radio and the press, came into being, with a journalist, Jim Carr, as first executive officer. The council's first target area was home accident prevention, but it also worked very successfully to improve public acceptance of polio immunization in the Salk vaccine campaign that began in July 1956. By the close of the 1970s, its staff had expanded from three to thirty and its annual budget from twenty thousand dollars to two hundred thousand.[35]

Health Promotion in Australia

In January 1978, in a time of budgetary constraint and concern about rising health care costs, the federal health minister, Ralph Hunt, announced an inquiry to be headed by Professor Lindsay Davidson, principal of the School of Public Health and Tropical Medicine (SPHTM), into programs on health education, promotion and prevention, especially those "motivating people to take a personal and active role in their own health status."[36] The Davidson inquiry showed that it was well aware of growing WHO interest in health promotion and recent inquiries carried out in the United States (the *Report of the President's Committee on Health Education,* 1973), in Canada (the report to the Canadian minister of health and welfare, Marc Lalonde, entitled *A New Perspective on the Health of Canadians,* 1974), and in Britain (*Prevention and Health: Everybody's Business,* 1976). It also showed itself aware of the limitations of the individualistic, "lifestyle" approach to health promotion, especially its failure to recognize the social determinants of disease. It recommended that national objectives for health promotion be established by the federal government; that a national health promotion center (within which a center for research and a teaching unit would function) be created by the Federal Health Department in association with the SPHTM at the University of Sydney (it was to be almost two decades before a center was funded by the commonwealth at the Department of Public Health and Community Medicine, the University of Sydney); that the commonwealth finance a special projects grants scheme with priority to be given to research (or educational programs) on premature mortality and morbidity from chronic diseases and on mass-media program development; and that total spending on health promotion be doubled each year for three years from the existing meager level of $2.04 million.

Elsewhere, Davidson and colleagues pointed out that the Australian government was currently spending $447 per capita annually on health care but only four dollars per capita on prevention. Reviewing the health education manpower situation, they encountered a dismal scene. Health promotion could not be called an occupation, let alone a profession. Three broad areas of employment existed: health education sections of state and territory health departments; other organizations, like the Family Planning Association, which still did much public education work; and doctors or researchers who had become involved in the educational side of their field of specialization, such as research physicians who also worked in coronary heart disease education.

For health educators as such, career prospects were very poor and salaries commonly low. Training opportunities were equally limited. An associate diploma had been offered at Claremont Teachers College, Western Australia, since 1975 and a diploma and a bachelor of education degree at Sturt College of Advanced Education (CAE), South Australia, since 1974. Degrees or graduate diplomas were to be available from 1979 at Canberra CAE, ACT (bachelor of applied science); Burwood State College, Victoria; Sydney Teachers' College, NSW; Kurringai CAE, NSW (bachelor of arts degree); and Kelvin Grove CAE, Queensland. Hitherto, training had tended to be predominantly in-service or short-course in style. Moreover, the existing and proposed academic courses were intended to produce school or community educators. There was need for master's-level courses to produce graduates with skills in policy development, planning and evaluation, or specialized competence in areas like mass communications. With professional health educators comparatively few in number, Davidson and colleagues saw potential in health promotion being done as part of their wider work by the much more numerous general practitioners, nurses and pharmacists (see table 4.3).

They noted that the Royal Australian College of General Practitioners was training doctors in health promotion under the federally funded Family Medicine Program. They thought that a doctor specializing in health promotion might become a part of group practices or that health educators might be placed in group practices or hospitals and see patients on referral from doctors. They observed that pharmacists, who were traditionally consulted by many people about medical problems, were well placed to carry out health promotion work and that nurses (and physiotherapists and occupational therapists), with more time to spend with patients than doctors had, were also in a prime position to do similar work.

Looking at the health authorities in the different jurisdictions, they identified Queensland (except for the absence of sex education from schools) and

Table 4.3
Estimated Numbers of Health Professionals in NSW, 1978

Health Education Officers	45
Community Educators	140
Health Inspectors	1,050
General Practitioners	4,000
Community Nurses	1,400
Pharmacists	5,400
Total	12,035

Source: L. Davidson, S. Chapman and C. Hull, *Health Promotion in Australia 1978–79* (Canberra: Australian Government Publishing Service, 1979), 49.

the ACT as having the most advanced health education programs. It saw these as demonstrating the following virtues: pursuit of specific behavioral changes rather than changes in broad behavioral complexes; centralized, sustained and coordinated education and promotion programs rather than local and short-lived ones; planned interventions rather than ad hoc responses to public demand; use of the methodologies of epidemiology and social science rather than reactions coming from a "service" orientation; and outcome evaluation of all programs rather than occasional process evaluation. They also recognized that particular programs in other states were following paths of methodological virtue. The contemporary prevention program being mounted in the North Coast region of NSW was a coordinated attempt to encourage health lifestyle change using all local electronic and print media and community health facilities. A professional journalist and advertiser were employed full-time on the media aspects of the program and were particularly concerned with antismoking material. In Victoria, the state Anti-Cancer Council was praised for its educational work within its specialized area, especially its use of epidemiological findings on cancer prevalence and the efficacy of treatments, as well as from research on psychological and sociological factors in prevention, to guide its health education work. It spent $286,000 of $1.6 million income on education in 1978, an unprecedented proportion on education in Australia.

Davidson and colleagues noted that the NHMRC had an ongoing interest in health education and promotion. Two committees were directly involved: the Health Education (Standing) Committee, which advised the Public Health Advisory Committee, a key committee, on health education matters; and the Community Health Promotion (Standing) Committee, formerly the Preventive Medicine in Community and General Practice (Standing) Committee. The renaming of the latter committee indicated a more specific focus on health promotion. The NHMRC had recently made various recommendations concerning health promotion: health and human relationships education in schools; liaison between health, welfare and education departments in health education matters; support for postgraduate degree training in health education; concern about the high incidence of alcohol-related health problems; and postgraduate courses in alcohol studies for medical and other health professionals.[37]

The Davidson inquiry pointed to the ludicrously small expenditure on health promotion, especially when compared to spending on commercial advertising of potentially harmful products like alcoholic beverages. Noting that differences in accounting procedures between state and federal governments, as well as definitional problems about the limits of health promotion, made it impossible to give precise figures, the inquiry estimated that in 1977–78 federal grants to the states under the National Drug Education program totaled $750,000. Direct spending by the Federal Health Department on health and drug education was $254,000, while expenditure under the CHP grants program on health education projects was $1.036 million. These figures may be compared with spending in Australia in 1977 on advertising alcoholic drinks of $14.8 million, on tobacco of $12.5 million, and on analgesic drugs of $2.8 million.[38]

A national health education conference, the first in twenty-three years, was held in Canberra in association with the Davidson inquiry. Representatives of health departments, hospitals, nongovernment organizations, academic medicine, education and sociology from around the country attended. The conference made a number of recommendations, many of which were taken up by the Davidson inquiry: that increasing expenditure on health care be contained by health promotion; that the federal government fund a national health education program, on the grounds of both health advancement and cost containment; that education departments give more priority to health education in schools; that a national health education organization be formed, with a secretariat in Canberra and funding from the Federal Health Department; that a national institute for health promotion be established to carry out research, act as a clearinghouse for information, and advise on research and training matters; that high priority in resource allocation be given to training of health educators; and that existing courses be upgraded to match the best overseas ones.[39]

The only immediate fruit of the 1978 Davidson inquiry was the Fraser government's commitment of five hundred thousand dollars to a national health promotion program. The federal health minister, Ralph Hunt, declared himself at a press conference in May 1979 a convert to individually oriented health promotion: "I have become more and more convinced that continued concentration on traditional curative medicine, with its associated high costs both for the government and the individual, can add little to improving the nation's health status. I believe this can be achieved only by motivating individuals to take a responsible attitude for their own personal health care."[40] Most of the new program's funds were spent on "Help Yourself to Better Health," a media campaign encouraging individuals to change their lifestyle. This was followed by information services and campaigns, plus market research studies. As Nancy Milio, an American health promotion expert familiar with Australian conditions, noted, it amounted to using health promotion as a marketing technique rather than a coordinating of community building—health as "a magic bullet" rather than "a continuous flowering." This approach made no use of the legislative and fiscal strategies discussed by Davidson and colleagues as means to overcome structural constraints on health improvement.[41]

The NHMRC began looking at a national strategy for health promotion. In 1982, the NHMRC's Community Health Promotion and Education Committee committed itself (as one of its three principal tasks for the triennium) to the development of goals for health promotion. These were to be broad ones against which specific projects and research could be viewed by health educators and other health professionals planning coordinated activities. In September 1984, the committee produced *Towards a National Policy on Health Promotion;* the full NHMRC, noting that many countries were now establishing national, measurable goals, endorsed the paper and forwarded it to the Australian Health Ministers' Conference. It recommended that the document also be sent to state and territory health authorities.

The NHMRC defined health promotion in a comprehensive way, moving beyond the limitations of an individualistic approach. It saw health promotion as any combination of education; community development; media and marketing; professional involvement; legislative, fiscal and administrative measures; environmental control; technological change; and social reform. It identified a number of areas in which national goals needed to be set: alcohol abuse, accident prevention, dental health, drug abuse, emotional health, environmental protection, family planning, immunization, nutrition, occupational health, physical fitness, sexually transmitted diseases, smoking, town planning, toxic agent control and vector-borne disease.[42]

The Australian Medical Association Federal Council's Standing Committee on Health Education and Promotion, formed in 1980, produced a report on health education in 1981. The AMA's primary preferred approach was production of literature for doctors and the public on particular issues, such as alcohol-related health problems. While the public relations value of the exercise was clear, the report did show a commitment, if a limited one, to harnessing the medical profession's knowledge and experience to the developing field of health promotion. The stirring of interest at the federal level in the late 1970s and the work of the AMA and the NHMRC a little later did indicate some movement toward emergence of health promotion as a significant concern of major political and professional-interest players in health policy. But as public health doctors Stephen Leeder, of Newcastle University's Faculty of Medicine, and Terry Dwyer and Julian Gold, of the Commonwealth Institute of Health at Sydney University, glumly noted in late 1983, an effective framework was needed: "The field of preventive medicine, and of public health generally, suffers from lack of direction." This was not solely due to a shortage of trained people but "rather to the absence of a framework on which national action can be based." Efforts to reduce the prevalence of hypertension or smoking had to be set in a context of national goals. They pointed out that associated with Canada's national health insurance scheme was a Health Promotion Directorate responsible for strategic planning of health promotion activities. They called for a similar body to be set up in connection with the soon-to-be-introduced Medicare scheme.[43]

The problem was not only a lack of central direction but the limited range of health promotion strategies being employed. A survey of health promotion in NSW found that almost two-thirds of over 4,600 programs in the second half of 1983 aimed for long-term psychological and social well-being, while more than one-third tried to do primary prevention; 92 percent employed educational approaches, using print and audiovisual material. Evaluation was inadequate—54 percent had no idea whether or not they were successful.

In 1984 a report to the NSW minister of health was made on health promotion and education. It viewed health promotion as a balance between encouragement of individual behavior change and creation of supportive environments, with use of multiple strategies from media campaigns to development of government policy. Yet its recommendations focused on specific behavior changes, like lowering smoking prevalence. It looked to mass marketing rather than efforts to influence policy, and it saw individuals as passive consumers rather than citizens involved in shaping the development of services. The recommendations were much influenced by the 1984 South Australian health promotion program, which, a 1985 review said, displayed a strong entrepreneurial approach. However, it also said the $1.64 million spent might have been more effectively deployed. An antismoking media campaign costing $365,000 had achieved nothing, and even a thirty-five-thousand-dollar immunization campaign, which raised the overall rate of immunization, did not do so for disadvantaged groups. Moreover, evaluation was carried out only in terms of marketing, not epidemiological impact. The 1985 review changed the South Australian program. But women's health centers in Adelaide had already for some years been responding to the complexity of health promotion by combining educational approaches with community development strategies and by working at the same time with individuals, small groups and community organizations like trade unions. They thus pursued a range of activities, from providing services for individuals to attempting to influence government policy.

South Australia, led by a committed Labor minister for health, Dr. John Cornwall, introduced in the late 1980s a primary care health policy and a social health strategy that encouraged attempts to apply new public health ideas in various settings. Community and women's health centers grew in number. A "healthy cities" project was developed. Mental health and other health services tried to apply new public health concepts. One of the more ambitious developments was the creation by the Health Commission in 1988 of four experimental health and social welfare councils, which were to promote community participation in decision making, accountability of the health and welfare systems, and community education. They were also to encourage local efforts to prevent health and social problems. A 1991 evaluation said the councils had indeed involved local citizens and achieved some successes—notably a 1992 community consultation and planning process concerning mental health care involving the southern metropolitan area, and the resulting establishment of a mental illness advocacy scheme to represent mentally ill persons. The scheme survived the demise of the councils that followed loss of funding in 1995.[44] John Cornwall himself accurately described the social and political difficulties faced by a new public health approach to health improvement:

> The magic bullet approach . . . is much simpler than a necessarily complex approach based on the more accurate notion that health is the consequences of many and varied public policies interacting with the individual. . . . At a political level the public policy approach lacks support because it produces results in the long term and less visibly than the short-term crisis intervention of heroic medicine. Addressing questions of poverty, education, housing, nutrition and income maintenance to overcome the problem of very low birthweight babies is not possible in a sixty-second television news segment. . . . It also implies a consensus on equity of important health-producing goods and services which we have not yet achieved.[45]

In Victoria, the 1985 Ministerial Review of Community Health Services saw health promotion as dealing with health education of individuals and groups, yet also with strategies (whether legislative, fiscal, organizational or environmental) involving bridges between various state departments, different levels of government, and community organizations. Following the regionalization of health administration, District Health Councils provided structures through which to implement the social view of health promotion, which the review supported. The councils could employ the range of health promotion approaches—educational, community development, and advocacy with community and government bodies—that the review endorsed.

In mid-1986, another ministerial review reported to the health minister, this time directly on health education and promotion in Victoria. Chaired by Dr. Nigel Gray, director of the state Anti-Cancer Council, which had a fine record of specialized health promotion work, the review committee, using the language of HFA by the Year 2000, set up the following goals: first, "equity in health" (reduction of social inequalities in health status); second, "to add life to years" (as full a life as possible, whatever the health state); third, "to add health to life" (reduction of disease and disability); fourth, "to add years to life" (reduction of untimely deaths). Attempts to change individual behavior had to recognize the wider context of that behavior—that is, changing lifestyles involved recognition of the need to change the social, cultural, economic, physical and political environment.

The committee made a number of general recommendations, including one for an increase in funding for health promotion and education from the current 0.16 percent of the health budget to 1 percent by 2000; development of a statewide policy, indicating priorities; a health promotion advisory committee for the health minister, a strong central health promotion unit, and regional teams; formal and informal intersectoral collaboration between such departments as Health, Agriculture and Education and relevant university units; legislation to support policy; specification of goals and measures of effectiveness for services, the focus to be where greater health gains were to be made (thus more on alcohol and tobacco and less on illicit drugs);

and improvement of preservice and in-service training of health promotion professionals. The committee observed that in Victoria health promotion was not well established as a profession and that few people were designated officially as health educators. Moreover, the bodies carrying out the work were working autonomously, and a central clearinghouse for information was needed. Worse, there was little formal evaluation of health education activities.[46]

Western Australia—which, as we have seen, was, like Queensland, a pioneer of organized health education work—continued to be one of the more enterprising states. In the 1970s, health education officers had been appointed in the regional centers of Busselton, Mandurah, Lockridge, South Hedland and Geraldton, and later at Kwinana and Claremont. A 1978 review committee proposed that the Health Department take over the longstanding Health Education Council's work. This transfer took place in 1980.

In the early 1980s the campaign against smoking was stepped up. With the election of a Labor government in 1983, the health minister introduced a bill to prevent promotion of tobacco products and their sale to youth. Antismoking education funding was to be increased. Passed by the Lower House, the bill failed in the conservative Upper House. However, Parliament agreed to higher taxes on tobacco in 1983. The new tax revenue provided two million dollars per annum for the department's Health Education Unit to run a smoking and health project, open a health promotion center in Perth, and appoint eight more regional health education officers. The new funds were a considerable advance on the twenty thousand dollars a year for health promotion hitherto provided by the Health Department, although by 1989–90 the new special funding had been diverted to consolidated revenue. Befitting its new affluence, health promotion's standing within the department was upgraded in 1984 when the Health Promotion and Education Division was established. In 1986, following some years of compiling a database on the health status of Western Australians, the health authorities published *Our State of Health*. This led to a prioritizing of health promotion work, as a result of which regional health education officers were required to spend 80 percent of their time on five priority areas: tobacco, alcohol, nutrition, Aboriginal health, and control of infectious disease. So active had the state become in health promotion by the later 1980s that the federal health minister, Neal Blewett, could say, "WA leads the Commonwealth in health preventive campaigns. I am tremendously impressed by what the Government is doing here."[47]

We noted above that government-sponsored legislation to prevent tobacco advertising was defeated in the Western Australian parliament in 1983. The year before, a private member's bill to ban such advertising had also been defeated. Both had foundered because of the concerns of the powerful sports and arts lobbies. Sports and the arts received considerable financial support from the tobacco industry, which in return received thereby much advertising exposure. A creative solution to this problem was devised jointly in Victoria by Dr. Nigel Gray, David White (the health minister), and his adviser, Peter Warland. The solution was to prevent advertising and at the same time levy a new tobacco tax to fund sports and arts activities. It was clear from market research that the community would accept the new tax and the ban on advertising if revenue from the tax was used in this way.

The Victorian Tobacco Act of 1987 phased out advertising and established the Victorian Health Promotion Foundation (VicHealth). It disposed of twenty-eight million dollars a year from the wholesale tax on tobacco products. This may be compared with an annual health budget in Victoria of $3.2 billion. The foundation over the next five years encouraged a range of health promotion strategies from integrated campaigns and social marketing to community organization and health education. It provided funding for sports and arts activities to replace tobacco industry sponsorship. Within the first two years sport in Victoria became almost totally free of tobacco industry involvement. The foundation allocated 20 percent of the budget each year to the research program, which involved grants for large biomedical, behavioral and public health research projects, grants for smaller public health projects, and public health overseas fellowships. In five years, the program spent about $35.6 million on about 150 research grants. Particular concern was paid to socially disadvantaged groups—Aborigines, adolescents, the young unemployed, recent immigrants, disabled persons, women and the aged.[48]

Foundation SA, the South Australian Health Promotion Foundation, came into being in mid-1988 to provide alternative sponsorship for sports and the arts to that offered by the tobacco companies. Initially disposing of six million dollars a year from state tobacco licensing fees, it had funds totaling nine million dollars a year by 1993–94. In its first two years, with larger sports and arts organizations not eager to carry messages about health in return for funding, and with some politicians and some parts of the media hostile, the foundation had a rough passage. But by the early 1990s it had become an accepted feature of the state's health scene. In campaigns it cooperated with major voluntary health bodies like the National Heart Foundation, as well as the South Australian Health Commission. At first unwilling to fund local health promotion initiatives, it came to see that these were unlikely to develop without external support and in any case would reinforce its statewide media campaigns. So the community grants program was developed to work alongside the major campaigns. While partly inspired by the Victorian Foundation, it emerged as something somewhat different. This was because it was born of legislation passed after a long, often hostile parliamentary debate in the form of a Sports Promotion, Cultural and Health Advancement Trust and partly because the legislation did not divide expenditure between activities. After establishment, the foundation decided to give priority to spending on tobacco sponsorship replacement, because that had been the impetus behind the act, apportioning 60 percent of funds to sports and recreation sponsorships, 20 percent to cultural sponsorships and 20 percent to health promotion. Health promotion bodies, not unnaturally, continued to be unhappy with this division of funds. Having selected five preferred health areas (smoking, alcohol, nutrition, injury prevention and blood pressure), the foundation carried out media campaigns. These were organized by its own sponsorship officers rather than by giving funds to health agencies (as was done in Victoria and Western Australia), in order to link sponsorships with media campaigns. By the early 1990s, the foundation was delivering four to five major public awareness campaigns each year as well as funding local activities all over South Australia. Further, it administered three hundred sports and arts sponsorships each year while at the same time supporting most health agencies' yearly awareness campaigns.[49]

The Australian Capital Territory also set up a Health Promotion Fund. Unlike those in the states, it was not autonomous, being part of the Territory Health Department. It had similar objectives, however: to support health promotion programs, especially by nongovernment bodies; to replace tobacco industry sponsorship of sporting and cultural activities; to sponsor activities where they delivered health promotion messages; and to promote social, behavioral and market research supportive of these aims. By the early 1990s it was receiving just under a million dollars a year from the wholesale tobacco tax revenue.[50]

In Western Australia, the Tobacco Control Act of 1990 had two primary aims: to phase out tobacco industry sponsorship and advertising and to establish Healthway, a Health Promotion Foundation, which began to operate in February 1991. The foundation used at least 30 percent of its about eleven million dollars per annum income in sponsorship of sporting bodies and 15 percent sponsoring arts organizations. A range of programs was developed—health promotion projects, health promotion research, sports and arts sponsorship, racing sponsorship, and tobacco company sponsorship replacement. Healthway reinforced an already well-established health-promotion presence in the western state. Thus, the Health Department's health promotion services branch had been involved in a range of programs for some years, and in particular had run large-scale "Quit" (smoking) campaigns since 1984. Western Australian universities were producing a stream of professionals with skills in health promotion planning, evaluation and research. Healthway provided funding for the Health Promotion Development and Evaluation Program (HPDEP) of the University of Western Australia, which trained health agency personnel in marketing, sponsorship, program planning and evaluation. HPDEP also carried out evaluations of health projects funded by Healthway as well as of the work of Healthway itself, thereby building accountability and feedback into Healthway's operation.[51]

On taking office in 1983, the Hawke federal Labor government was, as mentioned earlier, much preoccupied in the health area with the implementation of Medicare. Medicare was an important part of the "social wage," under the Labor Party's February 1983 Accord with the Australian Council of Trade Unions. The accord was central to Labor's income and prices policies, which aimed at promoting economic growth in an era characterized by high inflation and high unemployment.[52] But Labor did initiate new policy in the public health area. In early 1985, Dr. Neal Blewett, the federal health minister, established the Better Health Commission (BHC), under the chairmanship of Associate Professor Derek Llewellyn-Jones of the Obstetrics and Gynaecology Department, Sydney University. The BHC was Australia's response to its WHO obligations under the Health for All by the Year 2000 policy. It was a historic turning point in health policy, as Dr. Blewett recognized: it "represents the first concerted national effort to change the basic direction of health policy in this country. For far too long, the emphasis on health care in Australia has been on illness treatment rather than prevention. Not enough attention has been paid to the encouragement of a healthy environment and lifestyle."[53] On another occasion, Blewett wrote, "But governments have a . . . far more important role to play than simply underwriting the health insurance arrangements. Governments must promote better health and influence individuals and families to make behavioural or lifestyle choices to improve their health."[54]

With a budget of only $250,000 and a life of one year, the BHC did not look initially like a major policy initiative. Some observers saw it as a cosmetic measure. Some within government circles saw it as a way by which Blewett could overcome any negative reaction to his recent dispute with the medical profession in New South Wales over Medicare. One member of the BHC, Stephen Leeder, then professor of community medicine at the University of Sydney, has recalled how the idea of "better health" was derided by people in health circles. The appointment of commissioners from the media, sport and trade unions (as well as health administration and academic medicine) was seen as "lunacy writ large."[55] But the BHC received an extension of life and one-third of the $1.5 million allocated for health promotion. Derek Llewellyn-Jones was not satisfied with the five hundred written submissions the BHC received, so the commission visited all state and territory capital cities, plus Alice Springs in the Northern Territory and Townsville in Queensland, taking oral evidence.

A three-volume final report was tabled in federal Parliament in late 1986. The BHC said that health had not improved as much as it might have, for various reasons: there was no national focus on prevention; there were no national goals or strategies to achieve those goals; state and territory funding of prevention was small and erratic, and research into prevention was inadequate and fragmented; medical students were not being trained in health promotion; and the use of the media was too limited and sharing of information was constrained. It proposed national goals and associated targets in three areas—cardiovascular disease, nutrition and injury. They were chosen because they were significant health problems but also because different approaches were needed in each area and could thus be demonstrated. Cardiovascular disease showed how risk factor modification might reduce it. Nutrition was both a social and individual phenomenon, having multiple health outcomes; and injury was an example of a health problem the solution of which required action outside the health sector as such.

The BHC urged creation of a national health promotion body to oversee pursuit of its proposals and to be funded from several sources—a 1 percent increase in tobacco and alcohol excise, 1 percent of the Medicare taxation levy, general revenue appropriations, and tax deductible donations. Among its national strategies for better health, the only identifiably new public health proposal was that for a national community development fund to assist local communities, especially disadvantaged groups, in advocacy and participation projects. Most of the rest were essentially lifestyle education strategies, like school health education.

The BHC also proposed some important public health infrastructure initiatives: establishment within a university of a national, multidisciplinary, postgraduate "center of excellence" for public health training and research; creation of a national center for health statistics; and that all prevention projects funded by federal and state governments be required to include evaluation criteria. The commission noted that it had not proposed action in the very important health areas of drug abuse, HIV/AIDS or occupational health because the federal government had already set up national strategies for each: the National Campaign Against Drug Abuse, for which twenty million dollars had been provided by the commonwealth in 1985–86; the National AIDS Strategy, for which the commonwealth had provided $8.6 million in the same year; and the National Occupational Health and Safety Commission, which in December 1985 had become a statutory body nationally responsible for occupational health.[56]

The BHC report was endorsed by the Australian Health Ministers' Conference in 1986. In early 1987 it created, to function under the auspices of the Australian Health Ministers' Advisory Council, the Health Targets and Implementation (Health for All) Committee (HTIC), chaired by Stephen Leeder. The HTIC was to devise strategies to attain the goals and targets established by the BHC but also to add goals and targets in the areas of the health of older people and of cancer. The committee did not deal with women's health or Aboriginal and Torres Strait Islander people's health, because they were being dealt with in separate policies. The committee's report, *Health for All Australians*, observed that two basic principles informed its work—improving the health status of the whole population and reducing the inequalities in health status among social groups. It drew attention to recent public health infrastructure initiatives taken by the Hawke federal government: establishment of the Australian Institute of Health (later the Australian Institute of Health and Welfare) for development of better national health statistics; creation of the Health Advancement Division in the Commonwealth Department of Community Services and Health for development of health promotion strategies; and various public health education and research initiatives. I will look at the development of public health infrastructure later in the chapter.

The HTIC drew up Australia's first set of national health goals and targets, and these reflected overseas practices, especially those of the United States, in setting national goals and targets. The report identified twenty-eight goals and sixty-five targets in three major areas—population groups, major causes of illness and death, and risk factors. It made wide use of new public health terminology, but the focus was very heavily on prevention. It used an epidemiological, goal-oriented approach in its health advancement strategy and set targets in various illness categories. Its national priorities for the proposed National Program for Better Health, to commence in 1988, were determined by concern for the seriousness of the problem, lack of current action and the feasibility of effective action. The priorities were control of high blood pressure, improved nutrition, injury prevention, the health of older people; the primary prevention of lung and skin cancer; and the secondary prevention of breast and cervical cancer. The main barriers to better health were identified as: orientation of the health system to treatment, complacency on the part of bureaucrats and politicians about prevention; compared with attitudes to acute care; financial constraints; the impact of federalism on coordination of health administration; lack of clarity about the role of intersectoral action in health promotion; and the effect of poverty on capacity to improve health. Structural changes needed to remove these barriers were prevention, emphasis on health promotion and reduction of health inequalities between social groups in all health systems; improved training of health professionals in prevention and promotion; encouragement of community involvement in decision making about health; financial incentives for general practitioners to undertake promotion and prevention work; and federal-state financial arrangements that would better support promotion and prevention.[57]

Endorsement of the report by the Australian health ministers in 1988 was the first occasion on which high-level, political approval was given to a national plan to use health promotion to advance health status. The ministers pledged forty-one million dollars, half coming from the commonwealth and half from the states and territories, to be spent over three years on a National Better Health Program (NBHP). This would "spearhead Australia's drive toward health promotion with special emphasis on the development of national strategies in priority areas not being addressed elsewhere on a national basis."[58] When the NBHP was evaluated in 1992–93, it was found that the program had had considerable impact on health promotion infrastructure—so much so that without it some states would have still lacked health promotion services. It was also found that real progress had been made in the five priority areas: injury prevention, health of older people, primary prevention of lung and skin cancer and secondary prevention of breast and cervical cancer, prevention of high blood pressure, and nutrition. The five areas were at different stages of development, as action in each area under the NBHP recognized. In nutrition, the focus was on developing healthy public policy, where in injury prevention action took place at an earlier developmental stage, with the focus on collection of data, because reliable information as the basis for preventive programs was lacking. The comparatively modest NBHP could not in itself produce the organizational change, change in intersectoral relationships, or modifications in individual and community knowledge and behaviors necessary to fulfil the national health goals and targets. However, it brought home the potential in an approach that established measurable outcomes, created priorities and provided leadership at the national level.[59]

The NBHP and the National Health Promotion program were replaced in 1992 by the National Health Advancement Program. The sum of $6.1 million was provided to refine national goals and targets, build health impact assessment into national policy for ecologically sustainable development, create a national food and nutrition policy, and develop an injury prevention strategy. In the same year, the Federal Health Department asked Don Nutbeam, professor of public health (health promotion) at the University of Sydney, and colleagues to identify goals and targets for 2000. They were specifically instructed to include a social view of health in their proposals. They thus were able not only to identify factors determining social inequalities in health but to set up goals and targets to deal with them.

They proposed goals and targets across four areas—morbidity and mortality, healthy lifestyles and risk factors, health literacy, and healthy environments. The first two built on the earlier set of goals and targets, but the last two represented a move toward a new public health approach. As one commentator noted, it was "a tremendous step forward in encouraging people to consider issues such as transport and housing, and not just doctors and hospitals, when they think about health."[60] In February 1993, the Australian Health Ministers' Advisory Council (AHMAC) issued its "Sunshine Statement." This document called upon the health system to be considerably more oriented to health outcomes, and it supported the setting of goals and targets based on the framework proposed by Nutbeam and his colleagues.

The Nutbeam review enjoyed mixed fortunes. It acted as a catalyst for incorporation of a commitment to develop national goals and targets into the Medicare Agreements between commonwealth and states/territories in 1993. A report followed—*Better Health Outcomes for Australians* (1994)—on the process of developing goals and targets in the four national priority areas of cardiovascular health, cancer control, injury prevention, and mental health (a fifth, diabetes, was added soon after). The 1994 report pointed out that cardiovascular disease was the leading cause of death and that cancer was the second most common cause, while injury (including suicide and road trauma) was the main cause of death of males and females aged one to forty-four years; further, at least 20 percent of adults and 10 to 15 percent of young people had mental health problems at any given time. However, the report failed to address adequately the issue of the social, economic and environmental determinants of health, which had featured so prominently in the review by Nutbeam and colleagues. Healthy environments went into the "too-hard basket." The report recognized they were "a vital component" of efforts to promote greater equity in health, but it went on to admit that the issue of healthy environments was not addressed in its goals and targets process, and that some other way of ensuring that it was addressed would have to be found.[61]

In 1993, a distinguished epidemiologist and leading figure in Australian public health, Tony McMichael, ruminated in print about the achievements of the new public health in Australia over the previous decade. Mortality from heart disease, stroke and chronic respiratory diseases had markedly declined. But he doubted whether socioeconomic gradients in health had been reduced, and in particular that Aboriginal health had improved. He cautioned that in the domain of real-world population health change was readily observed, but causation could be inferred only with great difficulty. Goals and visions were legitimate as the inspirational part of public health, but cities did not become healthy simply by "ideologically fortified declaration." A senior public health person was heard to ask a plenary speaker at the 1993 Public Health Association conference whether it was really known if national health promotion strategies worked.[62] I will look further at the question of the effectiveness of health promotion programs later in the chapter.

PUBLIC HEALTH EDUCATION, RESEARCH AND PROFESSIONALIZATION

I noted in *The People's Health*, volume 1 the emergence in Australia in the late nineteenth and early twentieth century of a cadre of professionally qualified public health doctors, specialists in public health with postgraduate qualifications. This development may be seen as the first stage in the history of public health professionalization in this country. The second stage was marked by the opening of the national School of Public Health and Tropical Medicine (SPHTM) at the University of Sydney in 1930. For almost sixty years thereafter, a steady stream of doctors from across the country graduated with diplomas in public health or tropical medicine. From 1978, the new degree of "master of public health" could be taken in public health, tropical medicine or occupational health. Unlike the graduates of 1933–77, candidates were not necessarily medical. In any case, the school had always run nondiploma courses for a range of people from various occupations—

engineers, health inspectors, food technologists, occupational health nurses and armed services personnel; and also for lay persons, especially Christian missionaries going to work in the Pacific or in remote regions of Australia. The staff of the school had carried out both laboratory and field research in locations in Australia and overseas. Work was done in entomology, cell biology, parasitology, toxicology, nutrition, bacteriology, medical anthropology, epidemiology and preventive, tropical and industrial medicine.[63] Moreover, undergraduates in medicine, architecture, education and engineering were taught at the school. The third stage in the history of professionalization of public health developed in the 1980s against a background of uncertainty about the future of the school at Sydney University.

A committee to review the school had been set up by the federal health minister, Dr. Doug Everingham, in 1973. It recommended in 1975 that the school rename itself the Australian Institute of Health, forge appropriate links with other tertiary education and research institutions, and develop, as a matter of priority, three areas of research—health services, health education and preventive medicine, and health surveillance. But this ambitious program was not pursued. The school's academic and research capacity over the next ten years suffered from the fact that it was part of the Federal Health Department, the issue of transfer to the University of Sydney remaining unresolved. In that time, funding for research in clinical and basic sciences through the NHMRC was much improved by the Fraser government. Yet national research support for public health and epidemiology was not comparably improved. By the time of the Hawke government, public health research was nevertheless flowering in some centers outside Sydney—in Perth in the NHMRC Research Unit in Epidemiology and Preventive Medicine under Bruce Armstrong, in the University of Newcastle Medical School, and in the Human Nutrition Division of CSIRO under Basil Hetzel. The Commonwealth Institute of Health (CIH) itself was not underperforming; it had attracted research funding of $4.3 million (besides maintenance funding).

A pioneering health economist, Dr. John Deeble, had become an adviser to Minister Blewett on the implementation of Medicare. He had already established a small Health Economics Research Unit at the Australian National University (ANU) in 1977 and was keen to expand its work especially in the health statistics area. The Federal Health Department was interested in his heading a Bureau of Health Economics within the department, but he preferred an academic setting. Blewett suggested combining Deeble's unit and the CIH, with the Sydney branch of this new Australian Institute of Health continuing to train public health personnel while research, especially in health economics and other social sciences, would be located in Deeble's branch at the ANU in Canberra. During the 1984 federal election campaign, Prime Minister Hawke made an omnibus promise to central North Queensland electors to develop research in tropical health at James Cook University in Townsville in tropical Queensland, a promise some facetious observers saw as driven by a "scientific" rationale that would require an Institute of Antarctic Medicine to be located in Australia's southernmost capital, Hobart. Universities in other parts of the country clamored for support for new facilities. The idea developed among the federal minister's advisers to call in an external independent expert to review national public health and tropical health research and educational requirements—that is, to provide what Blewett was later to call a "conceptual framework," after which the federal government could settle administrative and financial arrangements.

Dr. Kerr White, consultant in public health to the Rockefeller Foundation and former deputy director of health sciences of the foundation, was known to such senior members of the Federal Health Department as Dr. Ron Wells. Kerr White held strong views on the need to heal what he saw as the schism between medicine and public health in the United States, which had developed in the early twentieth century when population health and the science of epidemiology had become institutionalized in separate schools of public health. He was keen to bring public health and epidemiology back into medical schools. However, not all in the United States agreed with him. Leading American public health figures like Dr. Milton Terris feared that medicine's appropriation of epidemiology (as clinical epidemiology) would shift the focus onto clinical concerns and away from population-level social and economic determinants of health.

Kerr White had had some experience of Australia, as he had been here in 1984 at the invitation of the South Australian government to investigate the functioning of the South Australian Health Promotion Unit. The Rockefeller Foundation itself had provided substantial funding for the Asian and Pacific Centre for Clinical Epidemiology at the University of Newcastle, which was connected with the Department of Community Medicine, headed from its inception by Professor Stephen Leeder, who was soon to become professor of community medicine at Sydney University's Westmead Hospital Clinical School and later dean of the Faculty of Medicine at Sydney. Stephen Leeder had recommended Kerr White to Bernie McKay, head of the Federal Health Department.

Many staff at the SPHTM (it had now reverted to its old name) had opposed incorporation into Deeble's Australian Institute of Health and the possibility of their transfer to Canberra. The school's staff was suspicious of the Kerr White review, as were others in public health. Some viewed the exercise as essentially an excuse to dismantle the SPHTM. Leading public health figure, Ian Webster, professor of community medicine at the University of New South Wales, expressed publicly his disquiet about Kerr White's review. He pointed to the history of the Rockefeller Foundation's involvement in community medicine, with its emphasis on promotion of centers of excellence for education and research, from which public health benefits were to trickle down to a passive community; although Rockefeller had begun to change to "a growth from below" approach involving the community, Kerr

White's approach to reform of public health research and education in Australia was still elitist.[64]

Kerr White's independent review (also known as "Australia's Bicentennial Health Initiative"—the bicentenary of British colonization of Australia was to be celebrated in 1988) was presented to Health Minister Blewett on 10 January 1986. It was publicly released on 29 January. The conceptual basis of the review lay in two assertions—"population-based" thinking had to permeate the health sciences and services, and epidemiology had to permeate the training of clinicians in medical schools so they might reclaim a "population-based" perspective that had been too long exiled in schools of public health. Various concrete recommendations were made: creation of an Australian Academy of Health (similar to the Institute of Medicine in the United States) to provide "timely consideration" of national health problems (a budget of $1.5 million a year); the Australian Institute of Health strengthened to provide policy analysis for the federal minister (a budget of half a million dollars a year); a new National Centre for Health Statistics to supply reliable national statistics (so underpinning policy analysis and development, with a budget of two million a year); and a new National Centre for Technology and Health Services Assessment to develop methods to assess health outcomes from individual and collective interventions ($1.5 million annually).

In addition, since most submissions and interviewees, as well as the consensus of a seminar convened in Sydney, supported the view that the SPHTM had "outlived its usefulness," all funds going to the SPHTM should be redirected to new institutional and organizational initiatives; a new National Centre for Epidemiology and Population Health should be set up at the Australian National University, with an epidemiologist having a laboratory or clinical background as director and with research and graduate training in public health, especially epidemiology, as its function (two million dollars annually for six years); at least four million a year should be provided for academic staff appointments initially at Adelaide University, Sydney University's Westmead Hospital Community Medicine Department, and at Newcastle University; at least a million dollars annually should be set aside for salaries for departments in institutions other than the aforenamed universities, which offered undergraduate and postgraduate public health courses; about two million dollars a year should go for fifty scholarships for training in public health disciplines, to be administered by the proposed Health Development Committee of the NHMRC

The Medical Research Committee of the NHMRC, the recommendations continued, should become the Health Research Committee, with at least four of its seventeen members and at least two of its eight medical researchers to be from population-based disciplines like epidemiology or sociology, and at least 15 to 33 percent of research funds to be for population-based projects; funding of NHMRC research grants scheme should be immediately increased to seventy million dollars a year; a Health Development Committee should be created, with a majority of members from public health disciplines and with a mandate to finance problem-oriented, developmental projects out of funding of fifteen million dollars a year; the Queensland Health Department should establish an Epidemiological Surveillance Unit in Townsville; the Queensland Institute of Medical Research should become the Queensland Institute of Health Research with expanded block-grant support and possibly transfer of appropriate staff from the SPHTM; a unit of the institute should be located at the Australian Institute of Marine Sciences, Townsville, to carry out marine-based disease research, and the School of Tropical Veterinary Sciences at James Cook University, Townsville, should be assisted to strengthen immunology and epidemiology; scholarships should be provided for clinicians and nonphysicians to attend MBA courses, including a new health services module, at the Australian Graduate School of Management of the University of New South Wales so that a cadre of highly skilled health services managers might be trained (Westmead Hospital's Department of Community Medicine or the proposed Centre for Epidemiology and Population Health at ANU might provide staff for the health services module); finally, as a bicentennial health objective, alcohol-related traffic accidents and deaths should be reduced by 30 percent, with a million dollars provided for this work.[65]

With Kerr White's authority and strong support within the Federal Health Department from the secretary, Bernie Mackay, and others like Blewett's advisers, in favor of closure of the SPHTM, a number of major new initiatives were taken. Blewett, who was from South Australia—where, as we have seen, the community health-social health perspective was particularly strong—was already well disposed to public health development. Moreover, as a member of the center-left faction of the Labor Party, he enjoyed the support of Prime Minister Hawke at this time. In 1987, a Public Health Research and Development Committee (PHRDC) (to parallel the long-established Medical Research Committee) was created within the NHMRC in order to corral funding for public health research projects and postgraduate training. The MRC already funded clinical and laboratory research in medicine. Sidney Sax and John Deeble lobbied strongly Bernie Mackay and the minister to have the PHRDC established. This was a considerable advance for public health in national research support. But it is worth noting that PHRDC funds were only a very small proportion of what went to the MRC—in 1990 a budget of $3.8 million, compared with seventy-nine million.[66]

In 1987, the SPHTM closed, and its public health functions and public health staff went to the University of Sydney. The staff formed the Department of Public Health of the Faculty of Medicine. The Australian Institute of Health, which was originally a small bureau in the Federal Health Department launched in 1984, became in 1987 a statutory authority under the community services and health minister's portfolio. Its mission was to provide a better national health database through the collection and analysis of health statistics. It was by the close of the 1980s developing a national death index, a national cancer statistics clearinghouse, and a national nosology reference center, as well as compiling national Aboriginal health statistics. It took over the work of the National Committee on Health and Vital Statistics, financed (together with the states) the National Injury Surveillance and Prevention project, funded the National Perinatal Statistics Unit at Sydney University (now at the University of New South Wales) and the Dental Statistics and Research Unit at Adelaide University, and acted as the secretariat for the National Health Technology Advisory Panel, the function of which was to coordinate evaluation of new technologies in health. The National Centre for Epidemiology and Population Health (NCEPH) was set up at ANU as part of the Public Health Education and Research Program (PHERP). ANU had earlier been keen to obtain an undergraduate medical school (in addition to the long-established John Curtin School of Medical Research), but this had gone instead to Newcastle University. When set up, NCEPH was under the temporary directorship of the eminent demographer Professor Jack Caldwell. The permanent headship was filled by Professor Bob Douglas, a medically qualified epidemiologist from Adelaide. (More recently, Canberra has become host to one of Sydney University Medical School's clinical schools, which is attached to Canberra Hospital.)

NCEPH offered the master of public health (MPH) degree, while Sydney, Adelaide and Monash Universities expanded existing MPH programs under PHERP. The University of Western Australia introduced an MPH course, while Queensland University in association with the Queensland Institute of Medical Research provided master's and diploma-level courses in tropical health and assumed national responsibility for research and education in tropical health. James Cook University of North Queensland brought into being a Tropical Health Surveillance Unit. Newcastle University increased its postgraduate training capacity in clinical epidemiology and biostatistics. All these new developments were also funded under PHERP. The federal government promised twenty-six million dollars for 1986–88, a maximum of $41.5 million over seven years, for the PHERP training initiatives.[67] The MPH program at Sydney University, which closed with the closing of the SPHTM, rose phoenixlike under PHERP. By the early 1990s it was the largest public health training program in Australia. PHERP funding was distributed as shown in table 4.4.

It is noteworthy that most of these new educational facilities were developed within faculties of medicine, reinforcing medicine's control of public health, even though Kerr White himself had looked to multidisciplinarity in public health research, and though the historical record of support for public health from medical faculties had left much to be desired. Kerr White had proposed that three centers—Westmead, Newcastle and Adelaide—be

Table 4.4
Allocation of Public Health Education and Research Program Funding

Institution	Base Allocation A$	1990–91 Allocation A$
Australian National University	1,500,000	1,866,913
University of Sydney	1,850,000	2,302,529
University of Newcastle	210,000	261,368
University of Queensland	984,000	1,224,695
Queensland Institute of Medical Research	500,000	622,304
James Cook University	400,000	497,844
University of Adelaide	2000,000	248,922
University of Western Australia	200,000	248,922

Source: G.C. Salmond, ***Independent Review of the Public Health Education and Research Program in Australia: Report to Hon. Brian Howe M.P., Minister for Health, Housing and Community Services*** (Canberra: Commonwealth Department of Health, Housing and Community Services, 1992), 43.

supported to develop public health education. But state health departments and other universities lobbied hard, and a much more decentralized arrangement of public health education eventuated. The growth of educational facilities was marked. Where only two postgraduate courses in public health were available when Kerr White carried out his review in 1986, four years on more than twenty were in operation. By 1993, universities receiving the special education funds had enrolled in their public health courses more than eight hundred students. Universities not receiving the special federal largesse also offered courses, so that a total of three thousand students were enrolled in such courses in any given year. Indeed, in 1992–93, twenty-one institutions ran twenty-nine master's of public health or related courses. There was a good deal of relief in public health teaching circles when in the budget of August 1993 the federal Labor government provided nine million dollars a year on an ongoing basis for public health education, to be offered to consortia of institutions in the different states so as to avoid duplication of courses and other waste of resources.[68]

In 1990, the Public Health Association of Australia produced a report on the public health workforce describing three major groups. Members of the first group were specialists working on the frontier of public health in research, teaching and consulting; there was a need for more specialists in biostatistics, environmental health, epidemiology, health economics, health promotion and toxicology. Those in the second group were practitioners with a generalist postgraduate qualification, often an MPH. They usually acted as service providers for the community; there was an increasing demand for training courses for this group. Members of the third group were general health and associated workers—about three hundred thousand in number—who also carried out public health work, sometimes or regularly.

The PHRDC of the NHMRC provided something like a national mechanism for the development of public health research. But such a mechanism was clearly lacking for development of the public health workforce. In 1992, George Salmond, sometime New Zealand director-general of health, carried out a review of PHERP for the federal Labor minister for health, housing and community services, Brian Howe. Having found that PHERP had met its general objectives, Salmond proposed some changes. He recommended that in each state or territory public health networks be created, using PHERP funds to do so; that funding through PHERP be distributed now on a competitive basis; and that universities, state health departments, hospitals and industry cultivate more cooperative relationships. As we have noted, the federal government in 1993 indicated that it would continue to support the PHERP program, funding up to eight centers plus a national center for international and tropical health.[69]

The strengths of PHERP in 1987–92 had been that it had underpinned the evolution of a small number of larger, multidisciplinary groups that, while not large by the standards of American schools of public health, offered wider coverage than would otherwise have been possible of public health disciplines, and that it had also locked universities into support of public health education. The weaknesses were that with a specific date for termination, a good deal of unnecessary uncertainty was created about continuation of the program; that being narrowly focused on education, especially the MPH, PHERP unwittingly limited growth of research programs and careers, which loss was not compensated by the PHRDC funding program. In the period 1993–99, competitive funding encouraged the growth in the number of centers participating, so that the comparatively small overall funding was spread even more thinly across sixteen centers. This probably had the effect of weakening research capacity in the large centers. Multi-institutional consortia, following Salmond's proposals, developed in Sydney, Melbourne, Brisbane, Adelaide and Perth. National tertiary education funding policies (especially since the 1996 advent of the Thatcherite Howard coalition government) which have seen reduction of federal funding and pushed competition between universities, have worked against collaboration in order to avoid duplication of teaching. Moreover, the thinner spread of funding has tended to produce duplication, particularly in core disciplines like epidemiology. It is also possible that these forced "marriages" at state level have inhibited the emergence of national consortia for education and research made feasible by Web-based information technology. On the other hand, students have benefited from more flexible learning arrangements and movement between universities, developments that would have been less likely to have taken place without PHERP.

Although PHERP was able to promote considerably the growth of a specialized public health workforce—producing by the late 1990s at least thirty doctorates and several hundred masters or diplomas of public health—it failed to encourage introduction of public health into undergraduate or postgraduate training of allied health professionals, like doctors or nurses. Further, focusing on education, PHERP failed to nurture research capacity. No adequate career structure for public health researchers was developed. The recent organizational changes to the NHMRC, and in particular the disappearance of the PHRDC when the MRC and the PHRDC were merged for the triennium of 1997–2000 into a single Research (Public Health and Medical) Committee, raised questions about the future of public health research support. They have a potential to negate whatever gains in research capacity have been made.[70]

The PHRDC had, of course, grown out of Kerr White's review of 1986. Established as a new principal committee of the NHMRC, equal in status to the MRC, the PHRDC had as its first chairman veteran public health figure, Dr. Sidney Sax. Its second chairman, Professor Ken Donald from the University of Queensland Medical School, was concerned that proposals to reorganize the NHMRC after the Bienenstock review of 1993 would disadvantage public health and public health research support. His defense of the PHRDC and separate funding for public health research was to no avail. In his view, the Public Health Association failed to support his defense of the PHRDC either out of a failure to understand the issues or out of basic acceptance of the organizational change. Initially, the PHRDC was to support research with regard to national priority areas that it adopted from the BHC—nutrition, and prevention of cardiovascular disease, injury, cancer and mental health. It stimulated interest in the priority areas by holding a series of workshops at which consumers, health administrators and researchers assembled. In 1991, it decided to abandon the focus on priority areas, but Aboriginal health continued to be a research priority.

In 1989–94, PHRDC funds rose from $2.61 to $6.594 million, with the bulk spent on research (70 percent in 1994) and most of the rest on fellowships and scholarships (24 percent in 1994). In this period, fourteen development program grants for three to five years at the rate of a hundred to two hundred thousand dollars a year were approved. Subjects of research were mostly related directly to priority areas—for example, diet and exercise in heart disease prevention; diabetes, obesity and cardiovascular disease in Aborigines and Torres Strait Islanders; and sunscreen and other interventions to prevent skin cancer. Some related indirectly—for example, women's health programs and workplace health promotion. In the order of 124 project grants (and ninety seeding grants) were approved. These went to universities, research institutes, state health agencies, hospitals, Aboriginal health services and cooperatives. The MRC provided about ten million dollars a year of additional funding for public health research.[71]

PHERP was supposed to promote not only production of well trained public health workers but to help encourage development of public health occupational opportunities and links between practitioners and academic institutions. New South Wales led the way in fulfilling these wider objectives in relation to the public health workforce. The Salmond review of PHERP in 1992 noted "a spectacular improvement" in public health activity in the previous few years; the NSW Health Department had established a network of public health units based on the health system's area health boards, which in turn were supported from the center by a strong public health core unit. To help staff the network the department ran "an excellent" training program for public health officers, many of them graduates of the MPH program at the University of Sydney. In this and other ways the service network was closely linked academically with this university's Department of Public Health.

In 1990, a new public health service infrastructure had been set up when fourteen public health units had been established in the Health Areas and Regions of New South Wales. These dealt with local problems ranging from infectious disease outbreaks to assessment of the local population's health needs. A training program was also established to produce a workforce. The first recruits—six public health officers—were inducted in 1990 for a three-year course of competency-based training. At first open only to medical graduates, the program was quickly made available to nonmedical graduates as well. All recruits had to have an MPH or equivalent degree plus a minimum of three years of health service experience. Recruits occupied various supervised training placements and also attended formal training sessions. Graduates of the program were awarded a graduate diploma of applied epidemiology, and the program was accredited with the state Education and Training Accreditation Board and the Australasian Faculty of Public Health Medicine. Originally, the emphasis in competency was on quantitative epidemiological skills; however, by the late 1990s more weight was being placed on management and policy development. The program's graduates came to occupy many senior posts within the New South Wales Health Department and in other health sectors in NSW and other states. In 1997, the Health Department began to provide scholarships for Aboriginal and Torres Strait Islander people to study public health at Newcastle University. Those completing such studies were eligible to join the Public Health Officer Training Program and were expected to contribute importantly to the advancement of Aboriginal health in New South Wales.[72]

A senior public health figure, Professor Tony Adams, said of the post–Kerr White educational and workforce development that it indeed was "a flowering of public health" that in turn made the Public Health Association of Australia, public health's professional body, "a force to be reckoned with."[73] The Public Health Association (PHA) and its predecessors made notable contributions to the development of public health in policy advocacy and formation, especially at the federal level. Indeed, the formation of the PHA itself is part and parcel of the general renaissance of public health during Neal Blewett's long tenure as the federal health minister, 1983–90.

Tony Adams himself played a pivotal role in the foundation of early public health professional organizations. Having taken an Harvard MPH in 1961, taught in community medicine at the University of Kentucky and done research in the School of Hygiene and Public Health at the Johns Hopkins University, 1962–64, Adams returned to a senior lectureship in the SPHTM at Sydney University, 1965–73. In 1974 he commenced what became a distinguished career in public health administration, first in New South Wales and then in the Federal Health Department, 1974–97.

After his American experience, Adams was dismayed at the paucity of epidemiological research being done in Australia. As a member of the long-established American Public Health Association, he was keen to see something like it created in Australia. In August 1968, Adams convened a meeting of about sixty people at the SPHTM where it was resolved to establish an organization to promote the study of community health and epidemiology and to appoint a working party of Professor Basil Hetzel, Doctors A.I. Adams, S. Sax, M. McCall and S. Boyden, and Mrs. R. Inall to set up the organization. Doctors T.A. Welborn and K. Cullen were asked to join the party, which met on 15 August and resolved a number of issues. It was decided that the new body, to be known as the Australian Society for Epidemiology and Research in Community Health (ASERCH), would not become a subsection of any established organization, such as the Australian Institute of Urban Studies or the Australian College of General Practitioners, because none could meet the specific needs for which ASERCH was established. Affiliation with the International Epidemiological Association would be sought. While the national body would hold an annual scientific meeting, state or local chapters might meet more often. At the first formal meeting of ASERCH at the University of Adelaide in August 1969, the fifty-one persons present elected Professor Douglas Gordon as chairman, Tony Adams as secretary and Professor Basil Hetzel as treasurer. Links with people in other countries of Oceania were to be encouraged. As well as regional convenors for each Australian state and the ACT, convenors for New Zealand (Professor C. Dixon) and Papua New Guinea (Dr. R. Scragg) were appointed.[74] By 1970, individual membership had climbed to 118. There was one institutional member. By 1971, 132 individual members were on the books.[75]

In the late 1960s, a Western Australian Public Health Association, driven by Bill Davidson, Jack Flood and colleagues from the state Health Department, and a New South Wales Public Health Association, started by Sandy Douglas, Con Ryan and others employed by the state Health Department (mainly public health doctors and nurses, and environmental health officers), were established. Sandy Douglas became president, and Tony Adams became secretary of the Australian Public Health Association, an amalgamation of the five existing state bodies, in 1969. Efforts were made to establish branches in other states and territories. Tony Adams was at this time secretary of the APHA and of ASERCH. Around the same time, the idea of combining the state Public Health Associations and ASERCH was discussed, but the epidemiologists did not think that the public health workers would share their core concerns and vice versa, so nothing came of the proposal at this stage. In May 1972 ASERCH held in Perth a conference that had a fourfold focus—medical care, the economics of medical care, screening procedures and health care for Papuans and for Aborigines. But at its annual meeting in August, the focus was on social health as the concept of community health services was explored.[76]

In 1974, a working party reported on the future of ASERCH, as it became clear that people from disciplinary backgrounds other than epidemiology and public health medicine (such as sociologists and other social scientists) would become more significant. The working party proposed that the organization become as multidisciplinary as possible and that a drive for new members be started; the relationship with the APHA be defined; that the relationship with New Zealand be investigated; and that the training functions of ASERCH be explored. The Royal Australasian College of Physicians was already looking at the future of training in epidemiology. ASERCH itself decided to consider training and recognition of epidemiologists and community health workers, both medical and nonmedical. At the annual general meeting of ASERCH at Otago University, New Zealand, in May 1975, the name of the dociety was changed to "Australian and New Zealand Society for Epidemiology and Research in Community Health" (ANZSERCH).[77] By mid-1976, ANZSERCH membership had grown to over three hundred. The Victorian branch had already effected a working amalgamation with APHA, involving joint meetings and a joint newsletter. Two years later, ANZSERCH had increased its membership to 550, with active branches in five states and a branch in New Zealand. A journal, *Community Health Studies,* under the able editorship of Dr. Neville Hicks, was in being. This publication from the outset covered epidemiological, social science and health policy approaches to public health. After a good deal of consideration of the question of training and accreditation, the society had decided to play only an informal role in these areas, leaving it to universities to provide training. With the emergence of the MPH program at the SPHTM in 1978 and the appearance of more doctoral theses devoted to epidemiology and community health, this informal role seemed adequate.[78]

ANZSERCH and APHA amalgamated as ANZSERCH/APHA. With the addition of 407 members of APHA, the joint organization had a total membership of 1,233 in 1981. In 1983 the outgoing president, David Christie, was pleased to report that the organization was being more frequently approached for expert advice on matters concerning epidemiology and community health. But not all was well; epidemiologists Stephen Leeder, Bruce Armstrong and David Legge formally complained about the "level of epidemiologic activity" in ANZSERCH/APHA. They looked to the formation of a specialist epidemiological association, while recognizing that the strength of the existing body lay in its broad disciplinary coverage. In 1984, interim guidelines were adopted for formation of special interest groups within ANZSERCH/APHA. This development went a good way toward meeting specialist needs within the broad unity of the organization's commitment to population health. An attempt was made to change the name of the organization to "Australasian Society for Health Research" in 1985. The Western Australian branch was particularly unhappy with the proposed new name, because about half its members were nonresearchers—public health and health education practitioners. The motion for change of name was lost. A separate attempt to change the name to "Australian and New Zealand Public Health Association" also failed.[79]

In 1985–86 the organization's involvement in expert committees and in building of links with like-minded national and international bodies continued. ANZSERCH was represented on, or in, the Public Health Committee of NHMRC; the National Committee on Health and Vital Statistics; the National Workshop on Medical Education and Workforce; and the Statistics and Surveillance Standing Committee of the National Occupational Health and Safety Commission. It had links with the World Federation of Public Health Associations, the Federation of Australian Technological and Scientific Societies, and ASH. The special interest groups within the organization were epidemiology, health services research, health statistics, international health and medical anthropology. The epidemiologists decided to create an Australian Epidemiological Association, to be affiliated with ANZSERCH.

At the annual general meeting in August 1986, a motion was carried to change the name of the organization to "Public Health Association of Australia and New Zealand" (PHA/ANZ) in the near future. There was strong support for the move. The executive of the PHA/ANZ in 1987 comprised the president, Professor Stephen Leeder; vice president, Dr. Frances Cunningham; secretary, Dr. Neil Thomson; treasurer, Mr. Lindsay Graham; and Dr. Fran Baum, as editor of *Community Health Studies*. ANZSERCH had been receiving federal funding for some time under the CHP grant system. Federal money now made possible the setting up of a federal secretariat in Canberra, in the mode of so many national nongovernment bodies wishing to influence commonwealth policy and actions. At the same time, a full-time executive director, Ms. Margaret Conley, was appointed. She had been for two years an adviser to Health Minister Blewett and was keen to take on a new challenge. New Zealand moved toward creation of a separate but closely linked Public Health Association, with the blessing of the PHA/ANZ. (From 1988, the PHA was the Public Health Association of Australia

[PHAA].) The journal *Community Health Studies* had in 1986–87 introduced special issues or supplements on important public health subjects—the Better Health Commission, aged care and smoking. It planned to bring out special issues on HIV/AIDS and on community development.[80]

By the end of the 1980s, PHAA was consolidating in some areas and opening up new activities in others. Organizationally, consolidation was occurring as new special interest groups in health promotion and in women's health were formed to add to the existing ones of Aboriginal health, health services research, health statistics, international health, medical anthropology and the political economy of health. Branches existed now in the six states and the ACT, and the struggle continued to establish one in the Northern Territory. In NSW a North Coast chapter had been formed. There were hopes for further chapters in the industrial cities of Newcastle and Wollongong. Participation in public debate through press releases and media contacts was making the PHAA and public health itself more visible. Public health advocacy was pursued through lobbying of ministers and shadow ministers, and through formal submissions in connection with such public health issues as the AIDS green paper and the Industries Assistance Commission inquiry into food processing and packaging. The PHAA involvement in national government and nongovernment health committees and working parties was growing. Representatives sat on the NHMRC's Public Health Committee and PHRDC, the National Better Health Council, the Commission of Worksafe Australia, the Australian Health Ministers' Advisory Council, the National Heart Foundation, the National Healthy Cities Program, and the Australian Cancer Society. Internationally, close ties were maintained with the New Zealand PHA and the Canadian PHA. The executive director was president-elect of the World Federation of Public Health Associations.[81]

In late 1990, Professor Charles Kerr of the Department of Public Health, University of Sydney, took over as editor of the association's journal. The Sydney team brought out the last issue of *Community Health Studies* in the format of the Adelaide publication. The first issue of 1991 came out in a new format with a new title, the *Australian Journal of Public Health*. At the changeover, the journal had a readership of 1,400 PHAA members, forty-four New Zealand subscribers, and 226 overseas subscribers, mostly libraries and institutions in the United States, Canada, the United Kingdom, Germany, France, Spain, Sweden, the Netherlands, Brazil, Israel, Kuwait, Hong Kong, Japan, Mexico and New Guinea. *Community Health Studies* had been located in the Department of Community Medicine at the University of Adelaide from its first issue in 1977. Members of the department and of the Foundation for Multidisciplinary Education in Community Health, a joint initiative of the University of Adelaide Faculty of Medicine and the South Australian Institute of Technology, had been part of the editorial group at different times. The journal, influenced by the social health outlook of the Adelaide editors, did much to build a concern for the social and political context of health in addition to the long-standing epidemiological concern of the association and its predecessors.[82]

In the early 1990s the association's political involvements expanded as the Standing Committee on Public Affairs (SCPA), under the astute direction of Dr. David Legge, began to formulate policy resolutions for adoption by the PHAA. The first ones were on abortion and on Aboriginal health. Professor Tony McMichael, president from 1989 to 1990, observed that public health was ultimately about social management and change, and that it had to address large-scale problems involving social values as well as public policies: HIV/AIDS control was beyond clinical medicine and demanded a health promotion response; and environmental problems like climate change raised the issue of the ecological sustainability of the dominant market orientation of the economy and also had enormous health implications. Yet, a recent federal government discussion paper on ecologically sustainable economic development showed no awareness that environmental degradation threatened health. The Australian Medical Association's recent public support for public health was welcome, but it understood this to mean one-dimensional interventions like taxing cigarettes to reduce consumption. The association had to educate the media to understand that public health was a much larger thing than the AMA's narrow, medical conception conveyed.

The PHAA contributed to various national reviews—the Triennial Review of the NHMRC, the National Review of Health and Vital Statistics, the 1991 review of PHERP, the Review of Funding of Peak Organizations, and the Review of Public Health Training. Greater national immunization coverage was a public health issue preoccupying the association at this time. The association sponsored the second national conference, in 1991, on immunization; it reviewed all the difficulties of applying well-established health technologies like effective vaccines, public health's "magic bullets"—as the president, Dr. Jane Hall, noted in 1991. The PHAA had adopted in October 1991 an immunization policy that noted that immunization levels were inadequate to control all acute, preventable, childhood infections; it urged the federal and state governments jointly to form a National Task Force to develop targets for coverage, quality assurance procedures and evaluation programs.

By 1992, there were 1,631 PHAA members from a variety of disciplines, and the association had compiled twenty-three policy statements. A Policy Statements Book was published in 1991 so that the association's stands on various issues were easily available. The SCPA reference group, comprising representatives of all branches and special interest groups, identified four priority policy areas: Aboriginal health, health care financing, health inequalities and environmental health. The international role of the PHAA was growing, especially in the Asian and South Pacific regions. The association worked with the Indonesian Public Health Association to strengthen this organization and undertook training responsibilities in Vietnam, helping that country develop a public health association.[83]

In 1992–93, PHAA under new legislation was to have a place on the council of the NHMRC and, among committees of inquiry and working parties, was represented on the National Health Goals and Targets Working Parties and the Joint Working Party on the Health Effects of Passive Smoking. It was also pressing for greater federal funding for public health research, which it saw as inadequate compared with what went to biomedical research. The 1992–95 strategic plan of the PHAA now specified eight objectives: provision of national leadership on public health issues, promulgation of public health policies, development of forums for debate of public health issues, promotion of public health in Australia's region and in international forums, expansion of public health's funding base, fostering excellence in the public health workforce through training and career development; and strengthening the association.

Readership of the *Australian Journal of Public Health* was 1,750 members plus almost three hundred subscribers, most of whom were libraries, universities, colleges and hospitals in Australia and overseas. In 1992 there were considered to be too few papers published on cardiovascular disease and on environmental health. By 1993 the deficiencies had been put right. The major content areas by number of papers were environmental health (ten), cardiovascular disease (nine), alcohol and other drugs (nine), primary health care (eight), injury and safety (seven), aged care (six), HIV/AIDS (six) and health services (six). In terms of the methodology used, forty-seven papers were mainly quantitative and twenty-eight mainly qualitative.

In 1994–95, Stephen Leeder returned to the presidency after an absence of six years. He observed how many new people had in this time joined the PHAA, guaranteeing its continuing vitality. Despite the diversity of backgrounds, they were united in a strong moral commitment to improving the health of Australians (for some, also, the health of overseas populations). By 1995, membership had grown to almost 1,800. This may be compared with the much larger membership of seven thousand of the historically influential Australian Medical Association. But the PHAA was using its less generous resources well, focusing on a few, significant problems and seeking to influence public opinion and public policy. One of its long-time strategies was the sponsoring of national conferences of experts on health issues looming large at any particular time. For example, there were the ongoing national conferences on immunization. We have mentioned the 1987 and 1991 conferences, and a third was held in 1993, focusing on the continuing poor vaccine uptake for preventable childhood infections; only Victoria and New South Wales had responded to the decade-old NHMRC recommendation that all states and territories introduce school-entry immunization requirements (by now updated to include childcare entry requirements). In 1994, a national conference on suicide prevention called for a national strategy to be devised, involving all groups with an interest in suicide prevention, including community and self-help bodies. In the same year, with tuberculosis resurgent in the United States and some other countries, a conference was convened on the public health issues of resurgent TB for Australia.[84]

REORIENTING THE HEALTH SYSTEM?

The "new public health," with its social view of health and basic principles of community participation, intersectoral action, population focus and promotion of health by multiple strategies, has been a major influence on public health professionals and public policy for at least a decade and a half in Australia. Some commentators have played down its impact on the health system, seeing it as having little effect on the economic, social and political structures that work against health advancement. Its concern for reduction of social inequalities in health, more emphasis on prevention, and equity of access to health services appear to be in conflict with the aims of the prevailing political ideology of economic rationalism—small government, market determination of resource allocation and preference for economic efficiency over social justice. But the new public health and the social view of health have a certain bamboo-in-the-wind resilience. The new publc health is part of a movement that is not dependent on a particular political party or social institution for its survival, though clearly translation of ideas into policy and action rely heavily on party and government support. As a movement and body of ideas, it has engaged the commitment of a group of able people—health practitioners, academics, health bureaucrats and some political leaders—since the 1980s. It has proven to be more than an intellectual and policy fashion. In the way of idealistic visions of human improvement, it has a moral energy and a certain subversive nature that may well allow it to weather the deep challenges of economic rationalism and uncontrolled globalization to national redistributive policies.[85]

Setting national health goals and targets in the last two decades has become an internationally popular means to try to reorient health policy toward an emphasis on public health prevention and health promotion. In the 1990s, the pursuit of targets, especially in the United States, the United Kingdom and Australia, was more systematic, with more explicit attempts to connect achievement of targets with health planning, management and funding. Attempts have also been made to involve all sectors of government in advancement of population health. As observed previously, the first country to try to develop comprehensive national health goals was the United States. In 1979, *Healthy People: The Surgeon General's Report on Health Promotion and Disease Prevention* identified fifteen priority areas where health gains might be expected and set up national goals for reductions in death rates or days of disability at the five life stages—infant, child, adolescents/young adults (fifteen to twenty-four years), adults (twenty-five to sixty-four years) and older adults (sixty-five years and over). In 1980, *Promoting Health/Preventing Disease* established specific measurable objectives for the fifteen priority areas—high blood pressure control, family planning, pregnancy and infant health, immunization, sexually transmitted diseases, toxic agent control, occupational health and safety, accident and injury prevention, fluoridation, surveillance and control of infectious diseases, smoking, alcohol and other drug abuse, physical fitness and control of stress and violent behavior.

Reviews of progress in 1986 and 1992 found that health had improved significantly in major areas, especially infant and child health. But there had been poor progress with the health of minorities, and there was a serious threat from HIV/AIDS. In 1990, after three years of consultation, the Department of Health and Human Services published a revised list of objectives for 2000, in *Healthy People 2000.* Its three hundred targets were divided among twenty-two priority areas. More detail was offered on how to reduce the difference in health status between the general population on the one hand and ethnic and low-income groups on the other. Progress was monitored in *Healthy People 2000 Review,* 1993. It revealed that 6 percent of objectives had been achieved and that in 36 percent there had been progress toward achievement, while in 15 percent movement had been away from targets. Priority areas with most progress were surveillance and data systems (six of seven objectives), cancer (eleven of sixteen objectives), and unintentional injuries (thirteen of twenty-two objectives). Those showing movement away from targets were occupational safety and health (four of fifteen objectives) and diabetic and chronic disabling conditions (five of twenty objectives). The overall importance of this strategy of goal and target setting is indicated by the fact that the secretary of health and human services and the president endorsed it. It is also indicated by the fact that state health departments took up the objectives and that federal agencies, beginning in 1981, set budgets in terms of the objectives.[86]

In the United Kingdom, after devolution of policy and management to the constituent nations, Wales was the first to attempt target setting. In 1989 the Welsh produced *Strategic Intent and Direction for the NHS in Wales.* This stated the long-term health goals to be achieved. Health gain became the litmus test for new investment and existing work, whether preventive, diagnostic, therapeutic or rehabilitative. Initially, ten priority areas were identified, and protocols for health gain were developed. These acted as indicators for future funding once they were connected to evidence of the effectiveness of particular health care services. In 1990, *Health for All in Wales: Health Promotion Challenges for the 1990s* was brought out. The "Health for All in Wales" strategy was widely discussed in a consultative process, and "plans for action" were developed. Current and future plans to implement the strategy were described. In 1992, with publication of *The Health of the Nation,* five key areas of action for health improvement were identified. Goals and targets, and strategies by which to attain them, were put in place. Health improvement was specified as a key concern of the National Health Service (NHS): "Improving health should be the prime concern of every NHS authority and health professional and manager in the NHS."[87] Primary care teams were given leading roles in the five areas of action, but the primary care focus was selective. With the British government intending to end free eye tests and dental examinations, neither dental nor eye health were included in *The Health of the Nation*'s target areas for health improvement. In Australia, it may be argued that the creation of health targets contributed to the coming into being of the first National Health Policy (1994) emphasising improvement of population health. Since the United States lacked a state-funded, national health insurance scheme like Australia's Medicare, the 1990 "Objectives for the Nation" acted as a catalyst for establishment of a national health agenda through identification of national health priorities and promotion of specific responses to the setting of such priorities.[88]

While, clearly, greater attention in the 1990s has been given in policy to trying to reorient the Australian health system toward advancement of population health, doubts must exist about the future prospects of the new public health. Before addressing these, I will briefly look at the related issue of the effectiveness of health promotion.

THE EFFECTIVENESS OF HEALTH PROMOTION

In 1995, the NHMRC produced a discussion paper that analyzed four examples of successful national health promotion interventions and attempted to identify factors contributing to their success. The interventions, or initiatives, were reduction in smoking prevalence, reduction in traffic injury deaths, reduction in premature mortality from cardiovascular disease, and reduction in the transmission of HIV/AIDS. In the case of smoking prevalence, the factors identified as contributing to success were a growing body of information about prevalence and why people smoke; advocacy groups that raised community and political concern, and elicited legislative and community action to reduce support for smoking; and multiple strategies—mass media campaigns, political advocacy, school education, individual and small-group counseling, legislation, tobacco taxes, labeling requirements, voluntary regulation and others—employed to reduce the prevalence of smoking. With reduction of traffic injury mortality, the factors were information on the extent of the problem and research into causes; active engagement of health professionals from advocacy of action by the College of Surgeons to health promotion to change driving behavior, and improvement of road conditions; multiple strategies combining educational and environmental approaches so that education led to voluntary behavior change (such as seat-belt use), which in turn led to legislation for compulsory behavior change; and partnerships among community, professional and private organizations, often outside the health sector, as with agencies responsible for road building, urban design and motor vehicle design.

In the case of reduced cardiovascular disease mortality, effective factors were action by the National Heart Foundation (and other nongovernment bodies) that raised public awareness, provided research findings on risk factors and, more recently, led to health promotion programs. The availability of good surveillance and research information on risk factor prevalence was critical. From the time of the Better Health Commission, national prioritizing of reduction of risk factors influenced health promotion efforts from the local to the national level. Commitment of funding for research and interventions over an extended period was necessary to bring down mortality over two decades. The combination of clinician's efforts to improve diagnosis, treatment and rehabilitation of high-risk groups and of public health workers' work in primary prevention to reduce risk-factor prevalence across the whole population was critical. Multiple strategies were required to reduce cardiovascular mortality. Indeed, all strategies proposed by the Ottawa Charter for health promotion were employed.

In the case of the containment of HIV/AIDS, research findings were continually used to inform policy-making and community-based education campaigns. Community-based peer education was central, with more general education being carried out by government agencies. Thus, in an exemplary fashion, community-based work was combined with government and professional expertise to achieve behavior change. From the outset, the goal of policy was clear—to persuade socially stigmatized groups (gay men, intravenous drug users and sex workers) to pursue "safe sex," since in the absence of a vaccine or cure, behavior change was the only way to contain the spread of the infection. Media campaigns were used both to educate and reduce stigma attaching to HIV/AIDS. Community-based care and support programs showed that care and education were interrelated. Empowerment of people affected by the condition and development of self-help groups like "People Living With HIV/AIDS" enabled them to act as educators as well as advocates for public support.

The factors making for success in these examples of national interventions can be assembled into three major groups:

1. Technical capacity, or best practice—knowledge, skills and information to identify the need for change, and to bring about change.
2. Policy and strategic direction—political commitment to, and means by which, to establish national agreement on goals, policy and delivery of effective health promotion.
3. Supportive structures—funding and other resources to support all work to advance population health.[89]

What is clear is that the causal chain linking action in health promotion and health outcomes is commonly complex and often problematic. Evaluation, then, has to be in terms of change in three types of outcome—improved personal health literacy, changes in public policies and organizational practices and changes in social norms and community actions. Past effort has gone into devising valid and reliable ways of measuring health behaviors, indicators of the physical environment, and changes in health service provision and use. Current effort is being directed into devising measures more responsive to the immediate effects of health promotion interventions. These include "measures of health literacy" like knowledge concerning the problem, self-confidence concerning tasks involved and behavioral intentions; "measures of social mobilization," like public endorsement of policy, community empowerment and community competency; and "measures of public policy and organizational practice" like enactment of legislation, changes to organizational structures and funding and other resource allocation. In health promotion, it is usually not possible to demonstrate a simple connection between intervention and the traditionally used indicators of health advancement—lower mortality and morbidity. Measures of effectiveness like those described above point to a move away in current best practice from a reductionist, behavioral approach to evidence of success, to a broader approach that allows for the complexity of links between eventual health outcomes and health promotion action.[90]

THE FUTURE OF THE NEW PUBLIC HEALTH IN AUSTRALIA

At the end of the 1990s, a neoconservative Liberal-National Party coalition government was in power at the federal level. It was bent on cutting public expenditure and privatizing services. Moreover, there were worrying signs that the focus of public health policy was moving away from a broad, "new public health" emphasis on the social, economic and political context of health to narrower, medical or behavioral concerns. Recent national initiatives were in areas like breast and cervical screening and immunization which, while valuable, yet smacked of a narrower, medical outlook rather than a new public health one. Substantial federal funding has gone into a reform strategy to encourage development of preventive and population-based work. in general practice. However, general practice is only a part of the primary health sector, albeit a significant part—about 80 percent of Australians, sixteen to sixty-five years of age, make at least one visit a year to a general practitioner. More significantly, the strategy does not embody new public health principles like community participation, use of multidisciplinary teams, intersectoral cooperation, health promotion and concern with communities rather than individuals.

The general practice strategy involved establishment of Divisions of General Practice and provision of project grants to assist general practitioners to integrate their work better with hospitals and community health services; provision of incentives to attract general practitioners to rural areas; a Better Practice program, which offered supplements to fee-for-service income; and a General Practice Evaluation program, which supported monitoring of the general practice strategy. The strategy's budget by 1995–96 was $238 million. The features that promoted public health were the encouragement of a population health perspective among general practitioners and the provision of means to achieve a degree of independence from the fee-for-service treadmill. A 1998 review of the strategy said that the new role in public health would demand not only more training but closer relationships with public health networks. Moreover, a great opportunity to promote closer integration of private general practice with state-funded, community health services (which themselves have suffered funding cuts in the 1990s, and particularly in Victoria and South Australia have seen service delivery emphasized over community development and advocacy) was foregone.[91]

From a new public health perspective, partnerships between a variety of players are integral to the advancement of population health. Historically, relationships between the commonwealth and states, and states and local government authorities, in health matters have often been fraught with difficulty because of the federal division of powers. The contemporary effort to coordinate the work of even more players is an even greater challenge. Creation of the National Public Health Partnership (NPHP) in 1997 presented opportunities for better collaboration and for coordination of policy and administration. The proximal origins of the NPHP lie in concerns expressed by the country's chief health officers and other national public health stakeholders, like the Public Health Association in late 1995 and early 1996, about developing a truly national approach to public health.

The reformers recognized that certain weaknesses had to be overcome. A series of vertical national health programs (for example, screening) had come into being in the 1980s and 1990s, as well as national strategies targeting particular diseases, risk factors, population groups and settings. The vertical programs introduced boundaries between the commonwealth and the states and territories, and between programs. Also, the principles of very successful strategies, like that for control of HIV/AIDS, should be applied more widely in public health. In some areas, such as health promotion, lack of clear responsibilities made for duplication of effort. The complexity of many public health problems like food-borne diseases and Aboriginal and Torres Strait Islander health meant national collaboration had to be strengthened. As health outcomes and allocative efficiency became the focus of the health system, the contribution of public health knowledge and skills to health advancement needed to be better articulated.

The NPHP offered a multilateral, intergovernmental framework for the cooperation required to overcome these weaknesses. It offered a chance to move toward a more systematic and strategic approach to public health. The hope was that it would provide a whole-of-system approach to replace the existing fragmented activities. It would encourage evidence-based policy and practice. It would enable each jurisdiction to clarify its role and then supply the appropriate infrastructure. The broad objectives of the NPHP, not surprisingly, are better collaboration of efforts, better coordination of public health strategies, and strengthening of public health infrastructure. The hope is that it will improve capacity to manage established problems like immunization and to respond to emerging issues like the spread of hepatitis C.[92]

The more distal origins of the NPHP lie in the commitment of the Council of Australian Governments (COAG) to reform of health and community services within a larger agenda of better coordination of commonwealth-state responsibilities. COAG was set up by the Australian heads of governments in 1992, when Paul Keating became Labor prime minister. Comprising the prime minister, premiers of states, chief ministers of territories and the president of the Australian Local Government Association, its prime task was to promote intergovernmental cooperation on reform of the national economy and structural reform of government. In April 1995, COAG agreed to go ahead with long-term changes to health and community services aimed at better meeting people's needs (by providing more choice, better information and continuity of care) and at providing more efficient services and containing costs (by planning for outcomes, investing in prevention, providing incentives for best practice and managing services near to the point of delivery). Long-existing problems in the health system were calling for resolution—such problems as inflexibility in programs, lack of balance between institutional and preventive services; administrative and service inefficiencies; cost shifting between levels of government; and difficulties with continuity of care as between acute and community care.

In October 1996, the Australian health ministers agreed to a National Public Health Partnership and recommended that the partnership be noted by COAG as an important move toward reform of commonwealth-state relations. The new federal coalition minister for health and family services, Dr. Michael Wooldridge, stated that he saw the partnership as a chance to put public health at the forefront of effective health care in Australia. The implementation of the NPHP was put in the hands of a partnership group that was itself a subcommittee of the Australian Health Ministers Advisory Committee. Working groups were set up on reform of legislation, health information, research and development, workforce development, planning, best practice and benchmark performance. One of the dangers facing the NPHP from a new public health viewpoint was the strong focus on state and commonwealth public health officers as the key players. There was a great need to be more inclusive of players from other sectors.[93]

Parallel with the development of the NPHP were bilateral negotiations carried out between the commonwealth, state and territory governments on the Public Health Outcome Funding Agreements (PHOFAs) for 1997–98 to 1998–99. The PHOFAs allowed "specific purpose payments" for eight existing national public health program areas to be "broadbanded" (pooled) to give states and territories greater flexibility to meet local conditions: HIV/AIDS Matched Funding Program, the National Women's Health Program, the Alternative Birthing Program, the National Education Program on Female Genital Mutilation, Breast Screen Australia, the National Cervical Screening Program, the National Childhood Immunization Program and the National Drug Strategy. Where the NPHP aimed to strengthen public health policy development by improving public health infrastructure, the PHOFAs aimed to achieve it by establishing more flexible, long-term funding arrangements for public health programs.[94]

An important focus of public health concern in Australia at the end of the twentieth century was, then, improving national collaboration in policy development and execution. An emerging area of concern of even more basic importance was that of social inequalities in health. In the following chapter, I will trace the development of public health's concern with the relation between social justice and health.

NOTES

1. J. Raftery, "The Social and Historical Context," in *Health for All: The South Australian Experience,* ed. F. Baum (Kent Town: Wakefield Press, 1995) 30; F. Baum, *The New Public Health: An Australian Experience* (Melbourne: Oxford University Press, 1998), 40.

2. J. Siddiqi, *World Health and World Politics* (London: Hurst, 1995), 193–97; M. Roemer, "Internationalism in Medicine and Public Health," in *Companion Encyclopedia of the History of Medicine,* vol. 2, ed. W.F. Bynum and R. Porter (London: Routledge, 1993), 1424–29; S.J. Kunitz, "Explanations and Ideologies of Mortality Patterns," *Population and Development Review* 13 (1987): 396–99.

3. Quoted in J. Ashton, "Health for All: The New Millennium," in *Progress in Public Health,* ed. G. Scally (London: F.T. Healthcare, 1997), 23.

4. G. Walt, *Health Policy: An Introduction to Process and Power* (London: Zed Books, 1994), 137–43; Ashton, "Health for All," 23; F. Baum, "Introduction," in *Health for All,* 3.

5. *Declaration of Alma Ata, adopted at the International Conference on Primary Health Care Alma Ata, USSR, 6–12 September 1978* (Geneva: World Health Organization, 1978), passim; G. Macdonald and R. Bunton, "Health Promotion. Discipline or Disciplines?" in *Health Promotion: Disciplines and Diversity,* ed. R. Bunton and G. Macdonald (London: Routledge, 1992), 9.

6. Quoted in M. Hogan, "Advocacy and Democratic Governance" in *Keeping It Together: State and Civil Society in Australia,* ed. A. Farrar and J. Inglis (Leichhardt, NSW: Pluto Press, 1996), 161.

7. Quoted in ibid., 162.

8. Ibid., 158–63; V. Burgmann, *Power and Protest. Movements for Change in Australian Society* (Sydney: Allen and Unwin, 1993), 3–10.

9. Baum, "Introduction," in *Health for All,* 3.

10. Macdonald and Bunton, "Health Promotion," 9–10.

11. Ibid., 8–11.

12. Baum, *The New Public Health,* 302–18.

13. Quoted in J. Welshman, "'Bringing Beauty and Brightness to the Back Streets': Health Education and Public Health in England and Wales, 1890–1940," unpublished paper, Centre for Urban History, University of Leicester, n.d., 5.

14. Quoted in ibid., 7.

15. Ibid., 2–9.

16. C. Webster, *The Health Services since the War,* vol. 1, *Problems of Health Care: The National Health Service before 1957* (London: Her Majesty's Stationery Office, 1988), 377–78.

17. C. Webster, *The Health Services since the War,* vol. 2, *Government and Health Care: The National Health Service 1958–1979* (London: The Stationery Office, 1996), 133–38, 244, 563, 674–80, 770.

18. I. Sutherland, *Health Education—Half A Policy: The Rise and Fall of the Health Education Council* (Cambridge: National Extension College, 1987), 234.

19. W.W. Holland and S. Stewart, *Public Health: The Vision and the Challenge* (London: Nuffield Trust, 1998), 131–32; C. Webster, *The National Health Service: A Political History* (Oxford: Oxford University Press, 1998), 160–61; P. Fisher, "The Reform of the Reform of the British National Health Service," *Journal of Public Health Policy* 20(2) (1999): 139–43.

20. Quoted in Holland and Stewart, *Public Health,* 141.

21. Ibid., 119–22, 141–42, 157–58, 184–85.

22. J. Duffy, *The Sanitarians: A History of American Public Health* (Urbana: University of Illinois Press, 1990), 214–16.

23. E. Fee, "Public Health and the State: The United States," in *The History of Public Health and the Modern State,* ed. D. Porter (Amsterdam, Atlanta: Editions Rodopi B.V., 1994), 244–45.

24. Quoted in ibid., 245.

25. L.W. Green and M.W. Kreuter, "Health Promotion as a Public Health Strategy for the 1990s," *Annual Review of Public Health* 11 (1990): 324–28.

26. U.S. Department of Health and Human Services, *Healthy People: The Surgeon General's Report on Health Promotion and Disease Prevention, 1979* (Washington, D.C.: Public Health Service, 1979), viii.

27. Ibid., 6–7, 21, 33, 43, 53, 71.

28. U.S. Department of Health and Human Services, *Promoting Health/Preventing Disease: Objectives for the Nation* (Washington, D.C.: U.S. Government Printing Office, 1988), 1–4.

29. Ibid., 1–4; M. Terris, "Epidemiology and Health Policy in the Americas: Meeting the Neoliberal Challenge," *Journal of Public Health Policy* 19(1) (1998): 21.

30. G.R. Palmer and S.D. Short, *Health Care and Public Policy: An Australian Analysis* (South Melbourne: Macmillan Educational Australia, 1994), 63–64.

31. See M.J. Lewis, "'Populate or Perish': Aspects of Infant and Maternal Health in Sydney, 1870–1939" (Ph.D. dissertation, Australian National University, Canberra, 1976), 10–11.

32. W.G. Armstrong, "Some Lessons from the Statistics of Infantile Mortality in Sydney," *Transactions of Australasian Medical Congress* (1905): 393–94.

33. See Lewis, "'Populate or Perish,'" 11.
34. G. Rodwell, "Lessons from the First World War: Drs Harvey Sutton and J.S. Purdy: Sydney's Health Week: 1921–1950," in *Individuals and Institutions in the History of Medicine,* Occasional Papers in Medical History Australia 9 (Sydney: Organising Committee of 6th Biennial Conference of Australian Society for History of Medicine, 1999), n.p.
35. C.D.J. Holman, R.J. Donovan and B. Corti, *Report of the Evaluation of the Western Australian Health Promotion Foundation* (Perth: Department of Public Health and Graduate School of Management, University of Western Australia, 1994), 4–5; D. Snow, *The Progress of Public Health in Western Australia, 1829–1977* (Perth: Western Australia Health Department, 1981), 116–20.
36. L. Davidson, S. Chapman and C. Hull, *Health Promotion in Australia 1978–79* (Canberra: Australian Government Publishing Service [hereafter AGPS], 1979), 222.
37. Ibid., viii–ix, 7, 13, 34–46, 48–49, 99–100, 109–24, 192–95.
38. Ibid., 93–94.
39. Ibid., 230–36.
40. B.S. Hetzel, *Health and Australian Society* (Ringwood: Penguin, 1983), 256.
41. N. Milio, "Promoting Health Promotion: Health or Hype?" *Community Health Studies* 10(4) (1986): 429–30.
42. C. Bridges-Webb, "Letters to Editor: The Nation's Health," *Medical Journal of Australia* 2 (1983): 604; National Health and Medical Research Council Community Health Promotion and Education (Standing) Committee, *Towards a National Policy on Health Promotion* (Canberra: Commonwealth Department of Health and Aged Care Library, September 1984), 2–4.
43. S.R. Leeder, T. Dwyer and J. Gold, "The Nation's Health. Goals for 1988," *Medical Journal of Australia* 2 (1983): 360.
44. Milio, "Promoting Health Promotion," 427–29; Baum, *The New Public Health,* 40–41, 323–24.
45. Quoted in Raftery, "The Social and Historical Context," 35.
46. Milio, "Promoting Health Promotion," 429; *Health Education and Promotion in Victoria: Report to Minister for Health, June 1986* (Melbourne: Victoria Health Department, 1986), 1–4, 12, 29.
47. Quoted in Holman, Donovan and Corti, *Report of the Evaluation of the Western Australian Health Promotion Foundation,* 5–6.
48. M. Daube, "Health Promotion Foundations in Australia," *Health Promotion Journal of Australia* 3(1) (1993): 3; R. Galbally, "The Victorian Health Promotion Foundation—Vic Health," *Health Promotion Journal of Australia* 3(1) (1993): 4–5; E. Cassell, "The Vic Health Research Program—The First Five Years," *Health Promotion Journal of Australia* 3(1) (1993): 16.
49. M. Court, "The South Australian Health Promotion Foundation—Foundation S.A.," *Health Promotion Journal of Australia* 3(1) (1993): 25–26: A. Wylie, "Increasing Community Participation in Statewide Health Awareness Campaigns: The Foundation South Australia Community Grants Program," *Health Promotion Journal of Australia* 3(1) (1993): 34.
50. K. Thompson, "ACT Health Promotion Fund," *Health Promotion Journal of Australia* 3(1) (1993): 70–71.

51. A. Carroll, "The Western Australian Health Promotion Foundation—Healthway," *Health Promotion Journal of Australia* 3(1) (1993): 42–43.

52. N. Blewett, "Healthy Public Policy," *New Doctor* 44 (1987): 17; F. Stilwell, *The Accord . . . and Beyond: The Political Economy of the Labor Government* (Sydney: Pluto Press, 1986), 159–60.

53. Better Health Commission, *Looking to Better Health,* vol. 1, *Final Report* (Canberra: AGPS, 1986), xii.

54. Blewett, "Healthy Public Policy," 17.

55. S. Leeder, "Better Health," in *The Tasks of Medicine: An Ideology of Care,* ed. P. Baume (Sydney: Maclennan and Petty, 1998), 238.

56. Better Health Commission, *Looking to Better Health,* vol. 1, vii–xv; Milio, "Promoting Health Promotion," 430; "'Tremendous Public Response to Better Health Commission,'" *Health Reporter* 3(3) (1986): 1; M. Wise and D. Nutbeam, "National Health Goals and Targets: An Historical Perspective," *Health Promotion Journal of Australia* 4(3) (1994): 9.

57. Health Targets and Implementation (Health for All) Committee, *Health for All Australians: Report to Australian Health Ministers' Advisory Council and Australian Health Ministers' Conference* (Canberra: AGPS, 1988), 1–21; Palmer and Short, *Health Care and Public Policy,* 216–17.

58. Quoted in Wise and Nutbeam, "National Health Goals and Targets," 10.

59. Ibid., 9–10.

60. Quoted in Palmer and Short, *Health Care and Public Policy,* 218.

61. *Better Health Outcomes for Australians: National Goals, Targets and Strategies for Better Health Outcomes into the Next Century* (Canberra: AGPS, 1994), 1–19; "Summary of the Australian Health Goals and Targets Process," *Health Promotion Journal of Australia* 4(3)(1994): 3; Palmer and Short, *Health Care and Public Policy,* 218; D. Nutbeam, "Creating Health—Promoting Environments: Overcoming Barriers to Action," *Australian and New Zealand Journal of Public Health* 21(4) (1997): 355–58.

62. T. McMichael, "Public Health in Australia: A Personal Reflection," *Australian Journal of Public Health* 17(4) (1993): 295.

63. D.J. Lee, *The School of Public Health and Tropical Medicine, 1930–1980* (Sydney: School of Public Health and Tropical Medicine, 1980), 66; J. Reid, "Public Health Education in Australia: Nobody's Child?" *Social Science and Medicine* 38(8) (1994): vi.

64. *Submission from Commonwealth Department of Health to Senate Standing Committee on Social Welfare: Inquiry into Evaluation of Adequacy of Australian Health and Welfare Services,* Commonwealth Department of Health, Canberra, July 1976, 8; Palmer and Short, *Health Care and Public Policy,* 167; J. Best, "Public Health—What Is This Thing Called . . . ?" *Medical Journal of Australia* 144 (1986): 93–97; Interview (Milton Lewis) with John Deeble, Canberra, 18 November 1997; Interview (Milton Lewis) with Margaret Conley, Canberra, 24 July 1997; Interview (Milton Lewis) with Stephen Leeder, Sydney, 6 March 1997; *In Touch,* March 1986, 1–5; I. Webster, "The Kerr White Report," *New Doctor,* 41–42 (1986): 58–61.

65. K.L. White, *Independent Review of Research and Educational Requirements for Public Health and Tropical Health: Report to Hon. Neal Blewett M.P., Minister for Health* (Canberra: Commonwealth Department of Health and Aged Care Library, January 1986), 4–14.

66. D. Fry, "Health Policy and the Need for Social Science Research," in *The Social Sciences and Health Research,* ed. J. Daly and E. Willis (Ballarat: Public Health Association of Australia, 1990), 5; Interview (Milton Lewis) with John Deeble, Canberra, 18 November 1997.

67. Interview (Milton Lewis) with John Deeble, Canberra, 18 November 1997; S. Chapman and S. Leeder, "Public Health Services in Australia," in *Oxford Textbook of Public Health,* vol. 1, ed. W.W. Holland, R. Detels and G. Knox (Oxford: Oxford University Press, 1991), 432–33.

68. Reid, "Public Health Education in Australia," viii–ix; S. Leeder, "The Stakes are High in Public Health," *Medical Journal of Australia* 159 (1993) 295–96; Palmer and Short, *Health Care and Public Policy,* 167–68.

69. Palmer and Short, *Health Care and Public Policy,* 168–69; G.C. Salmond, *Independent Review of the Public Health Education and Research Program in Australia: Report to Hon. Brian Howe M.P., Minister for Health, Housing and Community Services* (Canberra: Commonwealth Department of Health, Housing and Community Services, 1992), 39–40.

70. *Review of Public Health Education and Research Program: Main Submission to PHERP Review from the University of Sydney* (n.p.: Department of Public Health and Community Medicine, September 1998) [author's copy].

71. National Health and Medical Research Council, *Sixty Years of the National Health and Medical Research Council 1936–1996* (Canberra: AGPS, 1996), 141–43; Interview (Milton Lewis) with Ken Donald, Sydney, 8 March 1999.

72. L. Madden, "The NSW Public Health Officer Training Program," *In the News* 11(1) (1997): 7.

73. T. Adams, "Australia's Health in the 1990s," *Journal of Public Health Policy* 13(1) (1992): 99.

74. Minutes of Working Committee, Australian Society for Epidemiology and Research in Community Health (ASERCH), 15 August 1968, 1–3, Noel Butlin Archives Centre, Australian National University, Canberra [hereafter NBAC]; Minutes of First ASERCH Meeting, 20 August 1969, 1–2, NBAC.

75. Minutes of ASERCH, 14 August 1970, 1, NBAC; Minutes of ASERCH, 22 August 1971, 1, NBAC.

76. T. Adams, "History of PHA," unpublished note, October 1994, n.p.; Report of ASERCH Conference, 16 May 1972, 1–5, NBAC; ASERCH Annual Meeting, 19–20 August 1972, 1–2, NBAC.

77. Report of Meeting to Discuss Future of ASERCH, Melbourne, 23 October 1974, 1, NBAC; Minutes of Annual General Meeting, ASERCH, 22 May 1975, 2–3, NBAC.

78. Minutes of Australian and New Zealand Society for Epidemiology and Research in Community Health (ANZSERCH) Committee Meeting, 12 May 1976, 1, NBAC; Letter from I. Maddocks, vice president, ANZSERCH to R.P. Joske, Senate Standing Committee on Social Welfare, 30 July 1976, NBAC; Presidential Remarks at Annual General Meeting, ANZSERCH, 17 May 1978, NBAC.

79. Minutes of Annual General Meeting, ANZSERCH/Australian Public Health Association (APHA), 13 May 1981, 3, NBAC; Minutes of Annual General Meeting, ANZSERCH/APHA, 22 May 1983, 7, NBAC; 6 August 1985, 3–5, NBAC.

80. Minutes of Annual General Meeting, Public Health Association of Australia

and New Zealand (PHAANZ), 20 August 1986, 1–3, NBAC; 26 August 1987, 1–2, NBAC; Minutes of Annual General Meeting, Public Health Association of Australia (PHAA), 30 August 1988, 1–2, NBAC; Interview (Milton Lewis) with Margaret Conley, Canberra, 24 July 1997; Address by president (D. Christie), ANZSERCH/APHA, 1983, NBAC; Letter from S.R. Leeder, University of Newcastle, concerning Australasian Epidemiological Association, n.d. [early 1983?], NBAC.

81. Report of PHAA, 1988–89, 3–28, NBAC.

82. Report of PHAA, 1989–90, 9–10; 1990–91, 7, NBAC; J. Raftery, "Health Policy Development in the 1980s and 1990s," 53–54.

83. Report of PHAA, 1989–90, 3–11; 1990–91, 3–8; 1991–92, 4–13, NBAC; R. Hall and J. Richters, eds., *Immunisation: The Old and the New—Proceedings of Second National Immunisation Conference, Canberra, 27–29 May 1991* (Canberra: Public Health Association of Australia, Inc., 1992), 96.

84. PHAA Annual Report, 1992–93, 3–11; 1993–94, 5–8; 1994–95, 3–10, NBAC; *Participation in Health: 27th Annual Conference of Public Health Association of Australia, 1995,* 8, NBAC; *Immunisation: Doing It Better—Proceedings and Abstracts of 3rd National Immunisation Conference, Melbourne, 21–23 April 1993,* Public Health Association of Australia, 5–6, NBAC; *Suicide Prevention: Public Health Significance of Suicide—Prevention Strategies. Proceedings and Abstracts of National Suicide Prevention Conference, 1994,* Public Health Association of Australia, 102–4, NBAC; *TB: A Global Emergency. Public Health Issues for Australia. Proceedings of National Tuberculosis Conference, Sydney, 28–30 November 1994,* Public Health Association of Australia, 92–94, NBAC.

85. J. Raftery, "Health Policy Development in the 1980s and 1990s," 61.

86. U.S. Department of Health and Human Services, *Promoting Health/Preventing Disease,* 1–4; U.S. Department of Health and Human Services, *Healthy People 2000 Review, 1993* (Hyattsville, Md.: Public Health Service, 1994), 1–2; D. Nutbeam and M. Wise, "Planning for Health for All: International Experience in Setting Health Goals and Targets," *Health Promotion International* 11(3) (1996): 220.

87. Quoted in Nutbeam and Wise, "Planning for Health for All," 222.

88. Ibid., 222–24; Webster, *The National Health Service,* 179.

89. Health Advancement Standing Committee of NHMRC, *Health Australia: Promoting Health in Australia* (Canberra: NHMRC, 1995), 16, 20, 23, 25, 31, 38–39.

90. D. Nutbeam, "Health Outcomes and Health Promotion: Defining Success in Health Promotion," *Health Promotion Journal of Australia* 6(2) (1996): 58–60.

91. Baum, *The New Public Health,* 46–48; C. Silagy, S. Sommer and L. Piterman, "Preventive Care in General Practice," *Medical Journal of Australia* 156 (1992): 405.

92. "The National Public Health Partnership and Public Health Outcome Funding Agreements: How Are These Related?" *National Public Health Partnership News* 2 (1997): 5; "Discussion Paper on National Public Health Partnership," 1996, unpublished paper, papers of Professor Tony Adams, 4–6.

93. "Introducing You to the National Public Health Partnership," *National Public Health Partnership News* 1 (1997): 1–2; Public Health Division, Commonwealth Department of Health and Family Services, "The National Public Health Partnership: Commonwealth and State and Territory Cooperation," *Health Promotion Journal*

of Australia 6(3) (1996): 60–61; L. Rogan, "Tides of Change in Community Services: The Industry Commission and COAG as Case Studies," in *Keeping It Together: State and Civil Society in Australia*, ed. A. Farrar and J. Inglis (Leichhardt: Pluto Press, 1996), 141–46; Baum, *The New Public Health*, 54–55.

94. "The National Public Health Partnership and Public Health Outcome Funding Agreements: How Are These Related?" *National Public Health Partnership News* 2 (1997): 5.

Chapter 5

Public Health and Social Justice

SOCIAL INEQUALITIES IN HEALTH

The adoption by the World Health Organization (WHO) of the "Health for All by the Year 2000" strategy brought intranational and international inequalities in health status to the forefront of health policy. The European office of WHO set targets for the regional application of the strategy. These were endorsed by all members in 1984. Of the thirty-eight targets, the first was "equity in health," by which was meant reducing inequalities in health status between social groups and between countries by at least 25 percent. In Australia, the Health Targets and Implementation (Health for All) Committee's 1988 report to the Australian health ministers, *Health for All Australians,* put much emphasis on reduction of health inequities. It recognized that differences in health status existed as between social strata, races and genders. But it failed to suggest how these differences might be reduced, beyond more equitable access to health services.[1]

Public health concern with health inequalities has a long history. One of the leading figures of the early French hygiene movement, the physician Louis René Villermé (1782–1863), investigated mortality differences between poor and affluent areas of Paris in the 1820s. Of the twelve districts of the city he investigated, the lowest in per capita income—on average only thirty-six francs—experienced a 37 percent higher risk of mortality than the highest, in which district the average per capita income was 120 francs. Residents of the first-ranked district enjoyed decent housing, food and sanitary conditions and were not burdened by excessive labor. To reduce class differences in mortality, Villermé proposed better working conditions and more education for the lower classes.

The leading edge of social medicine and public health shifted to Germany in the 1840s. Radical German doctors, especially during the revolution of 1848, called for government action to reform health conditions. The most prominent—Rudolf Virchow, Solomon Neumann and Rudolf Leubuscher—believed that society had to protect the health of all the people and that the impact of social and economic factors on health should be scientifically investigated. In 1849 Neumann submitted a draft public health law to the Berlin Society of Physicians and Surgeons in which the following objectives were assigned to public health: the healthy mental and physical development of all citizens, prevention of all threats to health, and control of disease.[2] Dispatched by the Prussian government to impoverished Upper Silesia to inquire into a typhus epidemic that in 1847–48 was, together with famine, killing thousands, Virchow had reported that the fundamental solution lay in education, political rights, more employment, and higher wages. A state health service was needed to care for the poor. In 1847 Neumann had declared, "The majority of diseases which either prevent the enjoyment of life or kill a considerable number of people prematurely are not due to natural physical, but to artificially produced social conditions. . . . Medical science is by its very nature a social science, but until this is actually recognized and conceded to medicine, we shall be unable to enjoy its benefits and shall have to be satisfied with an empty shell."[3]

Where Virchow focused on inequalities in the distribution and consumption of social and economic resources, Friedrich Engels, the intellectual and political collaborator of Karl Marx, saw private ownership of the means of production under early industrial capitalism as the fundamental cause of the excessive burden of illness and mortality carried by the urban English working class. The conflict between the employer's quest for profit and the health and safety of employees meant that workers were unduly exposed at work to dust, chemicals, time pressure and debilitating body postures. Added to these stresses were general environmental pollution, poor housing, alcohol abuse and undernutrition. Writing about the situation in *The Condition of the Working Class in England in 1845*, Engels (who was not trained in medicine) cited vital statistics compiled by public health officers to demonstrate that urban mortality rates were inversely related to social class. In Manchester, mortality of working class children was much greater than that of children of "the higher classes." They suffered higher death rates from epidemics of measles, scarlet fever, whooping cough and smallpox.[4]

The failure of the 1848 revolutions in both Germany and France saw the defeat of radical politics in these two countries and the end of an interdisciplinary health program of social medicine that was then developing. In the last issue of *Medical Reform,* Virchow said, "The counterrevolution factually has conquered."[5] Virchow did not take up health reform again until his return to Berlin and the chair of pathological anatomy in 1856, and then in politically safe forms of action—sanitation projects and the provision of medical services for the poor. An elected member of the Reichstag over an extended period, he opposed Otto von Bismarck's conservative politics, but he never returned to the political activism and socialist radicalism of his early years. Engels's foray into the social origins of ill health (and social inequalities in health status) of the 1840s was not repeated, as he became caught up in the larger theoretical and practical life of Marxism.[6]

BRITAIN

There was a contemporary, if unrevolutionary, British interest in socioeconomic differences in health. In his *Report on the Sanitary Condition of the Labouring Population of Great Britain* of 1842, Edwin Chadwick, barrister and sanitary reformer, noted the average age at death of various occupational groups: "gentlemen and persons engaged in professions, and their families . . . 45 years; tradesmen and their families . . . 26 years; mechanics, servants and labourers, and their families . . . 16 years."[7] But Chadwick, Southwood Smith and the other sanitarians were not inclined to use social factors like poverty and debilitating work to explain differential mortality rates; they were focused on the hypothetical "miasma" as the agent of most diseases. They sought to rid the environment of it in a socially and politically undisruptive way—by a technical solution involving drains and sewers. They had powerful reasons for narrowing the ambit of public health in this way. Chadwick was secretary to the unpopular Poor Law Commission, at a time when social unrest and class conflict was growing intense. He was keen to reduce premature deaths in the laboring class so that the burden of poor relief for widows and orphans would become lighter on the propertied class. Southwood Smith was a liberal theologian and minister as well as physician, and he cleaved to an optimistic natural theology.

William Farr of the Registrar General's Department, as early as 1860, compared mortality in different districts in order to understand the environmental differences between more and less healthy areas so that health improvements might be achieved:

> With the growing knowledge that the greatest gaps between mortality of the upper classes and that of the general population occurred in infancy and childhood, there was strong concern within the statistical movement to obtain statistics on childhood mortality of the poorer classes. This concern was heightened when, with the marked improvements in adult mortality from 1840 onwards, there was virtually no change in infant mortality, which was annually responsible for the loss of 15 percent of births.[8]

In his analysis of mortality in England in 1861–70, Farr grouped occupations into the social orders of industrial society, with the aim of identifying social and biological influences, as opposed to the dangers of particular occupations. However, the first official classification by five social classes was established by T.H.C. Stevenson, superintendent of statistics, in 1911. Stevenson divided the population into five occupational classes: class I, professional; class II, intermediate; class III, skilled; class IV, partly skilled; and class V, unskilled. Standardized, all-cause mortality as recorded in the 1921 decennial supplement clearly increased with descending social class. With cause-specific mortality, the gradient was greater for some causes, like respiratory diseases and bronchitis, and less for others, like peptic ulcer. In the case of diabetes and appendicitis, the gradient was reversed, with classes I and II experiencing higher mortality than did the lower classes.[9]

As may be seen in table 5.1, mortality differentials between social classes increased in the period from the 1930s to the 1980s in England and Wales. This widening of differentials occurred even as the aggregate mortality rate declined. In the period from the 1890s to the 1970s, greater equality of access to and utilization of health care services in England and Wales did not result in more equality in levels of health across social classes, as can be seen in table 5.2.

From 1930, the inequality in male mortality across social classes increased. The introduction of the National Health Service seems not to have narrowed inequality. Indeed, the mortality ratios between classes III, IV and V, on one hand, and class I, on the other, increased. Similar results are seen with cause-specific mortality. For five of six diseases (leukemia, other cancer, hypertension, diabetes, respiratory tuberculosis and bronchitis), mortality ratios between classes I and V widened in the period after introduction of the National Health Service (NHS); bronchitis was the exception.[10]

Between 1911 and 1972, both neonatal (first month of life) and postneonatal (one to twelve months of life) mortality fell substantially, the first because of improvement in antenatal care and access to medical services in childbirth, and the second because of improvement in the socioeconomic environment of the child and in delivery of medical services. Every class shared in the secular decline, but inequality between classes actually increased. In 1911 the ratio of class V to I neonatal rates was 1.4; it was 1.7 in 1950 and about two in 1970–72. The inequality with postneonatal rates was greater over time; the ratio was 2.4 in 1911, 3.8 in 1950, and four to five in 1970–72. Since the size of population in class V has fallen and those in classes II, III and IV have grown, the trends for these classes are interesting. Where the neonatal trends are not distinct, the postneonatal trends show some reduction in inequality. Thus, the ratio of class IV to class I declined from 3.5 in 1921 to 2.4 in 1970–72, and similar narrowing occurred for classes II and III (see tables 5.3, 5.4).[11]

The nineteenth-century interest in the relationship between health and social class (and between poverty and excess disease and death) continued in the early 1900s in the work of Newsholme, Newman and others on class

Table 5.1
Mortality* of Men 15 to 64 Years by Social Class, England and Wales, 1930–82

Social Class		1930–32	1949–53	1959–63	1970–72	1979–80/1982–83
I.	Professional	90	86	75	77	66
II.	Intermediate	94	92	81	81	76
III.N	Skilled nonmanual	97	101	100	99	94
III.M	Skilled manual	97	101	100	106	106
IV.	Partly skilled	102	104	103	114	116
V.	Unskilled	111	118	127	137	165

*Standardized mortality ratios, all men = 100

Source: M. Marmot, M. Bobak and G. Davey Smith, "Explanations for Social Inequalities in Health," in *Society and Health*, eds. B.C. Amick III, S. Levine, A.R. Taylor and D. Chapman Walsh (New York: Oxford University Press, 1995), 177.

Table 5.2
Mortality† of Men by Social Class, England and Wales, 1890–1972

	Social Class				
Year	I	II	III	IV	V
1890–92	83‡				125
	(1.0)*				(1.5)
1900–1902	89				154
	(1.0)				(1.7)
1910–12	88	94	96	93	142
	(1.0)	(1.07)	(1.09)	(1.06)	(1.6)
1921–23	82	94	95	101	125
	(1.0)	(1.15)	(1.16)	(1.23)	(1.52)
1930–32	90	94	97	102	111
	(1.0)	(1.04)	(1.07)	(1.13)	(1.2)
1951	103	108	117	119	136
	(1.0)	(1.04)	(1.14)	(1.16)	(1.32)
1961	77	85	105	108	134
	(1.0)	(1.1)	(1.36)	(1.4)	(1.74)
1970–72	78	81	104	113	123
	(1.0)	(1.04)	(1.33)	(1.45)	(1.58)

‡Standardized mortality ratios
*Ratio of SMR of each class to SMR of class I is in parentheses
†Men aged 15 or 20 to 64 or 65 years

Source: J. Rogers Hollingsworth, "Inequality in Levels of Health in England and Wales, 1891–1971," *Journal of Health and Social Behavior* 22 (1981): 279.

differences in infant mortality, especially from diarrheal and associated conditions. It was taken up again in the economically depressed 1930s by John Boyd Orr, in *Food, Health and Income: Report on a Survey of Adequacy of Diet in Relation to Income* (1937); G.C.M. M'Gonigle and J. Kirby, in *Poverty and Public Health* (1936); and Richard Titmuss, in *Poverty and Population: A Factual Study of Contemporary Social Waste* (1937). Titmuss, in particular, showed that class differences in health were significant and that preventable mortality among the poorer classes was substantial. The clear implication was that the provision of health and social services for these social groups was inadequate and in need of improvement.[12]

The coming of the NHS in 1948 and apparent equality of access to health care put an end to concern about health inequalities until the 1970s. Indeed, a basic argument in support of the NHS in those two to three decades was that some kind of equality in health had been achieved. The very existence of the NHS, it might be argued, had precluded investigation into and debate about social and economic factors (other than health care) that influence health inequalities. Political awareness of geographical inequalities in

Table 5.3
Neonatal Mortality by Social Class, England and Wales, 1911–1970/72

	Social Class#				
Year	**I**	**II**	**III**	**IV**	**V**
1911	30.3‡	36.5	36.8	38.6	42.5
	(1.0)*	(1.2)	(1.2)	(1.3)	(1.4)
1921	23.4	28.3	33.7	36.7	36.9
	(1.0)	(1.2)	(1.4)	(1.6)	(1.6)
1930–32	21.7	27.2	29.4	31.9	32.5
	(1.0)	(1.3)	(1.4)	(1.5)	(1.5)
1939	18.9	23.4	25.4	27.7	30.1
	(1.0)	(1.2)	(1.3)	(1.5)	(1.6)
1950	12.9	16.2	17.6	19.8	21.9
	(1.0)	(1.3)	(1.4)	(1.5)	(1.7)
1964–65	9.2 (I–II)		11.8	13.2 (IV–V)	
	(1.0)		(1.3)	(1.4)	
1970–72†					
Males	8.9	9.7	10.7 11.0	12.7	17.0
	(1.0)	(1.1)	(1.2) (1.2)	(1.4)	(1.9)
Females	6.3	7.4	7.6 8.2	9.1	12.6
	(1.0)	(1.2)	(1.2) (1.3)	(1.4)	(2.0)

‡The top figure in each case is deaths per 1,000 live births.
*The ratio of the mortality rate in each social class to the mortality rate of social class I is in parenthesis.
†For 1970–72, the two categories of social class III data refer to nonmanual skilled and manual skilled occupations, respectively.
#Occupation of father of infant.

Source: J. Rogers Hollingsworth, "Inequality in Levels of Health in England and Wales, 1891–1971," *Journal of Health and Social Behavior* 22 (1981): 277.

health care facilities had existed at the birth of the NHS. Aneurin Bevan had opposed a local government health service, inter alia, because he did not wish to perpetuate a better service in the rich areas and an inferior one in the poorer. Richard Crossman, secretary of state for social services, 1968–70, resurrected concern about such geographical inequalities; this resulted in creation of a resource-allocation formula to distribute more fairly funds between hospital boards, and subsequently in the introduction of the Resource Allocation Working Party (RAWP) formula in 1977–78.

The Trades Union Congress (TUC), the union movement's peak organization, responding to a 1976 consultative document, *Priorities for Health and Personal Social Services,* pointed out that considerable differences in

Table 5.4
Postneonatal Mortality by Social Class, England and Wales, 1911–1970/72

	Social Class				
Year	I	II	III	IV	V
1911	46.2†	69.9	75.9	82.9	110
	(1.0)*	(1.5)	(1.6)	(1.8)	(2.4)
1921	15.0	27.2	43.1	52.7	60.1
	(1.0)	(1.8)	(2.8)	(3.5)	(4.0)
1930–32	11.0	17.8	28.2	34.9	44.6
	(1.0)	(1.6)	(2.6)	(3.2)	(4.1)
1939	7.9	11.0	19.0	23.7	30.0
	(1.0)	(1.4)	(2.4)	(3.0)	(3.8)
1950	4.9	6.0	10.5	13.9	18.8
	(1.0)	(1.2)	(2.1)	(2.8)	(3.8)
1964–65	3.5		5.4	7.6	
	(1.0)		(1.5)	(2.2)	
1970–72‡					
Males	3.5	4.1	4.6 6.2	7.3	14.6
	(1.0)	(1.2)	(1.3) (1.8)	(2.1)	(4.2)
Females	2.3	3.2	3.1 5.0	6.0	11.6
	(1.0)	(1.4)	(1.3) (2.2)	(2.6)	(5.1)

†The top figure in each case is deaths per 1,000 live births.
*The ratio of the mortality rate in each social class to the mortality rate of social class I is in parentheses.
‡For 1970–72, the two categories of social class III data refer to nonmanual skilled and manual skilled occupations, respectively; postneonatal mortality refers to infants aged one to eleven months.

Source: J. Rogers Hollingsworth, "Inequality in Levels of Health in England and Wales, 1891–1971," *Journal of Health and Social Behavior* 22 (1981): 277.

health status among classes continued to exist. The TUC demanded that efforts be made to reduce these inequalities. The RAWP report related the issue of equitable access to health care to the larger objective of reduction of health inequalities. But as the Radical Statistics Health Group (of the British Society for Social Responsibility in Science) observed, "Even if geographical variations were 'eliminated,' it does not follow that other variations would be."[13] Sir John Brotherston, chief medical officer of Scotland, called for action to reduce social differentials in health status as well as to improve Britain's overall health status. The United Kingdom had slipped from eighth to fifteenth in ranking of countries by infant mortality rate between 1960 and 1978. R.G. Wilkinson addressed a public letter to David Ennals, the secretary of state for social services, drawing attention to the large class differences in death rates. Ennals announced in a speech to the Socialist Medical Association in early 1977 that Sir Douglas Black, the chief scientist, would chair an inquiry into health inequalities. Other members of the Working Group on Inequalities in Health were Professor J.N. Morris, Department of Community Health at the London School of Hygiene; Dr. Cyril Smith, secretary of the Social Science Research Council; and Peter Townsend, professor of sociology at Essex University. Morris and Townsend, who had both worked with Titmuss, had considerable influence on the working group's thinking. Ideas that had been discussed in their publications were reflected in the recommendations made by the working group.

The Black group had been given the following tasks to carry out: to put together information on health status differences among social classes and on likely determining factors; to identify possible causal relationships and to assess policy implications; and to propose further research. There was little public discussion of the group's work during the life of the Callaghan Labor government. It would appear that it was seen officially as merely providing information for use within the Department of Health and Social Security (DHSS). But with Sir Douglas Black's retirement from his post of chief scientist at the DHSS and assumption of the presidency of the Royal College of Physicians, the group took a larger approach to its work. Redrafting and debate delayed the final presentation of the Black report until April 1980, after the fall of the Labor government.

As Charles Webster has pointed out, the report is a social science classic and may be seen as a more radical alternative to the contemporary report of the royal commission on the NHS, 1976–79, itself the first review of the health services since establishment of the NHS. The royal commission was concerned with "equality" of care within the health services; the Black report was concerned with "equality" in health status across society.[14] The Black report revealed that although the NHS, committed to equal access to care, had been functioning for over thirty years, notable differences existed in health status across social classes; for example, differences in mortality rates were such that "those in unskilled manual(labor) workers' families are four times more likely to die in their first year of life."[15]

The new secretary of state for social services in the Thatcher Conservative government, Patrick Jenkin, dismissing the public spending aspects of the report as "quite unrealistic in any present or foreseeable economic circumstances, quite apart from any judgement that may be formed on the effectiveness of such expenditure in dealing with the problems identified," did not endorse its recommendations.[16] He tried to restrict circulation of the report; only 260 duplicated copies were issued by the DHSS. Nonetheless, it was widely debated, and summaries were published by the TUC, in professional journals like *The Lancet,* and by public health workers. Two years later, a commercial publisher brought out an abbreviated version; it quickly turned into a best-seller. The Labor Party at its 1981 annual conference resolved that a Labor government should speedily implement the report's recommendations and that in the meantime Labor members of councils and health authorities should press for implementation of those with which local authorities could deal.

The Thatcher government continued to criticize the report. In spring 1981, Jenkin identified what he saw as the main defects: its inadequate explanation of the causes of health inequalities; failure to recognize the fact that lower-income groups obtain more NHS services than the average for the whole population; and that more spending on the NHS would not reduce health inequalities. In summer, the under secretary of state for health and social security, Sir George Young, repeated the first and last of these objections to the Black report, although he found the recommendations on prevention acceptable. The report's view of prevention, however, was considerably different from his, which focused on health education and individual responsibility for health. In 1985, the DHSS was still criticizing the reports: "The Government is not convinced that expenditure on the scale envisaged would necessarily be effective, even if it could be afforded."[17]

Although the Conservative government remained hostile in the 1980s, much research on inequalities, not infrequently underwritten by local authorities and voluntary bodies, was carried out. The WHO regional strategy of the mid-1980s had the effect of requiring the Thatcher government to deal with the question of inequalities again. But it responded to the WHO call for social equity in health in a narrow way—by identifying it only as geographical inequality in allocation of health service resources. Further controversy was stirred by the publication of the occupational mortality supplement to the 1981 census, for the data on social class were virtually restricted to the medium of microfiche so that the general reader would find them difficult of access. The reason given was that the data, particularly on social class V, were weak. But class differences might have been reliably mapped by combining classes I and II, and IV and V. Suspicion developed quite widely that the data had in effect been suppressed because they led to findings unattractive to the government. Public discussion of inequalities continued as more studies were published. In September 1986 a report, of which one of the authors was Peter Townsend, showed significant health inequalities between the electoral wards of the Northern Health Region.[18]

The Black group had found that lower social classes experienced poorer health at every stage of the life cycle. In 1970–72, if classes IV and V had had the death rates of class I, the deaths of seventy-four thousand people under seventy-five years would not have occurred. In the two decades to 1972, death rates of men and women thirty-five years and older in classes I and II had fallen, but the rates of those in classes IV and V had hardly changed, and in some cases had become worse. Social and economic factors outside health policy and mostly beyond the health care system's reach were responsible for the class gradient—income, unemployment, education, housing, transportation and lifestyle behavior. In any case, the members of the manual (labor) classes, who had greater need, used the health care system less. Among its proposals to remedy the situation, the group placed great importance on bettering the living standards of low-income people—a redistribution of economic resources to the poor—through such cash benefits as child, maternity and infant-care payments and a disability allowance, as well as development of antenatal clinics, day nurseries, better working conditions, community services and housing. It also emphasized greater development within the health services of prevention, primary care and community health work. In effect, it called for two areas of policy to be pursued: a "total and not merely a service-oriented approach" to health, and a "radical overhaul of the balance of activity" in health and community services.[19]

The group was careful not to make excessive claims for its analysis of the causes of inequalities, because insufficient research had been done. But it was firm in stating that material deprivation was a key factor, and it based its remedial action on that premise. Intellectual critics of the Black report attacked it on various grounds. First, social class V over time contained a declining percentage of the working population and so could not be used for comparative purposes. But for this reason the group had aggregated classes I and II, on the one hand, and classes IV and V, on the other, when comparing mortality rates. The result of the comparison for the two decades from the early 1950s was that for seven of eight ten-year age groups into which adults were divided, the class differences were clear. Second, it was objected that the nonworking population had not been dealt with by the Black group. But the report covered all population age groups—children, nonworking adults and the aged. Third, critics asserted that the report ignored the role of selective social mobility—the healthy are upwardly mobile, the unhealthy downwardly so—as a cause of class differences. However, the report acknowledged that cultural and genetic factors contributed. There was no "single or simple explanation of the complex data," but "we wish to stress the importance of differences in material conditions of life."[20] Subsequent investigations tended to support the view that factors related to social mobility "make only minor contributions to the observed class differences in health, and there is no evidence that their influence has increased."[21]

The time lag in production of official statistics had obliged the Black group to use much data from the early 1970s. What was happening to health inequalities in the 1980s needed to be investigated. In January 1986, David Player, director-general of the Health Education Council (HEC), engaged Margaret Whitehead to, first, review evidence on inequalities since 1980 and, second, comment on progress with the recommendations of the Black report. This was one of three major reviews commissioned, other two being a review of child health services over the decade since the Court report, and a review of progress with prevention since the 1976 DHSS report *Prevention and Health*. The three were seen to be concerned with themes central to health promotion, the primary responsibility of the HEC.

The Whitehead report, *The Health Divide,* appeared in March 1987. The Thatcher government's reaction was similar to its response to the Black report. Copies of the report had gone to regional and district health authorities, community health councils, and the academic and popular press. A panel of experts, including Sir Douglas Black and Professor Townsend, were scheduled to answer questions concerning the new report at a media briefing. But the chairman of the HEC, Sir Brian Bailey, canceled the briefing at short notice, stating that the full council would need to consider the "possibly controversial document." The panel went ahead with the briefing at another location.

The report elicited great media interest. Claims were made that the DHSS had urged the HEC chairman to cancel the briefing—claims, of course, denied by the department and the government. Government ministers responded to questions about action to correct inequalities by pointing to increased life expectancy and lower infant mortality. The issue of health inequalities received a good deal of attention in the two houses of Parliament. It was pointed out that inequality might increase even as general progress in health was achieved. As one peer noted, "Just as the gap between the richest and the poorest has increased within an overall increased national income[,] . . . so health inequalities have increased. . . . It is all part of the same pattern."[22]

The Health Divide showed that in the 1980s, whether the indicator of social class was occupation, house and car ownership or employment status, those in the lowest classes experienced much higher mortality rates. This social class inequality existed at each stage of life from birth to old age. Sickness rates were likewise patterned. Geographical inequalities also existed. Mortality was greatest in Scotland, and in descending order, the north and northwest of England, and the southeast and East Anglia. Further, inequalities existed within regions.

The study confirmed the claims of the Black group that inequalities among working age adults had increased from the 1950s. In 1971–81, nonmanual groups experienced a considerably greater mortality decline than manual (labor) ones. Semiskilled and unskilled manual (labor) groups used preventive services less than did professional and managerial ones, although they consulted general practitioners more. While some downward social mobility resulted from ill health, it alone did not account for the inequalities, which arose from lifestyle and living-condition differences. Since socioeconomic conditions influenced health-related behavior, policy had to allow for this rather than focusing on individual choice and responsibility alone. No policy action concerning the Black report proposals had been taken. Homelessness and the number of children in poverty had grown. Housing remained in short supply, and much of the stock of housing was in need of repair. On the positive side, local authorities were showing a new interest in public health, and many professional bodies had begun to demonstrate concern about health inequalities. Finally, the WHO Health for All strategy, with its devotion to equity in health, might be expected to keep the question of inequalities in the field of vision of future governments.[23]

Some social scientists, notably Raymond Illsley and Julian Le Grand, doubted the claim that the health divide had grown over time. They objected to use of occupation as indicator of living standard over time, because some occupations were allocated to different classes in the official statistics and because manual occupations had proportionally decreased, so that simply comparing classes I and V might give unreliable results. But *The Heath Divide* discussed research that allowed for these problems by looking at inequalities across all classes and weighting each class by its share of the population. Also, only occupations that could be consistently monitored across time were followed. Employing such approaches, researchers still found that the health gap had grown in 1931–71 and also in the period 1971–72 to 1979–83, when the gap between manual and nonmanual increased. A 4 percent movement in people from manual to nonmanual occupations, as well as changes in occupational classifications, failed to explain the growing inequality.

Illsley and Le Grand also criticized the focus on the population under sixty-five years, because in the period since the 1930s the proportion of deaths in this age group had declined. But further research showed that inequality also exists for the population aged between sixty-five and seventy-five years. The deaths under sixty-five, moreover, are important because most are preventible. Critics showed that variation in the age at death for the population as a whole had decreased. Some in the media wrongly interpreted this to mean that social class inequalities had declined, when it merely showed variation in the age at death of individuals had declined. Because since the 1920s the great child mortality from infections and respiratory diseases (falling mostly on the poor) had disappeared, variation in the age at death had decreased. Even so, contemporary degenerative diseases (killing in middle and old age) also fell disproportionately on the poor.[24]

Social-class differences in mortality continued to exist in the 1990s. For male, all-cause mortality in England and Wales, 1991–93, the gradient was as follows: class I, just under three hundred per hundred thousand men aged twenty to sixty-four years; class II, three hundred per hundred thousand; class III (nonmanual), just over four hundred per hundred thousand; class III (manual) and class IV, five hundred per hundred thousand; and class V, over eight hundred per hundred thousand.[25]

It was widely expected that with the coming to power of the Blair Labor government at the close of the 1990s, the issue of social inequalities of health would be directly addressed. Certainly, the Blair government in July 1999 issued a white paper, "Saving Lives: Our Healthier Nation," on how it proposed to "promote healthier living and reduce inequality in health." Called the first comprehensive government plan to attack the "main killers" (cancer, coronary heart disease and stroke, accidents and mental illness), the program involved the reduction by 2010 of the death rate: from cancer in those under seventy-five years by at least 20 percent; from coronary heart disease and stroke in the same population by at least 40 percent; from accidents by at least 20 percent, from serious injury by at least 10 percent; and from suicide and undetermined injury by at least 20 percent.

The new government listed a number of specific commitments to achieve these targets: twenty-one billion pounds for the NHS; reducing smoking as the single most preventible cause of ill health; integrating national and local government in health improvement; stressing health improvement as a key function of the NHS and pushing for high health standards for all the population. It would provide "healthy citizen" programs to encourage individuals and families to be more physically active, eat a healthier diet, and give up smoking. It specifically acknowledged that health inequality was widespread, whereas the Conservative government's "Health of the Nation" had failed to do so. Labour's "Saving Lives" promised that a range of initiatives in education, welfare-to-work, housing, transportation, and the environment would reduce inequality. For the first time, the NHS would ensure that health improvement was integrated into the local delivery of health care, with local authorities as partners in the planning of "health action zones" to end barriers in service provision and of "healthy living centers" to offer assistance in pursuing better health. To support health promotion, the Labour government promised to create a Health Development Agency, a statutory body that would advance the quality of public health provision; a skills audit and workforce-development plan to promote training for health professionals; public health "observatories" in each NHS region and disease registers to improve public health information and promote research; and a new Public Health Development Fund.[26]

However, as Professor Townsend noted when addressing a Public Health Association meeting in Australia, there was virtually no discussion in the white paper of the increasing inequality of income or of measures to raise the inadequate incomes of the poor, especially through social security benefits. While the Blair government was giving much more attention to health inequalities than preceding governments, serious questions remained unanswered about adequate incomes for the millions of unemployed and social security beneficiaries. The structural trends (as well as the effect of major policies) year to year needed urgently to be documented.[27] Reviewing international trends in economic inequality—those in Australia, Canada, Japan, New Zealand and the United States, as well as the countries of Western Europe—one expert observed that "the UK stands out for the sharpness of the rise in recorded income inequality in the second half of the 1980s" and that "this was unparalleled in the countries examined."[28]

Given the strength of Labour's commitment in opposition in the 1990s to reducing inequality, it was rather slow once in office to act to alleviate health inequalities. It decided to set up yet another inquiry into inequalities in health and to take no proper action until the inquiry had finished its work. Established in July 1997 and chaired by Sir Donald Acheson, a former chief medical officer, the inquiry published its report in November 1998. Its findings contributed to the development of the white paper "Saving Lives." The inquiry made thirty-nine recommendations—some "upstream" proposals relating to income, education and housing, and others "downstream," narrower in nature, such as promoting physical exercise. Unfortunately, since these recommendations were not prioritized, the importance of poverty as a determinant of health was somewhat obscured. In an attempt to provide some prioritization, Acheson identified the following recommendations as crucial: that all policies likely to affect health be evaluated for their impact on health; that families with children be given high priority; and that further efforts be made to improve the living standards of poor households. Implementation of recommendations, even when accepted, was not going to be speedy. From the outset, the government required the inquiry's recommendations to fit within the framework of its overall financial strategy. That strategy in its first two years of office was one of constraint on spending, in order to win the confidence of financial markets at home and abroad.

Health action zones (HAZs) had been identified by the Labour government as a key method for tackling health inequalities. Yet the first eleven were established only in April 1998. The amount to be spent on them was small—four million pounds in 1998–99. In any case, area-based (as opposed to people-based) policy has been shown to enjoy at best limited success in reducing health inequalities and poverty. This is because most "poor areas" contain a large number of "nonpoor" households. Poverty is not neatly distributed. Moreover, the success of HAZs depends critically on a high level of local expertise and enthusiasm. These will not be distributed at a high level across all HAZs.[29]

Morbidity and mortality rates are higher in the poorer classes of other economically developed countries. In the United States, analysis of a national sample of deaths in 1986 found that the age-adjusted mortality ratio of white males of the lowest educational level was over two and a half times greater than the ratio for those of the highest educational level. In Australia in the early 1990s, children with unemployed parents were 25 percent more likely to suffer from serious, chronic illness than children with at least one parent in paid employment. In Norway in a 1983 survey of adults twenty-five to sixty-six years, twice as many women in unskilled occupations suffered from cardiovascular disease as did professionals, and the proportion of unskilled men with chronic disease was 1.4 times that of those with high-status employment. A 1983 national morbidity survey in Italy revealed such health inequalities as that 25.7 percent of people with elementary education said their health was not good, where only 12.3 percent of the university-educated reported this. A 1984 French study using longitudinal mortality data found that unskilled males, forty-five to forty-nine years, experienced death rates four times greater than rates of those in high-status occupations. Examples could be multiplied from other economically developed countries.[30]

Unlike in the United Kingdom, vital statistics in the United States have not been routinely reported in terms of socioeconomic stratification; they have been stratified only by age, gender and race. Yet in the early twentieth century, a tradition of public health research on health in relation to economic status was initiated. The U.S. Public Health Service developed concern about the relation between working conditions and health after the introduction of workers' compensation laws in 1911. If national health insurance was to be introduced, information on the relative risks of illness of various subpopulations would be needed. In 1914, B.S. Warren and Edgar Sydenstricker collected data on the health of three thousand white, married garment workers and their families—garment workers were low-wage earners. Warren and Sydenstricker divided the study population in terms of annual income of the household head and found that health varied noticeably even with small differences in income. Thus, the poorest families had child mortality of 21 percent, whereas slightly more prosperous families suffered mortality of 12 percent.

Soon after, Sydenstricker joined Joseph Goldberger and G.A. Wheeler in a study of the aetiology of pellagra in southern millworkers. Earlier work pointed to pellagra's association with poverty, although whether the condition arose from infection or deficient diet was unclear. In order to test their hypothesis that it arose from diet, the researchers studied the quantity and type of food consumed by mill families. Family income was not a sensitive enough index of economic well-being, so Sydenstricker devised a single economic unit (based on adult male food consumption) in terms of which the requirements of other family members could be expressed, thus allowing for different sizes and compositions of families in relation to income. He also devised a more general unit based on the total cost of adult male maintenance. Sydenstricker carried out in 1921–24 a study of morbidity in an urban population—that of Hagerstown, Maryland. This involved data on the health and economic conditions of more than 7,200 white family members. The British remained convinced, however, of the superiority of the social class method over the Americans' income-status method, as T.H.C. Stevenson made clear. He suggested that income alone may not be a good guide to culture (education), which may independently influence mortality, as shown in the case of the clergy: "The income test . . . would certainly place them well down the list, yet their mortality is remarkably low. . . . But culture is more easily estimated as between occupations, than wealth, so the occupational basis of social grading has a wholesome tendency to emphasize it."[31]

The U.S. Children's Bureau, established in 1912 as a Department of Labor agency, carried out an eight-city study of infant mortality. The study revealed that the gap in mortality between the highest and lowest-income groups was considerable—64.3 per thousand births for those with annual incomes greater than $1,250, and 151.4 for those with $550 a year. The authors of the study concluded that the connection between income and infant mortality was independent of factors like race and nationality, breast or artificial feeding and frequency of births. Low income (plus intermediate factors like mother's employment, population density in housing and availability of health care) produced high infant mortality. While they recommended free antenatal and confinement care, infant clinics, sanitation and public housing, the bureau's researchers argued that a decent income was the best protection against a high infant death rate.

The National Tuberculosis Association, an influential voluntary health body, required data on mortality by occupation to mount TB control programs in workplace environments. The association sponsored a study by Jessamine S. Whitney in the late 1920s to provide for the first time mortality rates by occupation based on census figures. As a preliminary exercise, Whitney checked more than fifty-three thousand death certificates from a number of states to establish how adequate their information on occupation was. Whitney was enabled by the director of the census to work with the 1930 census data. Her final report included data for crude and age-standardized death rates of seven socioeconomic groups, fifty-three occupations, and seventeen causes of death; the age-standardized death rate of the total population—fourteen million men and 122,000 deaths—was 8.7 per thousand men. Four socioeconomic groups had lower rates: professionals, 7.0; proprietors, managers and officials, 7.4; clerks, 7.4; and agricultural workers, 6.2. The rates of three other groups were: skilled workers, 8.1; semiskilled, 9.9; and unskilled, 13.1. The highest rate was more than twice the lowest.

Against Sydenstricker and other Public Health Service researchers, Whitney also demonstrated that both the specific dangers of a given occupation and level of income were significant. For TB, the age-standardized mortality rate was 87.5 per hundred thousand men. But the range across and within occupational groupings was wide: 26.2 for professionals (but from 18.3 for lawyers to 30.7 for technical engineers); 43.2 for proprietors, managers and officials (but from 19.3 for bankers and brokers to 81.2 for restaurant employees); 65.8 for clerks (but from 28.4 for real estate agents to 97.9 for clerks); 46.5 for agricultural workers; 72.1 for skilled workers (from 34.6 for foremen in manufacturing to 143.3 for metal workers); 102.1 for semiskilled workers (from 91.9 for laborers not working in factories or construction to 227.3 for laborers in such industries).

Arguing that the effects of the economic depression of the 1930s were better reflected in disease prevalence than mortality, Public Health Service researchers undertook large-scale studies of morbidity by socioeconomic group. In 1935, the first National Health Survey was initiated. In it the health of 2.5 million people (white and "colored") in eighty-three cities was monitored for one year. Morbidity in relation to income and other social and economic conditions was mapped. The reports highlighted the significant role of socioeconomic factors in health status. However, by 1938, when the first analyses from the survey were published, the political climate was changing, as World War II loomed and conservatism began to replace New Deal reformism. Also, a generation of progressive researchers was dying. By the late 1940s, Cold War ideological constraints ended the concern with socioeconomic influences on health status. Tellingly, a 1943 report on vital statistics for the Bureau of the Census recommended the basic categories in which statistics be gathered as "age, sex and race," leaving it to special studies to examine the role of other factors like occupation. In 1948, the distinguished public health figure C-E.A.Winslow called, in an address on poverty and health, for health officials to consider seriously the effect of poverty—experienced by almost one-third of the population—on morbidity and mortality. He had no illusions about the contemporary ideological climate: "Even in an A.P.H.A. [American Public Health Association] audience I strongly suspect that there are those who are now saying to themselves, 'Why, this fellow is a Socialist! Or a Communist!'"[32] It was to be some years before health inequalities and the relationship between health status and race, gender, and income began to be seriously explored again.[33]

In 1973, E.M. Kitagawa and P.M. Hauser published a nationwide study of differential mortality in the United States. This showed that for males and females aged twenty-five to sixty-four years, death rates differed notably according to educational level, income, and occupation. Thus, the age-adjusted death rates of white males of low educational attainment were 64 percent greater than those of males with higher educational levels. For white females, the figure was 105 percent, while for nonwhite males and females, it was 31 and 70 percent respectively. Further, white males with the poorest education had higher mortality rates for every death cause where data was forthcoming, and white females of the same educational level experienced excess mortality for all causes other than breast cancer and motor vehicle accidents.[34]

In 1976, around a half of people aged forty-five to sixty-four years having family incomes below five thousand dollars were limited in their activities by chronic disability, but only around a sixth of the population with incomes of fifteen thousand dollars or more were so limited. In a similar fashion, those with low family incomes and aged forty-five to sixty-four years experienced more than three times as many bed-disability days per person as people with higher incomes—nineteen days compared with six days.[35] Essential hypertension (chronic high blood pressure) affected more than fifty million Americans by the 1970s. Studies of prevalence consistently revealed that hypertension increased with age for both black and white Americans. Similarly, for both men and women, it increased with age, but after forty-five years it was greater for women (black and white). The national prevalence by age and race in 1974 was as shown in table 5.5.

A gradual trend toward income equality had prevailed in the United States from the 1950s to the late 1960s. However, this was reversed by the early 1980s. In 1985, the top 20 percent of the population received 43.5 percent of national income (which was the highest level reached since 1947), whereas the bottom 60 percent received 32.4 percent. A national survey in 1984 found that one in five adults could not always afford food for the family. The Physician Task Force on Hunger in America found that twelve million children and eight million adults experienced hunger, to a large extent as a result of federal welfare cuts.[36]

In 1983–89, 66 percent of the total gain in net financial wealth in the United States went to the top 1 percent of the population and 37 percent to the next 19 percent, while the bottom 80 percent lost 3 percent. This trend toward greater inequality in distribution of wealth appears to have been associated with various adverse health outcomes.

R.G. Wilkinson has shown that in a number of industrialized nations, life expectancy is not well correlated with average income but that life expectancy increases as the income distribution becomes more egalitarian. He proposed that not only absolute income level but relative socioeconomic status may significantly influence health. This may account for the persistence of gradients in risk (so that even people high in socioeconomic status, but not at the top, have higher disease rates than people at the top) despite average incomes well above absolute poverty. Michael Marmot's study of ten thousand British civil servants revealed that over ten years, for men forty to sixty-four years, mortality in the clerical and manual (lowest) grades was about three and a half times as great as in the senior administrative (highest) grades. A mortality gradient thus paralleled the civil service hierarchy, with mortality increasing as one proceeded down the grades. Since no grade lived at the

Table 5.5
Hypertension, Prevalence per 100, by Age and Ethnic Group, United States, 1974

Age	All persons 17 years and over	White	Black
All 17 years and over	16.8	16.0	24.1
17 to 24 years	4.2	4.1	5.3
25 to 44 years	9.5	8.6	17.9
45 to 64 years	24.2	22.7	39.1
65 years and over	36.3	35.3	47.2

Source: P.L. Schnall and R. Kern, "Hypertension in American Society: An Introduction to Historical Materialist Epidemiology," in *The Sociology of Health and Illness: Critical Perspectives,* ed. P. Conrad and R. Kern (New York: St. Martin's Press, 1986), 84.

poverty level, absolute poverty could not be invoked to explain differentials, though marked income differences existed between the higher and lower grades. The mortality gradient existed in a number of conditions, some of which related to smoking. Even so, those in the top rank who smoked were much less at risk of death from smoking-related conditions. Marmot suggested that some general process connected with the existence of the occupational hierarchy might be operating to produce the differentials in health status. Primate (animal) studies have shown that rank in social hierarchies related to capacity to deal with stress (prolonged stress results in various illnesses). It is not clear, however, whether the higher mortality of Marmot's lower-rank civil servants was the result of more stress or the fact that they were less capable of dealing with stress, of their having less supportive work and domestic environments, or of their lower incomes. The four may well interact.

A study of the relation between income distribution variations among the fifty states of the United States in 1990 and variation in health outcomes, including variations in age-adjusted mortalities, found a similar pattern of substantial correlation between inequality of income distribution and adverse health outcome—a significant correlation ($r = 0.62$) between the proportion of total household income going to the less-well-off 50 percent of households and variations in death rates between the states. In the decade 1980–90, states that were more unequal in income distribution also experienced smaller falls in mortality.

Income inequality was associated with a number of other health outcomes. The strongest correlations existed with rate of homicide ($r = 0.74$) and violent crime ($r = 0.70$), per capita expenditure on medical care ($r = 0.67$), and percentage of live-born infants weighing less than 2,500 grams ($r = 0.65$). Further, states with greater inequality in income distribution experienced much higher rates of smoking, sedentary behavior, and disability, as well as larger per capita expenditure on police protection. While further studies of the association between variations in income distribution within a single country and health outcomes are needed, this study seems to suggest that, at the least, it would be advisable when the impact of economic policies is assessed to take into account the effects on health and associated costs.[37]

In this era of speedy economic and technological change and structural transformation of the global workforce, economic inequality within developed countries has grown. At the same time, internal migration and migration between countries has changed the ethnic mix of urban and rural areas, at a time when the structures of families and gender roles themselves are changing. Scholarly research in the United States on social inequalities has focused on individual status and "life chances." This has limited the capacity of resulting models to explain increasing health inequalities. A more structural approach, one that recognizes income inequality as a property of the population, not the individual, appears to be needed, even though it is still necessary to identify the behavioral, psychosocial and biological pathways through which inequality of income impacts on the health of individuals.

Widespread concern among American researchers about these questions led to the convening in 1994 of a conference on measuring social inequalities in health. Sponsored by the U.S. Public Health Service and the National Institutes of Health (NIH), the conference pursued four objectives: improvement of means for evaluating socioeconomic gradients in health; creation of measures to be used in federal data sets; clarification of the relationship of race/ethnicity, gender and age to social class, in order to modify measures in an appropriate way; and provision to researchers of a basis for implementing NIH guidelines on inclusion of women and minorities in research, as well as of familiarization with recommendations concerning taking into account the socioeconomic composition of study populations. While the conference was intended to improve data collection and analysis in the United States, the hope was that it might also help promote debate in other countries.[38]

AUSTRALIA

In 1990, life expectancy at birth for Australian women was eighty years, while that for men was 73.9 years. This put Australia ahead of the United Kingdom, the United States and New Zealand. Infant mortality was 8.2 deaths per thousand live births, a figure comparable to that of countries like the United Kingdom and Norway. Indeed, the Australian population is undoubtedly one of the most healthy on earth. Yet it also has notable inequalities in health status between population subgroups. The most notable is that between Aborigines and the Australian population as a whole; Aboriginal life expectancy at birth is fifteen to seventeen years less than that of the population as a whole, while infant mortality is three times the national figure. The contrast in adult mortality is most marked in individuals thirty-five to forty-four years of age. The death rate of Aboriginal men is over eleven times that of the total Australian male population, and that of Aboriginal women is about nine times that of the total female population.[39] The health inequality results from social and economic disadvantages that historically arose from the dispossession of indigenous Australians from the land and from the destruction of Aboriginal society.

In *The People's Health*, volume 1, we traced the fate of Aborigines in nineteenth century Australia. By the turn of the century, it was widely assumed even by governments that Aborigines were a dying race. The widely read *Bulletin* had observed in the 1880s: "The 'civilised black' . . . is a wretched creature. He is madly fond of drink. . . . He coughs, and everyone perceives he is in consumption. . . . In Victoria his case is not better. . . . In the south of Queensland the average blackfellow is just as depraved and miserable as in New South Wales."[40]

By World War I, all the mainland states had brought in legislation based on principles of protection and control. Where the "settled" states were mainly concerned with people of part-Aboriginal descent, the "frontier" states (Queensland, Western Australia and South Australia) and the Northern Territory introduced protective legislation for those of full Aboriginal descent but not so as to deprive European employers of their labor, without which the far-flung cattle and other enterprises could not have functioned. The Queensland Aborigines Protection and Restriction of the Sale of Opium Act, 1897, became the model for legislation applying in Western Australia (1905), the Northern Territory (1910) and South Australia (1911).

In the 1960s a new Aboriginal self-consciousness emerged, along with a resurgent activism. A growing number of non-Aboriginals supported the movement. The Federal Council for the Advancement of Aborigines and Torres Strait Islanders (FCAATSI) played a significant role in the campaign preceding the successful constitutional referendum of 1967 that endowed the commonwealth with power (concurrent with that of the states) to legislate for Aborigines and to count them in the national census. The referendum was to change the Aboriginal struggle from one for civil rights to one focused on autonomy. Indeed, only a few years later community-based Aboriginal bodies concerned with health care and legal services were set up. In 1965, a "Freedom Ride" through NSW country towns was organized by students from the University of Sydney—including one Aboriginal student, Charles Perkins—to bring attention to segregation of services and the poor living conditions experienced by Aborigines. The sight of Perkins confronting European officials inspired a new generation of militants.

In 1965, also, the Gurindji people's claims to their traditional land at Wattie Creek in the Northern Territory after leaving Wave Hill Station, a pastoral lease controlled by the wealthy Vestey family, evoked national non-Aboriginal support for the quest for land rights. Four years later, when the Yirrkala people objected to the commonwealth government's allowing the Nabalco Corporation to mine bauxite on their land without consultation, the struggle for land rights intensified. By the end of the 1960s, the longtime demand for equality with non-Aboriginals was being modified by the claim to recognition of the distinctiveness of Aborigines. The FCAASI had in 1966 included in its objectives the claim to recognition of Aboriginal and Islander people as "distinct cultural groups." Indeed, the reforming Whitlam federal Labor government, which came to office in 1972, was to make "self determination" central to federal policy, while at the same time doubling spending on Aboriginal programs. Understanding that governments are vulnerable to international criticism concerning approaches to colonized peoples, the Aboriginal movement from the 1970s resorted to the "politics of embarrassment" in international forums. It pursued strategies in the international as well as the domestic sphere, with visits overseas to seek support, including trips by left-wing activists to China and Libya.

The states with larger Aboriginal populations differed in the speed with which they had moved away from a control policy. In Queensland by the 1920s, when it had become clear that Aborigines and Islanders were not dying out, the Chief Protector of Aborigines, J.W. Bleakley, developed a new policy, the final goal of which was assimilation of Aboriginal people into the general population. The 1965 Aborigines and Torres Strait Islanders Affairs Act provided for various rights enshrined in the assimilation legislation of other states, but in other ways it continued the established policy of departmental control. With the 1965 act due to be renewed in 1971, Liberal-Country Party prime minister, William McMahon, and the Queensland Country Party premier, Johannes Bjelke-Petersen, agreed on the major elements of new legislation, including freedom to move off reserves, Aboriginal control of personal property and transactions, and more autonomy for reserve councils. But the 1971 act in the event included only some of the agreed objectives. With the act to expire again in 1977, an Aboriginal and Islander Commission was created to review matters. The federal minister for Aboriginal affairs called for full Aboriginal authority over reserves, full capacity to negotiate mining agreements, and vesting of titles to reserves in trusts. The commission report ignored such enlightened proposals, endorsing the established policy of assimilation and opting for gradual legislative advance. Premier Bjelke-Petersen indicated that land rights would not be forthcoming. The Land Act of 1982 made former reserve lands the subject of deeds of grant in trust. However, grants could be revoked by the state government and trusteeship of a community council removed.[41]

Western Australia was another "frontier" colony with a large Aboriginal population. Since the 1890s, when the colony had taken over Aboriginal affairs from the Colonial Office in London, the chief protector and his staff had exercised autocratic authority over Aborigines. In the 1950s, the Hawke state Labor government ended many controls on employment and the right to marry. In the 1960s, further liberalization took place. In 1971, the Tonkin government dismantled most of the remaining restrictions, including those still applying to liquor consumption. In mid-1974, the Western Australian Aboriginal Affairs Planning Authority was absorbed into the new federal Department of Aboriginal Affairs. The Whitlam government raised federal spending on Aborigines in the state from $2.5 million in 1971–72 to almost seventeen million dollars in 1974–75, although race relations in both the northwest and the southwest worsened, in part because of resentment about the improved funding of Aboriginal communities.

In the Northern Territory by the 1920s, the problems were no longer those of first contact but of how to preserve surviving Aboriginal populations. Under pressure from voluntary bodies concerned with Aboriginal welfare and from Christian missions, the commonwealth government called conferences involving such groups, as well as pastoralists (ranchers) and the Home Affairs Department, in 1929 and again in 1930. The main result was that policy became more protective and more restrictive. The Aboriginals Ordinance of 1933 retained penalties for miscegenation and made drinking or possession of alcohol an offense for Aborigines and "half-castes." The ordinance of 1936 provided for punishments for Aborigines and "half-castes" found on licensed premises, for suppliers of liquor, and for Aborigines caught drinking. An employer found to have had sexual intercourse with an Aboriginal woman might have his licence to employ Aborigines withdrawn.

The 1930s saw a new perspective in Aboriginal policy emerge, as more extensive anthropological knowledge and the obvious fact that the part-Aboriginal population was rapidly increasing finally overcame the long-existing view that the Aboriginal race would become extinct. In 1939 the federal interior minister, John McEwen, said that there would be a "New Deal" for Aborigines under federal control. World War II cut across this policy initiative, but it also promoted social change. With European labor limited, hundreds of Aborigines were employed as laborers by the armed services. The territory administration was impressed by the achievements of this corps of Aboriginal workers. The issue for Aborigines was no longer survival but equality of rights (as it would later be distinctiveness).

The Whitlam era of the early 1970s was to speed up this long, painful process. Various representative bodies—land councils, legal aid services, the Central Australian Aboriginal Congress and the National Aboriginal Congress—increased pressure for the granting of land rights. However, from 1974, the anti-Labor Country-Liberal Party (CLP) controlled the territory's Legislative Assembly. From 1978, when the Northern Territory gained almost full independence from the federal government, the CLP occupied the government benches. Aboriginal land claims became occasions for confrontation between the government and land councils.[42]

The Health of, and Health Services for, Aborigines

As in other Western colonies, the full benefits of Western medicine were not available to the Aborigines, as colonized people. Those working in the European economy were more likely to obtain medical treatment, because they had value to settlers and because they had a point of entry to the health care system.[43] Sick Aborigines in early-twentieth-century Western Australia who were not under contract to white employers were supposed to receive the same charitable treatment as provided for indigent whites. Few Aborigines were under contract, and most employers were lax about provision of health care. There was a continual tussle among the state Medical Department, the Aborigines Department, and pastoralists about who was responsible for paying for care. The Onslow District medical officer, Dr. Edwin Gurdon, in the 1900s refused to treat Aborigines for syphilis, which was believed to be rife on the frontier, because he was not paid for medicines and because they would not stay in contact for the two years of unpleasant mercury treatment considered necessary for a cure at that time. After 1915, when Western Australia (and other states) received federal funding—the first ever for national health services—to support free public treatment facilities for VD, Aborigines were excluded. J.H.L. Cumpston, federal director of quarantine and from 1921 founding commonwealth director general of health, told the chief protector that the "authorities had given no thought to Aborigines; they are not included in the scheme."[44]

When in 1910 the Australian Institute of Tropical Medicine—the first full-time medical research institute in Australia—was established by the commonwealth in Townsville, Queensland, its primary purpose was to help ensure the health of whites living in the tropics was preserved. The aim of policy was to quarantine, and where possible exclude, nonwhites, who were perceived as the carriers of threatening diseases. The institute's responsibilities were laid down thus:

> From the earliest days of colonisation European diseases were introduced in quantity among the early settlers; various tropical diseases were introduced by the Kanakas from the islands of the Pacific; and by the hordes of Chinese and other Asiatics that poured in before the days of Federation. . . . Three sets of disease conditions consequently present themselves for control: (1) those introduced from European countries; (2) those introduced from neighbouring tropical lands; (3) those indigenous to the country.[45]

Aborigines in Western Australia and Queensland suffering from VD were quarantined in special lock hospitals. In 1908, islands bordering Shark Bay, thirty miles from Carnarvon in Western Australia, were designated sites for lock hospitals. Until 1918, Aborigines with VD from all over the western, northwest, eastern and Kimberley divisions of this vast state were sent, forcibly if necessary, to the island hospitals, where they were detained for periods of one to twenty months for treatment, in some cases up to three years. In 1918, the inmates were removed to Port Hedland on the mainland, but the penal approach continued in this institution. In 1914, Fitzroy Island, off Cairns in Northern Queensland, was chosen as the site for a lock hospital for Aborigines from all over that state. But the coming of World War I halted progress with the proposal. After the war, cases were taken to Fantome Island Lock Hospital, from which discharges were few, because treatments were rarely successful.

Country hospitals and mission stations continued to provide treatment locally. In 1930, the Australian Board of Missions employed a venereologist at the Mitchell River mission. The next year the Hookworm Control Campaign Committee allowed its medical staff to survey Aborigines for VD and leprosy. In 1932, R.W. (later Sir Raphael) Cilento, director of tropical hygiene in the Federal Health Department, carried out a survey of Aboriginal camps between Townsville and Cairns on the Queensland coast and on the Atherton Tableland. He called for legislative control of the "crossbreed and alien coloured elements" living with Aborigines, because they spread "disease and vice." The following year he surveyed the health of Aborigines in the north of the state—in the districts of the Daintree River and Bloomfield River, Cooktown, Laura, Point Stewart, Coen and on missions at Cape Bedford, Lockhart River and Yarrabah. He discovered widespread food and vitamin deficiencies. He believed these were responsible for female sterility, infant mortality and susceptibility to respiratory infections.[46]

Except for valued workers like stockmen and female domestics, who received the same medical care—often rough-and-ready bush medicine—as whites, the central purpose of Aboriginal "services" in the Northern Territory was to protect Europeans from what were seen as "native diseases," especially VD, leprosy and TB (even though Europeans, Chinese or Macassans would have introduced the diseases). The main means of protection was segregation, by outlawing relations between white men and black women and by social "banishment" of town Aborigines to squalid fringe camps. During epidemics, the common procedure was to force Aborigines to leave town or, in Darwin, confine them to the Kahlin Compound. If necessary, diseased Aborigines could be forcibly detained for treatment. Restrictions applied as well to white sufferers of infectious disease, but they usually could obtain their own treatment. During the 1930 measles epidemic, Europeans hardly observed advice to keep children at home, but Aborigines were detained at the Kahlin Compound.[47]

When Port Darwin was occupied by Europeans in 1869, the area was very probably free of malaria, leprosy, tuberculosis and VD. The author of a modern study of tribal Aborigines in Arnhem Land in the 1970s has proposed that Aborigines in the immediate precontact period were "a healthy population capable of maintaining a fair degree of individual health," being free of severe respiratory complaints, heart disease, cancers, leprosy, malaria and VD, and having low blood-cholesterol levels.[48] The first reports detailing Aboriginal health were made in 1911 by M.J. Holmes and R.S. Burston, medical officers to the Aboriginal Department. They saw only small numbers (a total of perhaps fifty) in the Daly River area. The Aborigines were "well-nourished and of good physique," although syphilis and tuberculosis had already invaded the group. The practice of abortion by external manipulation of the abdomen, encouraged by the local Chinese, was resulting in widespread female sterility and ill health. In 1912, W. Baldwin Spencer, newly appointed chief protector of Aborigines, reported the same practice, observing that there was "wholesale prostitution" of urban Aboriginal women to "Asiatics" in return for opium and spirits. The administrator of the Northern Territory reported the next year that VD was prevalent among Europeans, Asians and Aborigines. Ulcerative granuloma, a venereal disease, appeared to be distributed among Aborigines all over the territory; sufferers from widely different areas were treated in Darwin after their despatch by local protectors (police were ex officio protectors).

In 1924, the chief health officer said that granuloma was far more common than syphilis or gonorrhea at the Kahlin Beach clinic in Darwin. Granuloma and gonorrhea cases remained a notable percentage of total cases treated at the Kahlin Beach Compound Aboriginal Hospital in the 1930s. Cecil Cook, territory chief medical officer, decided in 1937, in the face of the likely arrival of large numbers of troops as war clouds loomed, to reduce the risk of VD in Darwin by isolating forty infected mixed-race women in the quarantine station, a move reluctantly accepted by Cumpston, who feared adverse media coverage. By late 1938, the women were relocated to two isolation units built on the site of the new Darwin general hospital, itself on the site of the now-defunct Kahlin Beach Aboriginal Compound. Cook had moved Aborigines and mixed-race children to a new compound (to include a new Aboriginal hospital) at Bagot, outside the town. By 1940 with the arrival of military forces and a resulting acute shortage of accommodation, Aborigines were removed from the Bagot Compound and either repatriated to their home areas or sent to a new settlement across the harbor at Delissaville. Some men continued to work in Darwin, but all the women were moved out of the town.[49]

In 1919–20, Dr. Herbert Basedow was a member of three South Australian medical relief expeditions; on the last he visited the southern part of the Northern Territory. He reported that the incidence of syphilis and gonorrhea cases was high along the north-south transportation route. He noted a high incidence of infectious diseases as Aborigines changed from nomadic to unhygienic, fringe-camp lifestyles, and the high infant as well as general mortality resulting from malnutrition. Cattle destroyed traditional sources of food (and clean water), and government and cattle-station rations were merely flour, sugar, tea and tobacco. Basedow advocated declaration of reserves to keep white settlers off hunting grounds. In 1928, Dr. W.D. Walker of Adelaide toured the Alice Springs region. He found conditions little different from what Basedow had found almost a decade before. This is not surprising, as nothing had been done to assist Aborigines since Basedow's visits.

In 1933, "mixed-race" nurses were appointed to care for Aborigines at Darwin Hospital. The establishment of Katherine Hospital in 1931, the reopening of the Pine Creek Hospital in 1934, and greater use of Queensland hospitals at Camooweal, Wyndham and Cloncurry (for which the commonwealth paid fees) reduced demand for treatment at the Kahlin Beach Aboriginal Hospital in Darwin. Yet the standard of treatment and facilities for Aborigines remained inferior.

In Alice Springs, a galvanized-iron hut accommmodated the Alice Springs Aboriginal Hospital until a ward was provided at the Alice Springs General Hospital, which opened in 1938. The hut proved useless in dealing with recurrent epidemic disease. The first epidemic was a severe one involving gonorrheal ophthalmia. Fearing Aboriginal sufferers would spread it to whites, the government medical officer had them placed in a "barbed-wire compound." "Half-caste" people were excluded from the Australian Inland Mission hostel because of their part-Aboriginal descent, and from the Aboriginal medical hut because of their part-white descent. They received quite inadequate treatment at the Half-Caste Institution. Commonwealth financial stringency (in part because of economic depression) meant that the officially declared goals of improving Aboriginal health to a level where it no longer threatened the European community and of stopping the decline in Aboriginal population numbers could not be achieved. In 1935 Dr. Cecil Cook pointed out that where Queensland and Western Australia, the two states having large Aboriginal populations like the Northern Territory, spent two pounds and one pound per head, respectively, the commonwealth spent about seven shillings, or 0.35 pounds, per head.

Only in the first three decades of the twentieth century did major Christian churches establish mission stations in the Northern Territory: the Roman Catholics at Bathurst Island in 1908 and Port Keats, 1936; the Church Missionary Society at Roper River in 1907, Oenpelli in 1925, and Groote Eylandt in 1921; and the Methodists at Goulburn Island in 1916, Milingimbi in 1923 and Yirrkala, 1935. The Lutheran Church maintained at Hermannsburg the only mission to survive from the nineteenth century. In the interwar years, the missions gave more attention to medical care, but they believed government had the primary responsibility. Cook argued that missions exaggerated the extent and effectiveness of their medical care. Finally, in 1938 he managed to make government grants to missions conditional on the meeting of his standards in diet, health care and sanitation.

The mission societies did not regularly send medically qualified personnel to the Northern Territory until the 1930s. The Methodists were the first to start sending trained nurses, the first arriving in 1928. Epidemic disease repeatedly revealed the inadequacy of mission medical facilities; for example, the Methodists' work was halted by an influenza epidemic in 1926, and measles in 1929, followed by whooping cough. In 1936, the first purpose-built medical facility provided by the Methodists, a dispensary, was established at Milingimbi. But incapacity to isolate infectious patients properly remained a serious deficiency for all missions at the close of the 1930s.[50]

The missions legitimated their religious endeavors by providing for the most obvious medical needs of the Aboriginal people with whom they had contact but failed to deal with their general decline in health. Indeed, the congregation of Aborigines on missions cut across the peripatetic lifestyle that underpinned good traditional hygiene, reduced the quality of diet by denying access to bush foods, and changed activity patterns that had sustained fitness. The congregation in sedentary groups also encouraged diffusion of introduced infections. The few government health workers were largely concerned with containing diseases in Aboriginal populations that potentially threatened Europeans. Little attempt was made to understand traditional

Aboriginal approaches to ill health or traditional relationships with the land, which vitally influenced both diet and mental health. Understanding might have facilitated the integration of Western biomedicine. The overriding aim was always successful white settlement of the northern part of the continent.[51]

In the nonfrontier states, New South Wales and Victoria, Aboriginal populations were much smaller, and the tribal way of life had disappeared; most lived on government stations. By 1938, the NSW Aborigines Protection Board estimated that 805 people of full Aboriginal descent and 9,610 of part descent lived in the state. About 66 percent of them lived on twenty-one managed stations and sixty other reserves. The board was poorly funded. A 1937 inquiry heard evidence of appalling living conditions on some stations. Four-room dwellings housed two and three families. Poor hygiene, malnutrition and absence of medical facilities combined to reduce resistance to infections. Whooping cough, tuberculosis, trachoma and VD were said to be common in station populations. Moreover, Europeans in country towns were not happy about sick people from stations being placed in local hospitals. A 1939 health survey concluded that both tuberculosis and malnutrition were not serious problems but that the eye disease trachoma and dental caries were ubiquitous.

Aboriginal matters were not much discussed in the press or parliament of any state. When they did come up, it was the danger of the transfer of infections, especially VD, from Aborigines to whites that received particular attention. Lock hospitals, as noted, were created in the early twentieth century in Queensland and Western Australia. From 1911, in South Australia, examination of Aborigines and treatment in lock and public hospitals was compulsory. Legislation in New South Wales in 1936 provided for compulsory examination and treatment of Aborigines or persons of part-Aboriginal descent. The colonial secretary argued in support of compulsion that there existed a danger to the white community from gonococeal ophthalmia, which was then very prevalent in Aboriginal communities.

The NSW Aborigines Welfare Board annual reports of the 1940s and '50s show that epidemics of whooping cough, influenza, measles, mumps and scabies regularly swept through stations and reserves. However, some improvements were occurring. The newer houses came with bathing facilities, not provided in prewar dwellings. Baby Health and Bush Nursing Association nurses offered advice on diet and hygiene. From the early 1960s, medical officers of health made regular inspections of stations and reserves in their health districts.

In 1956, of a total population of 231 people of full descent, 6,388 "halfcaste" and 5,751 "lesser caste," 4,788 were inmates of Welfare Board stations and reserves. A majority of the rest occupied rented accommodations or their own homes in towns and cities, while a minority were condemned to live on the fringes of country towns in dreadful conditions. Health Department medical officers in 1963 believed that Aboriginal child mortality was double that of the white population. The Welfare Board defended itself by saying that it tried to improve water, sanitation and garbage-disposal services in fringe-dwelling communities and that medical officers of health regularly inspected station and reserve populations. When a 1968 state parliamentary inquiry into Aboriginal welfare criticized the board for the continuing poor living conditions on reserves, the board countered by pointing to the basic problem of inadequate funding.

In South Australia, in the 1940s, Aboriginal communities were surveyed for TB. Only a few positive cases were found. The surveys continued into the 1960s. Poliomyelitis was reported in the late 1940s and epidemics of whooping cough and gastroenteritis in children throughout the 1950s. In the 1960s, immunization against poliomyelitis, diphtheria, whooping cough, tetanus and influenza was routinely provided. In 1964 the Aboriginal Affairs Board asserted that better living conditions were cutting back the common illnesses of Aboriginal communities. All outback communities received health advice from visiting patrol or welfare officers, while the very young and the old were flown out of remote districts for treatment by the Royal Flying Doctor Service.[52]

In Victoria, from 1886 all healthy, part-Aboriginal people were excluded from government stations. Considerable savings were thus made on expenditure on the Aborigines Protection Board. Station populations continued to fall in number, and the board's activities were concentrated on the Lake Tyers facility. In 1958, the Aborigines Welfare Board replaced the Protection Board, which had operated since 1860. Aborigines were to have the same legal rights as Europeans in Victoria. The Welfare Board in its first report pointed to substandard living conditions to explain an infant mortality rate greater than that of the general community. By 1960, it was reporting that supplementary foods were being provided for children, and it was suggesting that a combination of poverty and ignorance was responsible for their poor nutrition. The board responded by employing a nursing sister to advise mothers on childcare and domestic hygiene. Five years later, it was reporting that dental caries, defective eyes, skin infections, heart disease, tuberculosis and nasal conditions were widespread and that infant mortality continued to be high because women lacked antenatal and postnatal care. By 1968, five nurses were employed in the visiting service. By 1971, many people who had been using the health care services of the Aboriginal Affairs Ministry used the health facilities in the general community. Two years later, the ministry's nursing service was absorbed by the Health Department as part of the policy of integration of Aborigines into the general community.

By the close of the 1960s, the Northern Territory had the largest population of people of full Aboriginal descent—about 45 percent of the national total—but the smallest proportion of part-Aborigines, about 20 percent. In the territory, 13 percent of Aborigines were town dwellers. Infant mortality was high but showed a tendency to decline: 143 per thousand live births in

1958–60 (the Australian rate was 22 in 1959) and 117 in 1965–68. Both infant mortality and age-specific rates were very high by international standards. The main causes of deaths of babies were "diseases of poverty"—gastroenteritis, pneumonia and malnutrition. Health services had clearly not been very successful in bringing down infant and child mortality. In any case, medical care would need to be underwritten by a significant increase in standards of living, hygiene and nutrition if rates were to be reduced to anything approaching acceptable levels.

Western Australia, like the Northern Territory, had a large population of full Aboriginal descent—8,121 to 10,121 (depending on data source) in 1961, compared to about twenty-one thousand in the Northern Territory. They had comparable crude death rates: in 1961–64, 19.9 per thousand population and 18.2 per thousand population, compared with Australia as a whole (exclusive of Aborigines), which in 1956–60 had a rate of only 8.8. The Aboriginal infant mortality rate in Western Australia was seventy-five per thousand live births in 1961–64, while that of the Northern Territory was more than 140 and that of white Australia was a mere twenty-two (in 1959). As in the Northern Territory, gastroenteritis/dysentery and pneumonia/influenza were the major causes of infant deaths. While infants from each jurisdiction faced the same risk of death from gastroenteritis/dysentery, those from Western Australia faced about half the risk of death from pneumonia/influenza confronted by Aboriginal babies in the Northern Territory. But the risks in both jurisdictions were much higher than those faced by white Australian infants, or even New Zealand Maori babies, as table 5.6 shows.

The standards of health services and the use made of them seem to have been better in Western Australia, as lower rates for two groups of chronic diseases (anaemia and malnutrition and tuberculosis) indicate. The rate for anaemia/malnutrition was thirty in Western Australia and seventy per hundred thousand population in the Northern Territory; the rates for tuberculosis were six and seventy per hundred thousand population, respectively.

Table 5.6
Infant Deaths, for Aborigines, Maoris and Non-Aboriginal Australians

	Gastroenteritis/ Dysentery	Pneumonia/ Influenza
WA full Aborigines	23 deaths per 1,000 births	15 deaths per 1,000 births
NT full Aborigines	26	28
Maoris	5	4
Non-Aboriginal Australia	0.5	1.6

Source: P.M. Moodie, ***Aboriginal Health*** (Canberra: Australian National University Press, 1973), 82.

The number of people of full Aboriginal descent in Queensland in 1961 was between 8,686 and 11,445, depending on data source. One study of nine mission and government settlements found a crude death rate of fifteen per thousand population and an infant mortality rate of 112 per thousand live births for 1962–66. However, the population on which the study was based included an unknown number of part-Aborigines. When the population was restricted to six settlements around the Gulf of Carpentaria (which were composed mainly of people of full Aboriginal descent), the crude death rate was 13.1 and the infant mortality rate eighty-six. Neither set of figures can be compared with those of the Northern Territory and Western Australia, because they are based on a small and selected proportion of the Queensland population. The leading causes of infant deaths in the study of Queensland mission and settlement populations were gastroenteritis, pneumonia and prematurity. The mortality pattern was thus similar to those in the Northern Territory and Western Australia.

The population of people of full Aboriginal descent in South Australia was 2,147 in 1961. For 1961–64, the percentage of total deaths in the first year of life (27 percent) was greater than in any other jurisdiction except the Northern Territory (31.4 percent in 1964–65). The leading causes of death were heart disease (19 percent of total deaths), gastroenteritis (17 percent) and pneumonia/influenza (13 percent). The number of people of full Aboriginal descent in New South Wales was even smaller, only 1,488 in 1961. The mortality patterns were not dissimilar: 26 percent of total deaths in 1960–65 were of children under one year; the leading causes of death were heart disease (28 percent of total deaths), pneumonia/influenza (13 percent) and gastroenteritis (12 percent). Neither Victoria nor Tasmania had populations of people of full Aboriginal descent.

Correlations seemed to exist between infant and child death rates and the extent of white settlement, the ratio of people of full descent to the total Aboriginal population, the ratio of those of full descent to the total population, and the proportion of people of full descent living on missions and settlements. An underlying "cause" might have been the degree of exposure of Aborigines to white rural society and the extent of acculturation in the more settled regions. While the data for part-Aboriginal populations is limited, it would appear that they experienced smaller infant and child mortality rates than did those of full descent (see table 5.7). Further, mortality indicators for Aborigines were almost all worse than those of New Zealand Maoris and American Indians, although it must be appreciated that the Maoris and Indian totals included larger proportions of part-Maoris and part-Indians than the Aboriginal populations included part-Aborigines.[53]

For historical reasons to do with the initial date and the spread of European settlement and the growth pattern of the European economy, the largest part-Aboriginal populations in the 1960s were located in Queensland (about thirty thousand), New South Wales (twenty-three thousand) and Western

Table 5.7
Death Rates, by Age Group, Aborigines, Australia, Maoris and U.S. Indians

Age	NT Aborigines, 1958–60	Australia, 1959	Maoris, 1958	U.S. Indians, 1959
Under 1 year	142.0 deaths per 1,000	22.0 deaths per 1,000	52.9 deaths per 1,000	56.6 deaths per 1,000
1–4 years	21.6	1.2	3.0	3.8
5–9 years	2.3	0.5	1.2	1.2
10–19 years	2.6	0.6	1.3	1.6
20–29 years	4.5	1.1	3.0	4.5
30–39 years	4.8	1.7	4.7	6.6
40–59 years	13.5	6.6	15.8	9.9
60+ years	61.5	51.5	65.7	50.0

Source: P.M. Moodie, *Aboriginal Health* (Canberra: Australian National University Press, 1973), 50.

Australia (twelve thousand). The 1961 census put the number of Aborigines in Sydney at 1,500, but independent "guesstimates" put it between ten and fifteen thousand. For fourteen Aboriginal stations in NSW for 1954–55 to 1963–64, the crude death rate was 11.6 per thousand. While it was impossible to obtain infant death rates directly, it was possible to obtain high and low estimates for nonmetropolitan Aborigines: 1950–54, ninety and seventy-two per thousand live births respectively; 1955–59, seventy-eight and sixty-six; and 1960–64, seventy-six and sixty-one. These figures indicate that this Aboriginal population had infant mortality rates three to four times those of Australia as a whole in these years (see table 5.8).

If accidents and homicides are set aside, Aboriginal excess mortality largely resulted from infections and neonatal deaths. From the 1950s, antibiotics could control most infections, and proper ante- and postnatal care could prevent most neonatal deaths. Clearly, the higher mortality experienced by Aborigines was due to a combination of low health status and inadequate nutrition, inadequate health services and underuse of such services as were

Table 5.8
Death Rates for Leading Causes of Death, NSW Aborigines, 1950–64, and Australia, 1961

Cause	NSW Aborigines per 100,000	Australia per 100,000
Pneumonia	147	27
Heart disease	133	256
Accidents	90	27
Gastroenteritis	86	4
Immaturity/other diseases of early infancy	79	13
Cardiovascular	66	114
Cancer	59	130
Birth injury	37	11
Nephritis	23	10
Congenital malformations	20	12
Malnutrition/anaemia	15	3
Automobile accidents	15	25
Pulmonary tuberculosis	16	4
Rheumatic heart disease	13	7
Infections of new born	12	2
Pregnancy/childbirth complications	9	1
Homicide	4.5	1.5
Suicide	3	12
All infective/parasitic diseases	49	9
All early infancy diseases	148	26

Source: P.M. Moodie, *Aboriginal Health* (Canberra: Australian National University Press, 1973), 109.

available. Improvement in the socioeconomic environment and access to appropriate health services was needed if this excess mortality was to be reduced.

Deaths from pneumonia, gastroenteritis and from accidents other than automobile and railway, and homicide and suicide, together with neonatal diseases, were extensive in the part-Aboriginal NSW population compared with those in the Australian population as a whole, but they were similar in extent to those in populations of full Aboriginal descent discussed earlier. Deaths from rheumatic heart disease and from nephritis were the end products of the long-term, toxic effect of streptococcal throat infections. Pulmonary tuberculosis deaths likewise resulted from infection caught years before. Both sets of deaths indicate failure to obtain early and proper treatment for initial conditions. The significance of the socioeconomic environment, rather than genetic or climatic influences, for the health of the part-Aboriginal population is seen in the fact that the population was less Aboriginal than European in heredity and that the population experienced the same climatic conditions as the much healthier white population. Further, the substantial mortality of one- to-four-year-olds and the particular causes of mortality for this age group indicated the impact of socioeconomic deprivation. In contrast, white children of this age were very healthy—indeed, so much so that until the first school medical examination, health authorities were little concerned with the health needs of these children.

Information on part-Aborigines in Queensland was limited to particular missions and settlements. Cherbourg (in the southeast of the state) and Palm Island (off the north coast) had predominantly part-Aboriginal populations, the first having in 1962–66 a crude general death rate of 16.5 and an infant mortality rate of 153, and the second rates of 14.4 and 106, respectively. Their infant death rates were considerably greater than those of the Gulf of Carpentaria communities of full Aboriginal descent discussed above. The latter had a collective infant death rate of eighty-six per thousand live births. The difference may have been due to the fact that communities of people of full descent were only a third of the size of the two part-Aboriginal institutional settlements, the fact that there was less close contact between health care workers and the much larger, part-Aboriginal populations, and the fact that these institutionalized populations probably contained more families beset by personal and domestic problems.

In Western Australia in 1967–68, Aborigines contributed disproportionately to infant and early childhood deaths. About 2.5 percent of the state's population, they experienced 20 percent of infant and 27.5 percent of deaths of one- to-four-year-olds. Where white postneonatal deaths represented 20 percent of white infant deaths, Aboriginal postneonatal deaths represented a massive 56 percent of Aboriginal infant deaths. Moreover, 43 percent of white one- to-four-year-old deaths resulted from infection but 92 percent of Aboriginal deaths in this age group. This Aboriginal infant and early childhood mortality pattern resembled that of white urban communities in the nineteenth century before the epidemiological and demographic transitions had occurred.[54]

Infant mortality rates of Aboriginal communities declined steadily in the 1970s, as did childhood mortality. But diseases virtually banished from the nonindigenous population—rheumatic fever, leprosy, childhood malnutrition, syphilis and trachoma—continued to impose a significant illness burden on indigenous people in the 1990s. Further, 20 percent of nonindigenes were older than fifty-five years, but only 6 percent of Aborigines. As the Aboriginal and Torres Strait Islander social justice commissioner, Mick Dodson, observed in his 1994 report, Aborigines remain the poorest, sickest, worst housed and most jailed part of the Australian population.[55]

As should be clear from discussion to date, the Aboriginal population is widely distributed, with 28 percent in capital cities, 50 percent in towns and rural areas, and 20 percent in remote areas. Urban Aborigines live mostly in NSW, Queensland and Western Australia, and rural and remote Aborigines live mainly in the Northern Territory, Queensland and Western Australia. Aggregate mortality and morbidity figures mask considerable heterogeneity of living conditions and historical experiences. Thus, the Pitjantjatjara and Yankunytjatjara, who live in the arid northwest of South Australia, have kept their land and culture yet lack adequate housing, water supplies and waste-disposal systems. However, the South Australian coastal tribes, who came into contact with Europeans much earlier, were decimated by violence and new infections. They were deprived of their land but took up European housing and education sooner than the remote desert tribes.

Total Aboriginal fertility rates fell in the 1960s and '70s from 5.9 children per woman (estimated) in 1966–71 to 3.1 in 1981–86. They remained at the latter level in the late 1990s. This was a level 40 percent higher than that for Australia as a whole (1.9 children per woman). But bearing of children among Aboriginal peoples begins at an earlier age, and stillbirths are much higher—11.5 as opposed to five per thousand births—while the low birth-weight rate is substantial, at 13 percent. Life expectancy at birth is much lower for Aborigines—55.2 years for males and 63.3 years for females, but for non-Aborigines 75 and 80.9 years. Aboriginal life expectancy has not increased for two decades, whereas that of non-Aborigines has grown markedly, in large part because of falling cardiovascular disease incidence from the 1960s. Populations with life expectancies of about fifty years commonly experience their excess mortality through childhood infectious disease, but among contemporary Aborigines a great deal of premature mortality results from adult heart disease. Falling infant death rates and infectious disease mortality since the 1970s have been balanced by growing excess adult mortality from chronic disease, accidents and violence.

Death rates from heart disease, hypertension and cerebrovascular disease are the main cause of death for Aboriginal men and women. They die as younger adults, at ages ten to fifteen years younger than members of comparable indigenous populations overseas. Automobile accidents, violence and suicide are the second cause of death for males and the third for females, and they are about four times greater than rates for the general population. Respiratory disease used to be the first cause of death and is now the second for women and the third for men. Cancer deaths are growing, while deaths from infections and parasites are declining, although the rate is twelve to thirteen times that for Australia as a whole.

While infant mortality has fallen notably since the 1960s, it remains two to four times that of white Australia. It is also, at twenty to twenty-five per thousand (1991), greater than that of American Indians (9.8), Maoris (eighteen), and Canadian indigenes (21.8). The gratifying fall in the neonatal rate very probably resulted from the growth of maternal and child health services, and the fall in the postneonatal rate from better nutrition and primary care and from air evacuation facilities for remote areas. Yet where infections caused 3.9 percent of white infant deaths in Western Australia (1991), they caused 28.6 percent of Aboriginal infant mortality. Lower infant death rates will result more from a better socioeconomic environment than from health interventions. Similarly, the maternal death rate remains unacceptably higher than that of the white population. Aborigines represent fewer than 3 percent of confinements but 30 percent of direct maternal deaths.

Illness in Aboriginal children, especially in remote areas, is still dominated by respiratory and gastrointestinal infections. Better living conditions have brought down the incidence and severity of the latter but have had less effect on the former. Concurrent or sequential infections impose heavy burdens in rural and remote communities. Cross infection is extensive, because of poor hygiene, high levels of bacterial carriage and overcrowded living circumstances. Nutritional disorders plague remotely situated Aborigines. Intrauterine growth retardation, low birth weight and faltering growth precede childhood undernutrition and nutritional difficulties during teenage pregnancies. In adulthood there follow diabetes and cardiovascular disease. A complex of factors produces poor nutritional status—remote location, high food prices and low income, high unemployment and substandard living circumstances, infections and coexisting illnesses. In some communities, like Cherbourg, comparisons of growth over the last three decades have indicated that present weight-for-age is at about international reference levels. But a study of hospitalized children in the Northern Territory revealed that high levels of malnutrition had not been reduced over the last two decades. The age-standardized Aboriginal mortality rate for diabetes is seven times the rate of nonindigenous Australia, and diabetes is a significant factor in premature mortality from cardiovascular disease and in chronic renal failure.

Trachoma, introduced by Chinese and Europeans, has decreased markedly in prevalence since the 1970s. It leads to blindness more rarely than in the past. Antibiotic use on a large scale has reduced its severity, but considerable prevalence reduction could be expected from improved living conditions. Professor Ida Mann, a Western Australian ophthalmologist, said as early as the 1930s, "If governments were to put the water on [that is, provide running water to homes], nobody would have trachoma."[56] Hepatitis B, which may lead to chronic hepatitis, cirrhosis or hepatic cancer, is widespread in rural and remote Aboriginal populations, even as it is becoming less common in urban populations.

The records of Aboriginal hospitals in northern Western Australia for the later 1930s show that cases of gonorrhoea and granuloma (donovanosis) were not uncommon. But infection with yaws and endemic (nonvenereal) syphilis rendered remote communities largely free of venereal syphilis, because of the cross-immunity conferred by these very closely related diseases. The postwar use of penicillin to root out yaws and endemic syphilis destroyed the cross-immunity.

In 1968 Garner, Backhouse, Moodie and Tibbs carried out a medical survey of eleven communities in the north of the Northern Territory and seven in the south. They warned that with 65 percent of adults in the sample lacking cross-immunity to syphilis and with growing opportunities for venereal transmission from developments like a more mobile population, venereal syphilis was a real threat. In 1974, notifications of syphilis increased sharply in the Northern Territory and remained markedly higher than those in other states: 317 per hundred thousand population in 1974, the rate rose to 883 in 1977 but was down to 283 in 1990. The national rate in 1974 was only seventeen; in 1977, 22; and in 1990, ten. The very high Northern Territory rates may be attributed to a large Aboriginal population (25 percent of the total), widespread screening, and high notification compliance. Aborigines are fewer than 2 percent of the national population but account for over 90 percent of syphilis infections; accordingly, state syphilis rates largely reflect the relative sizes of the resident Aboriginal populations. By the 1990s, gonorrhoea, syphilis, donovanosis and chlamydia were hyperendemic in Aboriginal populations in the Territory, north Queensland, and the Kimberley and Pilbara regions of Western Australia. In central and northern parts of the country, donovanosis was widespread. Reduction has been difficult because of low compliance with established treatment regimens. Oral treatment with Azithromycin, which has a long half-life in tissue, promises to reduce the level of treatment failure. Both ulcerative and nonulcerative sexually transmitted infections raise the risk of HIV/AIDS infection between three and five times. Moreover, HIV infection may make sexually transmitted infections like genital ulcers more prevalent; such is the epidemiological synergy between sexually transmitted infections and HIV.[57]

The incidence of HIV in the indigenous and nonindigenous populations is similar, but experts agree that there is a potential for an indigenous heterosexual epidemic because of the high and stable rate of sexually transmitted disease (STD) in the indigenous population, the younger age of STD cases, the higher proportion of female STD cases and other such factors. Homosexual contact is the primary means of HIV transmission, but the proportion of heterosexual contact cases is greater than in the nonindigenous population. There is wide variation of incidence between and within Aboriginal communities. While no HIV cases have been reported from the remote communities of central Australia, diffusion is likely to be speedy once it gains entry, because of mobile lifestyles and certain traditional practices carrying high risk of transmission. Rural and remote communities have poor health, with high levels of infections like tuberculosis and HTLV-1.

In large urban communities the risk profile is different; injecting-drug use among young people is a potent risk factor. In 1994, the National Sexual Health Conference for Aboriginal and Torres Strait Islander Gay and Transgender People explored gay and transgender risk issues. National policy has been slow to develop in this area. David Bradford, director of the Sexual Health Programme of the York Peninsula and Torres Strait Regional Health Authority, Queensland, had pointed out in 1994 that the threat of an indigenous epidemic had been predicted for some time. While there was wringing of hands, no real development of policies had occurred, except for targeted education programs in Aboriginal communities, which had had little effect on the high STD incidence. These high rates were in part due to community denial of the size of the problem, whether because of embarrassment, fear of persecution, or cultural taboos, and to the low priority accorded STD control in the face of the plethora of life-threatening medical problems like alcoholism, diabetes, hypertension and cardiovascular and renal disease.

The National Aboriginal Health Strategy, which was drawn up in the 1980s, had acknowledged that sexually transmitted infections were a serious health problem. However, it had insisted that health services controlled by the community were the key to HIV/AIDS control. When in the late 1990s a national indigenous Australians' sexual health strategy, 1996–97 to 1998–99, was developed by the federal government's advisory body on HIV/AIDS, the Australian National Council on AIDS and Related Diseases, the strategy supported a "horizontal" approach, to be pursued in a primary health care context. The reasons given were that indigenous involvement was critical if the response was to be relevant and effective. Further, individual components of the sexual health strategy, whether clinical or educational, had to be integrated with the indigenous response to health in general.[58] Announcing that the national HIV/AIDS strategy had been renewed for another five years—the fourth in fifteen years—the health minister in the federal Liberal-National Party government, Dr. Michael Wooldridge, said in mid-2000 that "the potential for the spread of HIV into Aboriginal and Torres Strait Islander communities continues to be of concern and the federal government is committed to working with communities to develop appropriate resources and strategies to prevent the epidemic."[59]

The impact of poor living conditions and hygiene continued to be seen in the endemicity of hepatitis B (HBV) in rural and remote communities, although, as noted earlier, HBV was on the decline in urban settings. As many as 73 percent of Aborigines in some remote locations in the Northern Territory have shown evidence of exposure to hepatitis. In the later 1980s, the HBV carrier rate in nonindigenous Territorians was less than 0.1 percent, a rate similar to that found in the rest of nonindigenous Australia. The relative contribution of sexual and needle-sharing transmission to spread of HBV among indigenes is unknown, but the potential is significant, given the very high HBV carrier rates in some communities. Most infection appears to take place perinatally, through transmission from mother to child, or early in life through "horizontal" transmission; overcrowding directly assists horizontal spread. The commonwealth provided, free from the beginning of 1987, universal vaccination for Aboriginal neonates.

Alcohol abuse is a major cause of premature mortality and excess morbidity. While a considerable percentage of Aboriginal people do not drink alcohol—an estimated 10 to 35 percent of males abstain, and of females 39 to 80 percent—a larger proportion of drinkers consume excessive quantities. "Binge" drinking is more frequently practiced than in the general community. As a direct cause of mortality, alcohol abuse is responsible for about 10 percent of deaths in Aboriginal communities. It contributes to violence, accidents, child neglect, violent crime and imprisonment. Alcohol was seen as significantly associated with deaths in police custody by the Royal Commission into Aboriginal Deaths in Custody in the early 1990s. Easy availability of alcohol in rural and remote communities contributes to abuse. For some time Aboriginal communities have pursued various types of self-help. Community interventions have included night patrols, dry (alcohol-free) areas, substance abuse programs, sobering-up shelters, drying-out "farms" and organized efforts to contain growth of licensed outlets.[60]

A great many communities endure social, economic and environmental deprivation, with low levels of education and income, poor community infrastructure, discrimination and high levels of unemployment, imprisonment and inadequate housing. This deprivation is the ultimate cause of the health inequality. By the late 1980s, the vast majority of Aborigines aged fifteen to twenty-four years had some schooling. Even in the Northern Territory more than 93 percent received some. But they quit school at an earlier age and were less likely to receive postsecondary education than other Australians. The royal commissioner on Aboriginal deaths in custody said in his 1991 report that education systems failed to provide equitable participation. The National Review of Education for Aboriginal and Torres Strait Islanders pointed out in 1994 that the education offered had to be regarded as appropriate by Aborigines themselves. However, high unemployment rates commonly result from lack not of skills but of job opportunities. The average Aboriginal unemployment rate throughout the country is three times the rate of non-Aborigines. The occupation distribution is greatly different, with Aborigines overrepresented in unskilled and semiskilled occupations. A much larger proportion derive income from social security benefits than do non-Aborigines. There is a wide range of socioeconomic status, from a few living in comparative affluence to the great majority in poverty, with the highest incomes in cities like Canberra, Melbourne and Hobart, and the poorest in rural and remote locations that have been seriously affected by rural economic recession.

Where 70 percent of Australians are home owners, about 26 percent of Aborigines are in this category. Indeed, housing inadequacy is a major social and health problem. In the early 1990s, a national survey found that while Aboriginal families accounted for 1.4 percent of total families, they represented 22 percent of families designated homeless and 38 percent of families occupying improvised housing (tents, caravans, boats or sheds). Overcrowding was four times the level of overcrowding in the non-Aboriginal population. Inadequate housing was worst in rural and remote locations. In the Northern Territory, 29 percent of families were homeless, with another 22 percent living in overcrowded conditions. Another indicator of inadequate housing is the degree of availability of "health hardware" to enable healthy living—water supply, waste disposal systems, washing facilities and toilets. A 1987 environmental health review of the Anangu Pitjantjatjara Lands in remote South Australia found that 50 percent of the people were not housed; 55 percent of hot water and 40 percent of cold water outlets were not working, and 57 percent of waste-water systems did not function. In yard areas, which was living space for many, 25 percent of taps did not work. Overcrowding was common. Individuals per house averaged 8.3. A 1992 national survey of infrastructure in rural and remote communities revealed that 34 percent lacked adequate water supplies. Better health can follow from better housing only if infrastructure is appropriately designed and reliably maintained.[61]

Poor living conditions have been identified by official inquiries as health hazards since the early 1970s. In 1973, the Whitlam government had introduced a National Plan for Aboriginal Health to raise Aboriginal health status to that of "their fellow Australians" within ten years. But in 1979 the House of Representatives Standing Committee on Aboriginal Affairs reported that the standard was intolerable. Creation of basic environmental facilities, particularly safe water supplies, was accorded first priority by the committee. The commonwealth announced in early 1981–82 that it would provide fifty million dollars over five years through the Aboriginal Public Health Improvement Program for basic facilities like water, sewerage and electricity. As early as 1983, a New South Wales task force on Aboriginal health, reporting to the state health minister, L.J. Brereton, noted that lack of information and consultation mechanisms for setting priorities, together with the size of the projects involved, caused implementation in that state to prove slower than anticipated. By the end of the 1980s many Aboriginal communities throughout the country still lacked safe and reliable water supplies, let alone other basic amenities.[62]

In 1987, the Federal Human Rights and Equal Opportunity Commission inquired into the social and material needs of Toomelah, an Aboriginal settlement of five hundred people on the New South Wales–Queensland border. The commission considered the community's most urgent need to be adequate and reliable water. Water rationing—bore water for two fifteen-minute periods a day—had been the rule for a decade. Aboriginal health workers claimed that inadequate water resulted in gastroenteritis; growth failure; respiratory disease; ear, nose and throat infections; skin sores; and stress. The commission concluded that provision of water and sewerage to Toomelah had been mismanaged and was inadequate, producing conditions that were intolerable. In the wake of the Toomelah report, the Race Discrimination Commission received complaints from numerous other Aboriginal communities and initiated inquiries into the water supplies of selected remote Aboriginal and Torres Strait Islander settlements in Western Australia, South Australia, New South Wales, Queensland and the Northern Territory. The findings were stark.

About twenty-one thousand Aborigines in 1989, residents of communities of thirty to a thousand people, lacked reticulated water supplies. Of these, 90 percent were in Western Australia and the Northern Territory. About nineteen thousand people had water supplies unable to meet reasonable demands; of these 75 percent were in Queensland and the Northern Territory. A minimum of a thousand people had water that did not meet the quality criteria of the 1980 NHMRC-Australian Water Resources Council guidelines. Another fourteen thousand (a figure that could have been as high as thirty thousand) had water not fulfilling quality criteria laid down in the 1987 guidelines. A 1992 Aboriginal and Torres Strait Islander Commission (ATSIC) national survey of the infrastructure of 907 discrete communities found a variety of problems, as table 5.9 shows.[63]

A World Bank expert panel in 1976 pointed out that it was difficult to quantify the relationship between a safe and adequate water supply and population health but that "other things being equal [which they never are]" it was "generally associated with a healthier population." The federal Race Discrimination Commissioner noted that while a safe and adequate water supply did not alone produce health improvement, it was "a vital step towards health improvement." ATSIC announced in 1992 that commonwealth funding of $232 million over five years would be used to raise health and infrastructure standards. But the royal commissioner inquiring into Aboriginal deaths in custody noted that this sum was less than 20 percent of what was estimated by the Aboriginal Health Development Group as necessary to raise standards.[64]

Table 5.9
Water Supply Aspects of National Survey of Remote Communities, Australia, 1992

State or Territory	Communities Surveyed	Groundwater as a Source %	Water Quality below NHMRC Guidelines %	Water Restrictions in Prior 12 Months %	No Water Supply Maintenance %	Insufficient Water for Next 5 Years %
NSW and ACT	67	10	6	34	13	22
Vic. and Tas.	2	50	50	50	0	50
Qld.	81	44	36	56	22	44
SA	96	84	22	71	8	36
WA	179	70	19	9	14	41
NT	482	66	46	30	13	51
Australia	907	63	34	33	14	45

Source: Federal Race Discrimination Commissioner, *Water: A Report on the Provision of Water and Sanitation in Remote Aboriginal and Torres Strait Islander Communities* (Canberra: Australian Government Publishing Service, 1994), 20.

Pursuing a comparative perspective on Aboriginal health, S.J. Kunitz reviewed the health status of indigenous peoples in Australia, Canada, the United States and New Zealand, all of which countries are Anglophone and have liberal democratic political systems. He found that in the 1980s Australian Aborigines had the worst and American Indians the best life expectancy at birth (see table 5.10).

He argues that where, as in the cases of the United States, Canada and New Zealand, the central government enters into treaties with indigenous peoples and is (rather than state or territorial governments) in charge of indigenous affairs, the health and welfare of indigenes have been better. It is noteworthy that after the commonwealth became more involved in Aboriginal health in the early 1970s, not only did services become more available but infant and child mortality fell considerably. There seems little doubt that effective, accessible preventive and curative services can have an impact on mortality patterns where infectious disease is significant, even when economic status is low and living conditions are poor.[65]

Kunitz and M.A. Brady proposed that in contrast to the Australian experience, the American Indian health service had been effective, and that three factors contributed to this pattern. The first is federal administration, which avoided state equivocation over responsibility. States in the United States, as in Australia, were competitors with indigenes for land and other natural resources. Second is the separation of health services from the U.S. Bureau of Indian Affairs since the mid-1950s, insulating them from policy struggles over natural resources. Third is the development over four decades of a professionally run health service that integrated primary, secondary and some

Table 5.10
Life Expectancy at Birth, for Indigenes and Non-Indigenes, the United States, Canada, New Zealand and Australia, 1980–85

	Indigenes		Non-Indigenes	
Nation	Male	Female	Male	Female
	Indians and Alaska natives		*Caucasian*	
United States (1980)	67.1 years	75.1 years	70.7 years	78.1 years
	Indians			
Canada (1982–85)	64.0	72.8	72.4	80.1
	Maoris			
New Zealand (1980–82)	63.8	68.5	70.8	77.0
	Aborigines			
Australia (1985)	54.0	61.6	72.8	79.1

Source: S.J. Kunitz, *Disease and Social Diversity: The European Impact on the Health of Non-Europeans* (New York: Oxford University Press, 1994), 25.

tertiary care, as well as alcohol and other drug and mental health services, with public health services—public health nursing, health education and environmental health programs. Underpinning the whole historical experience has been the fact of a treaty (or treaties) between the Indian tribes and the federal government. Whatever their limitations and historical breaches of "contract," treaties legitimized Indian land claims and rights to services.

It would seem that the absence of a treaty with Aboriginal Australia has deeply weakened the position of Aborigines and left them at the mercy of colonial and state governments. Even when the commonwealth began to intervene in health and welfare matters in the 1970s, the states continued to be involved in Aboriginal affairs. The ongoing conflicts have caused services to develop in a fragmented fashion. Further, relations between Aboriginal bodies and commonwealth and state governments have over the same period often been difficult. More specifically, relations between the independent Aboriginal medical services that developed from the 1970s and the commonwealth have commonly been soured by governments' wish to make the services accountable for public funding and the medical services' inclination to resist "control." The services have commonly competed with state health authorities for public funds.

Until the early 1970s, Aborigines obtained primary care through outpatient sections of public hospitals or by the private charity of general practitioners. Thus, they often looked for treatment only when they were seriously ill. Racism and cultural ignorance pervaded the services that treated Aborigines. In remote areas, nursing sisters on government settlements or attached to missions (and sometimes the Royal Flying Doctor Service) provided care. However, community-controlled medical services were established in cities to meet the real need, the first in Redfern, Sydney, in November 1971 (against the wishes of the state government) and then in Fitzroy, Melbourne, in early 1973. Run by an elected Aboriginal board and having Aboriginal staff, the centers were free and accessible. Using voluntary labor and community donations at first, they later received direct commonwealth funding—funding that was not channeled through the states. By 1979–80, medical services were receiving $2.9 million a year. Their number had grown by 1978 to eleven urban and three rural centers across the mainland states and the Northern Territory. By the 1990s, there were more than fifty community-controlled services. They have now become an established part of facilities for Aboriginal people.

Established before the Alma Ata Declaration's promotion of primary health care, these services fit well into the international concept, providing as they did not only medical care but community development and outreach programs. The Redfern center by 1974 distributed fruit and vegetables, provided vitamins, and offered emergency clothing and blankets to patients from rural areas. Aboriginal lobbyists soon made use of the principles of the 1978

Alma Ata Declaration and HFA by the Year 2000 in their political and ideological battle with the commonwealth and states to secure funding for the medical services. It is likely that commonwealth governments never wanted Aboriginal medical services to become a permanent feature, only conduits leading Aboriginal people into mainstream services. The result was that these separate services, by the early 1980s, attracted less than 5 percent of total national expenditure on Aboriginal health.

Their defenders used international endorsement of community participation to argue for separate services. They employed the broad WHO definition of health as complete physical, mental and social well-being to support the idea of an Aboriginal view of health, implying thereby a need for separate facilities to accommodate cultural differences from the white majority. They therefore saw Aboriginal medical services as long-term, not temporary, aspects of health provision for Aboriginal people. Indeed, even in 1973, at a Health and Community Development Workshop in Alice Springs, participants had opted for a broad definition of health that went beyond absence of organic disease. This broad definition "also includes having satisfying personal and spiritual relationships, children, and a minimum of violent conflict."[66] In their commitment to lay involvement and a broad definition of health, the Aboriginal services have long been at odds with state health departments, which see professional expertise as vital to programs, and health as being the absence of measurable disease conditions and as demonstrable by solid indicators like mortality rates. In contrast, the Aboriginal medical services have cleaved to a belief in the health-promoting involvement of lay members of the community in the running of the health services.

As Kunitz noted, these different conceptions of health and health services, stated in their purest forms, are as polarized as the WHO's own vertical and horizontal approaches to health improvement—vaccination campaigns against particular diseases versus across-the-board health advancement attentive to the psychosocial and cultural aspects of disease. Each has its characteristic strengths and weaknesses. Thus, horizontal programs will be better able to respond to problems like alcohol and other drug abuse, where the conception of the causal web can be so extensive that it may be difficult to design effective interventions. These differences are not insuperable; the institutionalized fragmentation of policy between commonwealth and states that seems to present more difficult obstacles to Aboriginal health advancement.

The commonwealth balked at assuming a predominant role. As early as 1980, a Fraser government review criticized the states' lack of enthusiasm for community-controlled services. It urged the commonwealth Health Department to assume responsibility for policy and funding over a three-year period, during which time relations with Aboriginal bodies could be put on a solid basis. The states would continue to obtain funds but under specific conditions. Not only was the advice ignored but in 1984 the new Hawke Labor government transferred health funding from the Federal Health Department to the Department of Aboriginal Affairs (DAA), which lacked expertise in primary health care and public health. In the course of the 1980s, attainment of objectives and setting of performance indicators became integral to funding. The National Aboriginal and Islander Health Organisation criticized the commonwealth's managerial assertion as a threat to community control of medical services. In 1989 the National Aboriginal Health Strategy come into being. Its provision for tripartite negotiations—commonwealth, states and Aboriginal Medical Services—did not allow for ATSIC (1990) to devolve allocation of funds (including part of the health funds) to its regional councils. A coherent commonwealth policy on Aboriginal health thereby became more difficult to achieve. Moreover, since the DAA, or ATSIC, during the 1980s and 1990s was carrying responsibility for health along with responsibility for politically controversial issues like economic development or land rights, the potential for health policy to be caught up with, and compromised by, these issues was great.[67]

As implied above, the American and Canadian experiences suggest that if the federal health authority is involved in the health of indigenous peoples, professional expertise is more likely to be brought to bear. Indeed, a number of Australian reports have called for professional involvement. In 1979, the House of Representatives Standing Committee on Aboriginal Affairs proposed that a technical advisory group be set up in the Federal Health Department. A task force set out for Aboriginal communities a variety of health care options, and it called for an independent evaluation of Aboriginal health services. Nothing was done. In 1986 it was proposed that the Australian Aboriginal Affairs Council support development of a national Aboriginal health policy; this initiative finally emerged as the National Aboriginal Health Strategy of 1989. Next, in 1990, the idea of an Office of Aboriginal Health for ATSIC was supported by federal and state ministers. Three years later, the Department of Prime Minister and Cabinet proposed that the NHMRC look at how to achieve equity in health for Aboriginal people and examine professional standards in Aboriginal health services, research, education and infrastructure.

Rising concern about competence in health matters produced debate in 1993 about what national body should have responsibility for Aboriginal health. NACCHO and the Aboriginal Health Resources Cooperative in New South Wales argued that the Federal Health Department could provide specialized support and "ministerial attention." The AMA, recognizing that ATSIC was trying to do a good job, called for more health experts to be employed. A 1994 evaluation of the National Aboriginal Health Strategy noted that ATSIC's capacity to deliver outcomes "has been weakened by a lack of expertise in health systems planning and policy development."[68] It wished to see "a workable expert National Council for Aboriginal Health involving commonwealth, state/territory governments, ATSIC and NACCHO to provide policy advice at the national level and oversight the implementation and development of the National Aboriginal Health Strategy."[69] Professionalism and professional competence can, on one hand, be employed ideologically to keep legitimate stakeholders like community representatives out of the decision-making process. But the idea of community control can just as easily be used manipulatively to advance the interests of political factions and powerful individuals.[70] Arguably, both are needed.

There is a problem, then, of a competent nationally cohesive administration. But more fundamentally, there needs to be a secure basis for ensuring that Aboriginal interests are not pushed aside by the claims of other sections of the population. The American and Canadian experiences suggest that formal treaties, imperfect as they have been historically in guaranteeing indigenous rights, do set standards over which litigation may take place, while reconciliation processes are under way. There is also a problem of adequate resources for Aboriginal health advancement. The 1998 Deeble report revealed that almost 80 percent of all services for Aboriginal people were under the control of state and territory governments and that total per capita expenditure on Aborigines and Torres Strait Islanders was only 8 percent greater than that for the national population. However, Aboriginal death rates are 300 percent greater than those of the population as a whole. Differential access to the commonwealth Medical Benefits Scheme and the Pharmaceutical Benefits Scheme means that the commonwealth spends only 63 cents per capita on the Aboriginal and Torres Strait Islander population for each dollar of spending on the population as a whole.

If the commonwealth were to spend another hundred million dollars per annum, with matching expenditure by the states, existing inequity in per capita benefits under the national health insurance scheme would be much reduced. As we have seen, living conditions—housing, water supply, waste disposal, education and income—especially in rural and remote communities, are commonly poor. Since these are known to have a large impact on mortality and morbidity, particularly where infectious diseases, substance abuse and injury are still significant, they must be addressed, even if the expenditure required may be of on even larger scale than that needed for health services. An intersectoral, "whole-of-government" approach will be needed.[71]

Immigrant Health

Another important social group with a health status different from that of the population as a whole comprises immigrants. Australia has been a land of immigration for over two hundred years. In the nineteenth century, most immigrants were English, Irish, Scots and Welsh. But since the 1850s Chinese (seeking their fortunes on the goldfields), since the 1860s Pacific Islanders (laboring in the sugarcane fields of Queensland) and since the 1890s Japanese (working in the pearl-diving industry in tropical Australia) have also come as immigrants. In 1901, the new commonwealth, pursuing the ideal of

"White Australia," excluded non-Europeans under the Immigration Restriction Act. This exclusion remained one of the national "settled policies" until the 1960s.

Until the 1940s, however, immigrants continued to be overwhelmingly drawn from Britain, with only a few from Ireland after it gained independence in 1921. There was some southern European migration, especially to Queensland in the period before the depression of the 1930s. During the Second World War, apart from a few Jewish refugees from Nazi Europe in 1930–46, migration virtually ceased, so that by 1947 fewer than 10 percent of the population were foreign born. But in 1947–72 there was massive migration from Europe, the noteworthy feature of which was a movement away from Britain as the dominant source of immigrants.[72]

After 1947 there were various waves of immigration, the two most important of which in their impact on ethnic health policy were those immediately following World War II and the Vietnam War. The first wave from Europe began after Australia agreed with the International Refugee Organization in 1947 to take displaced persons and refugees. Wars and political violence in Southeast Asia, the Middle East and Latin America, and the progressive abandonment of the White Australia policy from the 1960s, led to the second wave. Strict health screening protected Australians from diseases accompanying immigrants and ensured that the new settlers would constitute a reliable workforce as well as produce healthy Australian-born children. Not until the 1980s, however, did health and welfare services adequately meet the demands of the immigrant communities themselves. In the 1950s and 1960s immigrants arrived from the Netherlands, Italy, Malta, Austria, Greece, West Germany, Spain, Belgium, Switzerland, Finland, Scandinavia and the United States. The fact that young male workers were preferred and that all immigrants were carefully screened before departure meant that they were high in average standard of health and made little call on health services. Moreover, apart from sports clubs and places of worship, ethnic communities had not yet developed community organizations through which to articulate their health demands.

In the late 1960s and early 1970s, however, welfare inquiries revealed the comparative deprivation of immigrants in the areas of employment, housing and health care. Two major health system reforms of the Whitlam Labor government—Medibank (the universal health insurance scheme) and the Community Health Program—did much to overcome the health care disadvantages of migrants. But community groups like the NSW Mental Health Association began to lobby for specific services, as did the emerging ethnic lobby. Two lots of South Vietnamese refugees arrived with the end of the war in Vietnam in April 1975. A larger third group, the "boat people," came with inadequate or no health screening; its health status was lower than that of earlier arrivals. Many of the "boat people" were malnourished or carried tuberculosis, skin infections and intestinal parasites, and sometimes leprosy and sexually transmitted diseases. States began to set up medical screening programs for immigrants and to provide immunization services. The Galbally report to the federal government in 1978 recommended new services to compensate for inequities experienced by immigrants. Ethnic health workers and interpreters represented in the 1980s a significant improvement in access to health care facilities.

Beginning in NSW in 1976, ethnic affairs commissions were set up in South Australia (1980), Victoria (1983), Western Australia (1984) and Queensland (1990), signaling the advent of official recognition of multiculturalism or cultural pluralism. In the 1980s, certain states and territories developed ethnic health units and used ethnic advisers. In 1983, NSW reinforced multiculturalism by requiring all government departments to report each year on progress in ethnic affairs policy. In the 1980s and 1990s, the issue of mainstreaming versus provision of ethno-specific services was debated by health professionals and by the ethnic communities themselves. Historically, a social-welfare model of ethnic health policy, which focuses on cultural relations and implies an interest group view of policy, has prevailed. Absent has been a model focused on social inequality.[73]

Generally, immigrants experience lower death rates than Australian-born people, although the advantage diminishes with length of residence in Australia. Their mortality rates converge with those of Australian-born citizens over time. Also, for some diseases, especially some cancers, diabetes and infectious diseases, immigrants from certain countries do less well than the Australian born. As table 5.11 indicates, all immigrants had lower all-cause mortality rates than did Australian-born females and males. But some nationalities had higher ones for infectious diseases (listed on the table as Other Europe, Asia, and Other males and females); lung cancer (United Kingdom and Ireland males and females and Other Europe males); cervical cancer (Other Europe, Asia, and Other females); breast cancer (UK and Ireland females); motor vehicle accidents (Other Europe males, and UK and Ireland, Asia, and Other females); suicide (Other Europe males, and UK and Ireland and Other Europe females); homicide (Asia and Other males, and Other Europe, Asia, and Other females); and diabetes mellitus (Other Europe, Asia, and Other males, and Other Europe, Asia, and Other females).[74]

While the public health policy revival of the 1980s and 1990s saw attempts to address the social, economic and environmental determinants of health, the socioeconomic factors specific to ethnic communities have been largely ignored. A Better Health Commission report (1986) did acknowledge that social and economic distress, changes in diet and work-related health risk influenced immigrant health. But the *Health for All Australians* report (1988) virtually omitted consideration of structural determinants when it set out the goals of preserving the initial health advantages of immigrants by encouraging healthy lifestyles and environments, and addressing the special health needs of refugees as they arrived. The aggregate picture that the health of immigrants is better than that of the Australian-born tends to obscure the fact of socioeconomic status variation and widespread socioeconomic disadvantage in some communities. Unemployment rates tend to be higher. When in 1990 the Australian rate was 5.7 percent, the Vietnamese community rate was 12.5, the Lebanese community rate 23.9, and the Polish rate 11.8 percent. Some ethnic communities are disproportionately employed in manual work. Thus, 52 percent of Yugoslav-born males and 57 percent of Yugoslav-born females would need to cease to do manual work for the Yugoslav occupational distribution to approximate that of the Australian born.[75]

Health Status and Gender

In 1924, the age-standardized death rate for Australian males was 17.3 deaths per thousand population, and for females 13.9. Seventy years later they had fallen to 8.6 and 5.2, respectively, but the difference between them was exactly the same. However, the difference in terms of life expectancy at birth has widened—in 1920–22, 59.2 years for males and 63.3 years for females, and in 1994 seventy-five years and 80.9 years, respectively. Although women report more illness and use health care services more, the mortality differential is to their advantage. There is no expert consensus on the reasons for women's mortality advantage. Some have suggested that cultural and social expectations concerning tolerance for pain and stoicism in the face of suffering lead men to deny illness and decline to seek medical advice. They would accordingly report lower morbidity rates than women. As male attitudes and behavior change in the postfeminist era, men may be more willing to seek care earlier, and this may help reduce male death rates. A second argument has it that female biological resistance to disease is superior, as in part evidenced by the better survival rates of female fetuses and female infants' lesser susceptibility to infections. Women's greater morbidity rates can be in part attributed to reproductive lifecycle factors—menstruation, childbirth and menopause. In any case, cultural and social forces must have a significant impact, because in economically developing countries the gender mortality differential goes in the opposite direction. In developed countries, males disproportionately follow high-risk occupations, and risk taking is more generally an acceptable social norm for males; greater male mortality may be partly explained by these cultural and social differences between the sexes. One estimate in the early 1980s attributed about 90 percent of the excess of Australian male deaths (in the fifteen-to-forty-four-years age group) to accidents and suicide.

There is evidence of mortality differences by social class for women in the United Kingdom wherein mortality of women in nonmanual work is less than that of women in manual occupations. The differences are even greater for nonworking women. There is also some evidence of deprivation influencing health in a gendered way, in London. While disadvantaged people of both

Table 5.11
Mortality by Country of Birth, Cause and Gender for Population 15 Years and Older, Australia, 1992–94, Standardized Mortality Ratio

Cause	Australia	UK and Ireland	Other Europe*	Asia†	Other⊗
Males					
Infectious/parasitic	1.00	0.94	1.10	1.68	1.34
Cancers:	1.00	0.99	0.90	0.67	0.78
Lung	1.00	1.22	1.04	0.64	0.74
Diabetes mellitus	1.00	0.87	1.36	1.11	1.32
Cardiovascular diseases	1.00	0.90	0.88	0.65	0.91
Respiratory	1.00	0.99	0.59	0.57	0.63
Digestive	1.00	0.88	0.94	0.55	0.74
Motor vehicle accidents	1.00	0.93	1.02	0.72	0.92
Suicide	1.00	0.95	1.08	0.39	0.82
Homicide	1.00	0.92	0.98	1.06	1.16
All Causes	1.00	0.93	0.88	0.65	0.84

Females					
Infectious/parasitic	1.00	0.88	1.18	1.53	1.09
Cancers:	1.00	1.05	0.90	0.72	0.90
Lung	1.00	1.50	0.68	0.71	0.81
Cervix	1.00	0.85	1.16	1.17	1.03
Breast	1.00	1.11	0.88	0.66	0.96
Diabetes mellitus	1.00	0.85	1.86	1.64	1.14
Cardiovascular diseases	1.00	0.90	0.87	0.72	0.87
Respiratory	1.00	1.03	0.56	0.66	0.74
Digestive	1.00	0.99	0.80	0.71	0.75
Motor vehicle accidents	1.00	1.11	0.96	1.07	1.22
Suicide	1.00	1.34	1.57	0.96	0.97
Homicide	1.00	0.72	1.70	1.31	1.24
All Causes	1.00	0.96	0.87	0.74	0.87

*Continental Europe, including Eastern Europe, the former USSR and the Baltic States.

†Northeast, Southeast and Southern Asia.

⊗Middle East, Northern and Southern Africa, the Americas, New Zealand and the Pacific region.

Source: *Australia's Health, 1996.The Fifth Biennial Health Report of the Australian Institute of Health and Welfare* (Canberra: Australian Government Publishing Service, 1996), 31–32.

sexes report worse health, men are more influenced by material deprivation, women by social deprivation. Women in Western societies generally have a richer web of social relationships, and this may explain some of the female advantage in mortality. But there is also evidence of the health costs of caring and interpersonal closeness. In any case, gender roles and behavior are changing in ways sometimes detrimental to female health—for example, young women in Australia are now more likely to be cigarette smokers than young men—so the female mortality advantage may well erode significantly in the future.[76]

SOCIOECONOMIC STATUS AND HEALTH INEQUALITIES

We have seen that for 150 to two hundred years, major public health figures have from time to time taken up the issue of the social gradient in health status—the fact that lower socioeconomic status (SES) (or social class) tends to go in tandem with poorer health, usually characterized by high mortality rates. We have observed that in Australia, Aboriginality has historically been associated with very poor health and high mortality, in large part because it has also been associated with very low SES. We turn now to look at SES and health patterns.

As pointed out early in this chapter, professional interest in differences in socioeconomic status and correlations with differences in healthiness has a particularly long history in Britain. The modern revival of concern from the 1970s began there; it then spread to a number of developed countries, including Australia. A number of studies in Australia have helped establish that the pattern of health inequalities revealed in Britain and other countries also exists here. Whether defined by occupation, employment, education, income or place of residence, differences in SES have been linked with differences in health status. The conclusion would appear to be that social and economic conditions impact significantly on health: "The most disadvantaged groups within our society have the poorest health, highest rates of exposure to health-damaging risk factors, make the most use of primary and secondary health services, and make the least use of preventive services."[77]

Various explanations have been offered for the existence of social inequalities in health in developed countries. It has been suggested that the way social class has been measured exaggerates the health differentials—the artefactual explanation—because changes in the types of occupations make comparisons with occupational classification in periods earlier in the twentieth century impossible. But too many studies, using different indicators of class or socioeconomic status—such as education or income, or looking at retirees or females, not working males—have revealed the same association between health status and socioeconomic status. Social selection has been advanced as another explanation. People prone to illness move down the social scale or fail to move upward, so that low SES groups contain disproportionate numbers of unhealthy persons. Longitudinal studies following people from birth indicate that while health influences social status, the effect is not great enough to explain the social gradient. Social status determines health, not health social status, as the selection hypothesis would have it. Another explanation advanced has been that of differential access to health care services. The Black committee in the United Kingdom was asked to look at this but concluded health inequalities did not arise from unequal access. When mortality from causes amenable to medical care is examined, it appears that the decline in mortality from such causes is somewhat greater in social class I (the highest) than social class V (the lowest), perhaps reflecting unequal access. But the overall impact on mortality is small, because amenable causes represent a small part of the total, and the growing differential between classes is due to the falling nonamenable mortality of higher classes in contrast to an absence of decline in the lower classes. However, this finding concerning the limited role of inequities in medical care should not be used to support proposals to reduce funding for health care, because lower-class victims of the unequal distribution of ill health will continue to depend heavily on access to health care.

Another approach focuses on the role of early life experience—the origins in childhood of adult ill health. But it is difficult to assess the direct impact of early and subsequent life experience on health. Michael Marmot's Whitehall studies data show that height (which is influenced by genes and environment) relates to social status, as indicated by grade of Civil Service employment. Adult mortality is predicted by modest height independently of grade, so that this correlation reveals the ongoing effect of early life. However, Civil Service grade, itself reflecting contemporary social effects, is a predictor of mortality independently of height. Early life and contemporary influences are thus impacting on risk of mortality.

Because the social gradient in health status exists across many causes of death—lung cancer, coronary heart disease, cerebrovascular disease, chronic bronchitis, other respiratory disease, accidents and violence, for example, in the Whitehall data—it has been proposed that social class is linked with differing general susceptibility to disease. However, some cancers—brain, prostate, breast, colon, haematopoietic system, and melanoma—do not reveal the social gradient, thus calling the general susceptibility hypothesis into doubt. Yet both general and specific causes (like smoking) may be operating. Since the life experience of different social classes differ from the outset, cumulative effects on health may produce different general susceptibility to many diseases.

Differences in risk factors and health behaviors (lifestyle) explains social class differences only in part. In the Whitehall studies, those in lower grades of the United Kingdom Civil Service were more obese, more likely to smoke, and less likely to engage in physical exercise activities or to follow a good diet. Yet a social gradient in coronary heart disease mortality and incidence existed even when allowance was made for these behaviors. Nonsmokers showed a social gradient in mortality as marked as that for smokers. In any case, why do social inequalities in behavior exist? Smoking, for example, is related to social status. This itself is related to ill health, but not simply because of smoking behavior. As the Black report and the Australian National Health Strategy report of 1992 have shown, poverty—the lack of basic material resources—produces disproportionate ill health and mortality for lower social classes. It is a structural factor—something over which those caught in it have no personal control—given the existing distribution of income and educational opportunity.

Other investigators, while acknowledging the influence of material conditions, have given more weight to stress levels, social networks and social support, so that the emerging explanation of the social gradient relies on invocation of both material and psychosocial factors. As noted earlier in the chapter, Marmot's Whitehall studies, in particular, invoke psychosocial influences inherent in social position to explain differential mortality and morbidity. Moreover, this work looks to relative, not absolute material deprivation to explain the fact that the lower grades of the Civil Service had lower health status than the upper ones, even though they did not suffer absolute (or indeed extreme) deprivation in any sense. Addressing psychosocial factors, the Whitehall studies focused on job strain, low level of social supports and low level of control. Lower grades were relatively disadvantaged in relation to stress and degree of social support. Leonard Syme has independently argued that the lack of control over life arising from poverty, and indeed from relative deprivation, may partly explain differential health disadvantage. The second Whitehall study found that degree of control over, and nature of, work was more important than pressure (in the sense of being stressed by deadlines) in explaining the social gradient in coronary heart disease and other sources of ill health such as depression. Control over work meant latitude in decisionmaking and use of skills.[78]

We have already discussed the Acheson inquiry into health inequalities, 1997–98, and the Blair Labor government's response to its proposals. In the United States, the *Healthy People 2000: National Health Promotion and Disease Prevention Objectives* (1991) program identified three broad national goals, one of which was "to reduce health disparities among Americans." The other two were to increase the years of healthy life and to achieve universal access to preventive services.[79] In almost all cases, the disparities related to the large proportion of minority populations existing on or below the poverty line. But the *Healthy People 2000* program failed to deal with the need for a disproportionate allocation of resources to be provided for such populations which were the worst affected by health and social problems like hypertension, asthma, diabetes, violence, homelessness, HIV/AIDS, and low levels of immunization. *The Healthy People 2010* program has as one of its two aims—the elimination of health disparities over the next decade.[80]

The Australian research effort in the area of social inequalities in health showed a gradual upward trend in the 1970s and 1980s, and a marked upward trend in the 1990s (see table 5.12). The first of the modern empirical studies on the relationship between socioeconomic status and health appeared in 1971, although in an isolated study published in the 1940s, G.R. Bruns showed that the size of infant death rates of Melbourne suburbs in the 1930s correlated well with the socioeconomic standing of the suburb. To 1996, 202 studies were published in national and international journals. The largest proportion was published in the *Australian and New Zealand Journal of PublicHealth* (22.3 percent); the *Medical Journal of Australia* (17.8 percent); and *Social Science and Medicine* (7.9 percent).

In 1995–96, thirty-two papers appeared, being the largest number for any two-year period since 1971. This must be seen against the fact that in the same period more than two hundred papers (with SES indicators as descriptors) a month appeared internationally in health journals. Occupation-based measures of SES almost solely have been used in Australian studies because

Table 5.12
Number of Australian Empirical Studies on the Relationship between Socioeconomic Status and Health, 1971–96

Years	Number of Studies	Percentage
1971–72	4	2.2
1973–74	3	1.7
1975–76	6	3.4
1977–78	7	3.9
1979–80	13	7.3
1981–82	7	3.9
1983–84	16	8.9
1985–86	12	6.7
1987–88	10	5.6
1989–90	16	8.9
1991–92	25	14.0
1993–94	28	15.6
1995–96	32	17.9
Total	179	100.0

Source: G. Turrell, B. Oldenburg, I. McGuffog and R. Dent, *Socioeconomic Determinants of Health: Towards a National Research Program and a Policy and Intervention Agenda* (Canberra: Queensland University of Technology School of Public Health and AusInfo, 1999), 11.

information on other individual-level indicators of SES like income and education are not collected during the process of death certification and registration in Australia. Almost nothing is known therefore about how income and education are related to mortality. The great bulk of studies (individual and area-level) have been of urban populations so that it is unclear if rural inequalities are similar, and if they are due mainly to the presence of Aboriginal communities which are known to have poor health status. However, it is clear that people in lower socioeconomic groups have greater death rates for most significant causes of death, they endure more ill health, and they are less likely to use preventive services. Both women and men experience health inequalities at every stage of the life cycle. Moreover, these inequalities apply to psychosocial health, risk factor profiles, and health behaviors like smoking and diet. Yet, some major causes of mortality run counter to this trend. Breast cancer, colorectal cancer, and melanoma disproportionately affected people of higher socioeconomic status.[81]

Over the last two decades health in all age groups of the Australian population has advanced. Yet, social inequalities in health have increased. In 1985–87, mortality rates for men, twenty-five to sixty-four years, in the poorest areas were 55 percent greater for coronary heart disease, 60 percent greater for lung cancer and 73 percent greater for motor vehicle accidents than men in the least disadvantaged areas. In 1995–97, the differentials were 87 percent, 98 percent and 133 percent respectively. Women experienced the same increase in health inequality. In the mid to late 1980s, mortality of women, twenty-five to sixty-four years, in the most disadvantaged areas was 204 percent greater for diabetes, 66 percent greater for motor vehicle accidents, and 43 percent greater for asthma/emphysema than women in the least disadvantaged areas. In 1995–97, the differentials had grown to 249 percent, 121 percent, and 194 percent respectively.

The same social gradient operates for illness. Babies from low SES families are more likely to be premature or of low birthweight. Children from the same backgrounds experience greater rates of developmental retardation, worse dental health, more chronic ill-health, and higher rates of pedestrian injury. Adults of working age are more likely to have fair to poor health, to put up with more chronic health conditions, and to experience greater rates of serious occupational injury. Moreover, their risk factor profiles are worse—more likely to be obese, to experience higher, low-density, lipoprotein cholesterol levels (but lower levels of high-density lipoprotein cholesterol), high blood pressure and higher triglyceride levels, and higher absolute cholesterol intake. They have higher levels of hospital admissions and doctor consultations (reflecting their poorer health). But they use screening and other preventive services less, which may have implications for their rates of breast and cervical cancer. With virtually universal access to health care under the tax-funded national health insurance scheme, Medicare, inadequate health care is unlikely to be a major contributor to health inequalities.

One model useful for understanding relationships between health state and socioeconomic status involves identifying factors as "upstream" (macro), "midstream" (intermediate) and "downstream" (micro). Included in the macro factors are social and economic determinants like education, employment, occupation, income and housing. More remote determinants are national government policies concerning welfare and income distribution, which themselves are affected by the forces of the global, capitalist economy. Intermediate factors include psychosocial processes like stress, coping capacity and social support; health behaviors like diet, smoking and physical activity; and the health care system, which is critical in dealing with the problems of those worst affected by inequality. Micro factors include adverse changes to the functioning of individual's physiological and biological systems which produce illness and disease. Harmful psychosocial influences and health behaviors in the long-term produce the heavier burden of physiological and biological malfunctioning which leads to the poorer health status of lower socioeconomic groups. The multilevel model in principle provides at all three levels points of entry for policy interventions intended to reduce health inequalities.[82]

Policy interventions have to be applied at various levels as the evidence points to the fact that no one point of entry is paramount, although macro-level interventions clearly will act on the basic social and economic determinants of health. Further, the key determinants like housing, education, transport and employment lie outside the health sector. Intersectoral collaboration thus becomes vital in the quest to reduce inequalities. Interventions may be aimed at one or more of the following: new social and economic policies at the macro level such as training programs for unemployed people, especially the most vulnerable (youth, Aborigines and the disabled); improvement of living and working conditions in the traditional public health intervention areas—housing, sanitation, safe workplaces and a safe, nutritious, food supply; strengthening the social "fabric" by involving deprived communities in health-promoting activities such as planning urban renewal projects and promoting personal skills and network building to empower communities. WHO's Healthy Cities projects in various parts of the world, including Australia, is a prime example of working with communities; modifying harmful health behaviors by health promotion interventions which also provide for social support; empowering of disadvantaged individuals by improving their coping skills and social support; and maintaining the equity of the health care system by providing an economically, geographically and culturally accessible universal, tax-funded system; within the health care system, redistribution of resources to public health and health promotion activities including primary and community care programs. While a universal health care system appears to confer disproportionate benefits on higher socioeconomic groups, departure from universality disproportionately penalizes the most deprived groups.[83]

Canada has led the way in research on the social and economic determinants of population health in the 1990s. The work of the epidemiologists and economists of the Canadian Institute of Advanced Research on the concept of population health has stimulated debate in public health circles across the Western world including Australia. In the United Kingdom, as we have noted, research work on, and intermittent official inquiry into, the issue of social inequalities in health have been pursued since the 1980 Black report, even if policy action was delayed until Labor replaced the Conservatives in government in the late 1990s. Australian researchers have been pursuing research individually since the 1970s. Recently, a collective effort, supported by the commonwealth government, has been initiated. Moreover, high-profile clinicians' bodies have supported the call of public health researchers for action to reduce the steepness of the social gradient in health status. The Health Policy Unit of the Royal Australasian College of Physicians produced a publication on social and economic determinants of health: *For Richer for Poorer, In Sickness and In Health: The Socioeconomic Determinants of Health* (1999). In this, physicians are urged ". . . to act methodically in all areas of policy making to put what we know into practice. While the large burden of disease requires continuing investment in healthcare, we must move beyond alleviating damage once it has occurred and invest significantly in preventative health efforts."[84] A set of proposals are advanced concerning ways to reduce socioeconomic inequalities.

The Health Department of New South Wales recently established the Centre for Health Equity Training, Research and Evaluation. Although a neoconservative government has been in power at the commonwealth level since 1996, a number of Federal Health Department initiatives have been taken in the last couple of years concerning research on, and public discussion of, social inequalities in health, although no major policy developments have occurred. The commonwealth department commissioned the Queensland University of Technology School of Public Health to carry out a critical review of Australian research done in the area of health inequalities. This resulted in the School group producing *Socioeconomic Determinants of Health: Towards a National Research Program and Policy and Intervention Agenda* (1999).

Although the National Health Strategy (1992) addressed the issue of social inequalities, the first dedicated policy review published by the commonwealth department was *Health Policy and Inequality,* which came out in 1999. The publication reviewed the evidence, overseas and Australian, concerning the social gradient in health status. It gave too much weight, according to Najman and Davey Smith, to a psychosocial cause of health inequalities associated with the work of Michael Marmot, the degree of control felt by the individual over his/her work and life circumstances. Najman and Davey Smith point out that Marmot's control factor has not been found by others in replicated studies and that it might well be a result rather than a cause of inequalities.[85]

In 1998, the commonwealth Health Department commissioned the National Centre for Epidemiology and Population Health (NCEPH) at the Australian National University to carry out a feasibility study for a research and development collaboration on inequalities in health. It was to work with a reference group composed of representatives of the NHMRC, the Public Health Association and the Public Health Education and Research Program, as well as public health and social policy academics, to propose future developments. The Center sponsored a discussion paper and also consultations in conjunction with visits by distinguished overseas researchers, Leonard Syme, Emeritus Professor of Public Health, the University of California; Michael Marmot, Director, the International Centre for Health and Society, University College, London; and Fraser Mustard, Foundation Director, the Canadian Institute for Advanced Research. The consultations produced a consensus favoring action-oriented research emphasizing efforts to reduce inequalities. The commonwealth Department of Health and Aged Care gave a contract to NCEPH to create "an institute without walls." The collaboration was not to favor a particular research paradigm. It was expected to promote, nationally, research capacity in the area of social determinants of health and develop as well capacity to produce policy syntheses. Three areas of research were identified as priorities:

- The impact of early life experience and the differences between socioeconomic groups in the effect of cumulative disadvantages on health over the life cycle.
- Since evidence exists of the significance of social support for health, research into what produces a healthy community.
- The effect of primary health care on health status in the light of evidence that disadvantaged groups underuse preventive services.

Both socioeconomic and urban-rural differentials in health were to be investigated; at a later date, gender and ethnic differences. The interdisciplinary reach will extend to work beyond the usual mix of biomedical, behavioral and health-service determinants. Following the lead of Canada, regular policy syntheses will be produced to make available to policy makers, in appropriate form, research findings. In Canada, the process involves reviews of published and unpublished research material, interviews with experts, and analysis of data, after which a discussion paper is produced. In turn, this is reviewed by national and international assessors. Finally, policy makers join researchers to discuss translation into policy.

The Health Inequalities Research Collaboration is committed to helping improve the quality of data, including the development of a socioeconomic classification system for use by data collection agencies. It will promote longitudinal birth cohort studies and creation of a national record-linkage system. Such a system would facilitate connection of population health status, health services use and census data (especially on income and education). Small-area studies would permit inquiry into the relationship between community resources and health. The Collaboration hosted in mid-2000 the first conference of researchers in Australia on social determinants of health. Those at NCEPH connected with the Collaboration were keen to see a permanent body like the Canadian Institute of Advanced Research (CIAR), created by private sector effort in 1982, set up in Australia. This would take the research agenda beyond the collaboration's concern with health determinants to the broader issues of equity and distribution of income and wealth, which subsume the health inequalities issue. Independent of government and other interests, the CIAR, internationally recognized for the quality of its research work, seeks to promote synergies across the human sciences. It promotes debate among psychologists, biologists, physiologists, educationists, economists, statisticians, epidemiologists, paediatricians and policy scientists. Eight research programs are now being pursued—evolutionary biology, cosmology and gravity, earth system evolution, superconductivity, soft surfaces and interfaces, population health, economic growth, and human development. Population health, economic growth, and human development have formed the Human Sciences Cross-Program Linkages Group. The group has been addressing issues like the relationship between literacy and numeracy on the one hand and health on the other; individual and social wellbeing indicators for use in assessing progress; the impact of fairness in policies on health and wellbeing; and the effect of wealth on health. An Australian equivalent, pursuing a strategic view of social, economic and environmental change, would transcend the limitations of the Collaboration which arise from its direct creation by government and its strong focus on health policy.[86]

Public health in Australia as elsewhere is at a crossroads. It can take the broad road concerning itself with the social and economic determinants of health, and with health inequalities, human rights, and global environmental issues as they relate to health. Or it can follow a narrow path, focusing on individual risks of disease, disease prevention, and cost containment. With individualistic and market-oriented ideologies dominating public discourse about the state as well as government policy, the effort required to propel public health along the broad social road will be great. In the remainder of this volume we will review important, current preoccupations of public health, and try to answer the question, where to from here?

NOTES

1. P. Townsend, N. Davidson and M. Whitehead, *Inequalities in Health* (London: Penguin Books, 1988), 219; G.R. Palmer and S.D. Short, *Health Care and Public Policy. An Australian Analysis* (South Melbourne: Macmillan Educational

Australia, 1994), 216; F. Baum, *The New Public Health: An Australian Perspective* (Melbourne: Oxford University Press, 1998), 38.

2. B.C. Amick III, S. Levine, A.R. Tarlov and D. Chapman Walsh, "Introduction," in *Society and Health,* eds. B.C. Amick III, S. Levine, A.R. Tarlov and D. Chapman Walsh (New York: Oxford University Press, 1995), 4. G. Rosen, *A History of Public Health* (Baltimore: Johns Hopkins University Press, 1993), 228–32. M. Ramsey, "Public Health in France," in *The History of Public Health and the Modern State,* ed. D. Porter (Amsterdam, Atlanta: Editions Rodopi, 1994), 53–54.

3. Quoted in J. Trostle, "Early Work in Anthropology and Epidemiology: From Social Medicine to the Germ Theory, 1840 to 1920," in *Anthropology and Epidemiology,* ed. C.R. Janes, R. Stall and S.M. Gifford (Dordrecht: D. Reidel, 1986), 46.

4. Ibid., 45–46; H. Waitzkin, "The Social Origins of Illness: A Neglected History," *International Journal of Health Services* 11(1) (1981): 78–82, 97.

5. Quoted in Waitzkin, "The Social Origins of Illness," 85.

6. Ibid., 82–86; B.S. Turner, *Regulating Bodies. Essays in Medical Sociology* (London: Routledge, 1992), 130.

7. Quoted in M. Marmot, M. Bobak and G. Davey Smith, "Explanations for Social Inequalities in Health," in *Society and Health,* ed. B.C. Amick III, S. Levine, A.R. Tarlov and D.Chapman Walsh (New York: Oxford University Press, 1995), 176.

8. Quoted in C. Power, O. Manor and J. Fox, *Health and Class: The Early Years* (London: Chapman and Hall, 1991), 5.

9. J. Fox and M. Benzeval, "Perspectives on Social Variations in Health," in *Tackling Inequalities in Health: An Agenda for Action*, ed. M. Benezal, K. Judge, and M. Whitehead (London: King's Fund, 1995), 11–12; Power, Manor and Fox, *Health and Class,* 5; N. Krieger and E. Fee, "Measuring Social Inequalities in Health in the United States: A Historical Review, 1900–1950," *International Journal of Health Services* 26(3) (1996): 394.

10. J. Rogers Hollingsworth, "Inequality in Levels of Health in England and Wales, 1891–1971," *Journal of Health and Social Behavior* 22 (1981): 279.

11. Ibid., 276–78.

12. C. Webster, *The Health Services Since the War. Volume I. Problems of Health Care. The National Health Service Before 1957* (London: Her Majesty's Stationery Office, 1988), 14–15.

13. Quoted in P. Aiach and R. Carr-Hill, "Inequalities in Health: The Country Debate," in *Health Inequalities in European Countries,* ed. J. Fox (Aldershot: Gower, 1989), 46.

14. R.G. Wilkinson, "Dear David Ennals . . .," *New Society* 38 (16 December 1976): 567–68. C. Webster, *The Health Services Since the War. Volume II. Government and Health Care. The National Health Service 1958–1979* (London: The Stationery Office, 1996), 609–13; Aiach and Carr-Hill, "Inequalities in Health," 44–46.

15. Quoted in ibid., 46.

16. P. Jenkin, foreword (to Black Report) in Townsend, Davidson and Whitehead, *Inequalities in Health,* n.p.

17. Quoted in A. Scott-Samuel and J. Szalai, "Policy Issues in Health Inequality," in *Health Inequalities in European Countries,* ed. Fox, 66.

18. Aiach and Carr-Hill, "Inequalities in Health," 46–47; Scott-Samuel and Szalai, "Policy Issues in Health Inequality," 65–67; Townsend, Davidson and Whitehead, *Inequalities in Health,* 3–5.

19. Townsend, Davidson and Whitehead, *Inequalities in Health,* 2–3.
20. Quoted in P. Townsend, "Widening Inequalities of Health in Britain: A Rejoinder to Rudolf Klein," *International Journal of Health Services* 20 (3) (1990): 369.
21. Quoted in ibid., 363–69.
22. Quoted in Townsend, Davidson and Whitehead, *Inequalities in Health,* 9.
23. Ibid., 6–9, 221, 351–53.
24. Ibid., 13–15.
25. G. Davey Smith and Y. Ben-Shlomo, "Inequalities in Health: What is Happening and What can be Done?" in *Progress in Public Health,* ed. G. Scally (London: F.T. Healthcare, 1997), 75.
26. *Saving Lives: Our Healthier Nation* (London: The Stationery Office, 1999), viii–xi.
27. L. Macintyre, "Professor Peter Townsend–A Civil Society," *In the News* 13 (3) (1999): 3.
28. Quoted in M. Benzeval, K. Judge and M. Whitehead, "Introduction," in *Tackling Inequalities in Health,* ed. Benzeval, Judge and Whitehead, 1.
29. M. Shaw, D. Dorling, D. Gordon and G. Davey Smith, *The Widening Gap: Health Inequalities and Policy in Britain* (Bristol: Policy Press, 1999), 171–77.
30. Benzeval, Judge and Whitehead, "Introduction," 2–3.
31. Quoted in Krieger and Fee, "Measuring Social Inequalities in Health in the United States," 399.
32. Quoted in ibid., 411.
33. Ibid., 394–412.
34. S.L. Syme and L.F. Berkman, "Social Class, Susceptibility, and Sickness," in *The Sociology of Health and Illness. Critical Perspectives,* eds. P. Conrad and R. Kern (New York: St. Martin's Press, 1986), 28–29.
35. P. Conrad and R. Kern, "Who Gets Sick? The Unequal Social Distribution of Disease," in *The Sociology of Health and Illness. Critical Perspectives,* eds. P. Conrad and R. Kern (New York: St. Martin's Press, 1986), 24–25.
36. D.B. Dutton and S. Levine, "Socioeconomic Status and Health: Overview, Methodological Critique, and Reformulation," in *Pathways to Health. The Role of Social Factors,* eds. J.P. Bunker, D.S. Gomby and B.H. Kehrer (Menlo Park: Henry J. Kaiser Family Foundation, 1989), 35–36.
37. G.A. Kaplan, E.R. Pamuk, J.W. Lynch, R.D. Cohen and J.L. Balfour, "Inequality in Income and Mortality in the United States: Analysis of Mortality and Potential Pathways," *BMJ* 312 (1996): 999–1003. R.G. Evans, "Introduction," in *Why Are Some People Healthy and Others Not? The Determinants of Health of Populations,* eds. R.G. Evans, M.L. Barer and T.R. Marmor (New York: Aldine De Gruyter, 1994), 5–14.
38. N. Kreiger and N. Moss, "Accounting for the Public's Health: An Introduction to Selected Papers from a U.S. Conference on 'Measuring Social Inequalities in Health,'" *International Journal of Health Services* 26 (3) (1996): 385–86.
39. M. Whitehead, K. Judge, D.J. Hunter, R. Maxwell, and M.A. Scheuer, "Tacking Inequalities in Health: The Australian Experience," *BMJ* 306 (1993): 783.
40. "100 Years Ago in the Bulletin: Aborigines," *Bulletin,* 17 June (1980): 48.
41. M.A. Brady, "Difference and Indifference: Australian Policy and Practice in Indigenous Substance Abuse" (Ph.D. dissertation, Australian National University,

Canberra, 1999), 13–18; see M. Lewis, *A Rum State: Alcohol and State Policy in Australia* (Canberra: Australian Government Publishing Service [hereafter AGPS], 1992), 157–58.

42. See Lewis, *A Rum State,* 158–60.

43. D. Denoon, "Temperate Medicine and Settler Capitalism: On the Reception of Western Medical Ideas," in *Disease, Medicine and Empire: Perspectives on Western Medicine and the Experience of European Expansion,* ed. R. MacLeod and M. Lewis (London: Routledge, 1988), 121.

44. Quoted in M. Lewis, *Thorns on the Rose: The History of Sexually Transmitted Diseases in Australia in International Perspective* (Canberra: AGPS, 1998), 376.

45. Quoted in Denoon, "Temperate Medicine and Settler Capitalism," 125.

46. See Lewis, *Thorns on the Rose,* 374–79; Denoon, "Temperate Medicine and Settler Capitalism," 125–26.

47. S. Parry, "Disease, Medicine and Settlement: The Role of Health and Medical Services in the Settlement of the Northern Territory, 1911–1939" (Ph.D. dissertation, University of Queensland, Brisbane, 1992), 321–22.

48. Quoted in ibid., 340.

49. See Lewis, *Thorns on the Rose,* 379–82; Parry, "Disease, Medicine and Settlement," 34–42.

50. Parry, "Disease, Medicine and Settlement," 343–96.

51. Ibid., 399–401.

52. See Lewis, *Thorns on the Rose,* 382–85.

53. P.M. Moodie, *Aboriginal Health* (Canberra: ANU Press, 1973), 48–96.

54. Ibid., 97–116.

55. P. Miller and P. Torzillo, "Health, an Indigenous Right: A Review of Aboriginal Health in Australia," *Australian Journal of Medical Science* 17 (1996): 3–4.

56. Quoted in ibid., 7.

57. Ibid., 5–7; see Lewis, *Thorns on the Rose,* 387–97.

58. Miller and Torzillo, "Health, an Indigenous Right," 7; *The National Indigenous Australians' Sexual Health Strategy 1996–97 to 1998–99. A Report of the ANCARD Working Party on Indigenous Australians' Sexual Health* (Canberra: Commonwealth Department of Health and Family Services, 1997), 2–3; and see Lewis, *Thorns on the Rose,* 405.

59. *Sun-Herald,* 25 June 2000.

60. Miller and Torzillo, "Health, an Indigenous Right," 7–8; and see Lewis, *Thorns on the Rose,* 404.

61. *Enough to Make You Sick: How Income and Environment Affect Health,* National Health Strategy Research Paper 1 (Canberra: Commonwealth Department of Health, Housing and Community Services, 1992), 87–88; Miller and Torzillo, "Health, an Indigenous Right," 8–9.

62. National Aboriginal Health Strategy Working Party, *A National Aboriginal Health Strategy* (Canberra: AGPS, 1989), 7. New South Wales Task Force on Aboriginal Health, Report to the Minister for Health, Hon. L.J. Brereton, September 1983 (Sydney: no publisher, [1983]), 44–45.

63. Federal Race Discrimination Commissioner, *Water. A Report on the Provision of Water and Sanitation in Remote Aboriginal and Torres Strait Islander Communities* (Canberra: AGPS, 1994), 1–5, 17–19.

64. Ibid., 29; *Enough to Make You Sick,* 100.

65. S.J. Kunitz, *Disease and Social Diversity: The European Impact on the Health of Non-Europeans* (New York: Oxford University Press, 1994), 6, 27–31.

66. Quoted in Brady, "Difference and Indifference," 54.

67. S.J. Kunitz and M.A. Brady, "Health Care Policy for Aboriginal Australians: The Relevance of the American Indian Experience," *Australian Journal of Public Health* 19(6) (1995): 552–55; Kunitz, *Disease and Social Diversity,* 110–14; Brady, "Difference and Indifference," 34–36.

68. Quoted in Kunitz and Brady, "Health Care Policy for Aboriginal Australians," 557.

69. Ibid.

70. Ibid., 556–57.

71. I. Ring, "A 'Whole of Government' Approach Needed on Indigenous Health," *Australian and New Zealand Journal of Public Health* 22 (6) (1998): 639–40. R. McDermott, "Aboriginal Health Spending: More Needed, But Where?" *Australian and New Zealand Journal of Public Health* 22 (6) (1998): 637–38.

72. J. Jupp, "Two Hundred Years of Immigration," in *The Health of Immigrant Australia. A Social Perspective,* eds. J. Reid and P. Trompf (Sydney: Harcourt Brace Jovanovich, 1990), 8–14.

73. P. Garrett and V. Lin, "Ethnic Health Policy and Service Development," in *The Health of Immigrant Australia: A Social Perspective,* ed. J. Reid and P. Trompf (Sydney: Harcourt Brace Jovanovich, 1990), 341–70.

74. *Australia's Health, 1996: The Fifth Biennial Health Report of the Australian Institute of Health and Welfare* (Canberra: AGPS, 1996), 30–31.

75. Garrett and Lin, "Ethnic Health Policy and Service Development," 370–75.

76. *Australia's Health, 1996,* 5, 8; Baum, *The New Public Health,* 218–21.

77. E. Comino and S. Howell, "The Facts" in *Perspectives on Health Inequity* eds. E. Harris, P. Sainsbury and D. Nutbeam (Sydney: Australian Centre for Health Promotion, Department of Public Health and Community Medicine, University of Sydney, 1999), 37.

78. Marmot, Bobak and Davey Smith, "Explanations for Social Inequalities in Health," 195–206; M. Marmot, "Social Determinants of Health: From Observation to Policy," *Medical Journal of Australia* 172 (2000): 379–81; Baum, *The New Public Health,* 206–7.

79. U.S. Department of Health and Human Services, *Healthy People 2000 Review, 1993* (Hyattsville, Md.: Public Health Service, 1994), 1.

80. C.G. Healton, "The Shape of Our River," *American Journal of Preventive Medicine* 16 (35) (1999): 1. J.M. Dixon, R.M. Douglas and R.M. Eckersley, "Making a Difference to Socio-economic Determinants of Health in Australia: A Research and Development Strategy," *Medical Journal of Australia* 172 (2000): 541.

81. G.R. Bruns, "The Vitality of the People of Melbourne," *Australian Quarterly* 16 (1944): 66–80. G. Turrell, B. Oldenburg, I. McGuffog and R. Dent, *Socio-economic Determinants of Health: Towards a National Research Program and a Policy and Intervention Agenda* (Canberra: Queensland University of Technology, School of Public Health, Ausinfo, 1999), 32–33.

82. G. Turrell and C.D. Mathers, "Socioeconomic Status and Health in Australia," *Medical Journal of Australia* 172 (2000): 434–37.

83. B. Oldenburg, I.D. McGuffog and G. Turrell, "Socioeconomic Determinants

of Health in Australia: Policy Responses and Intervention Options," *Medical Journal of Australia* 172 (2000): 489–91.

84. Quoted in ibid., 489.

85. J.M. Najman and G. Davey Smith, "The Embodiment of Class-Related and Health Inequalities: Australian Policies," *Australian and New Zealand Journal of Public Health* 24 (1) (2000): 3. P. Hupalo and K. Herden, *Health Policy and Inequality* (Canberra: Commonwealth Department of Health and Aged Care, 1999), 2–15.

86. Dixon, Douglas and Eckersley, "Making a Difference to Socio-economic Determinants of Health in Australia," 541–43.

Chapter 6

At the Beginning of the New Millennium, Whither Public Health?

PUBLIC HEALTH, PARTICIPATION, AND HUMAN RIGHTS

The new public health approach emphasizes community participation in health administration and health policy development, as we noted earlier. The rise to prominence of the idea of community participation was not confined to health, however. In the 1960s and 1970s, in the political cultures of liberal democracies like Australia, the United States and the United Kingdom, popular participation in a larger proportion of private and public sector organizations seemed but a matter of time. A more participatory political culture seemed to be emerging. In the workplace, consultative arrangements, less hierarchical organizational structures and equal-opportunity policies were being pursued. In public administration, public-advocate offices, administrative appeals, fuller reporting, and decentralization were being developed. New community-based forms of service delivery appeared: community health centers, women's refuges, community schools, neighbourhood houses and rental housing cooperatives. In local government, services expanded, and elections were more widely contested as the stratum of government nearest the people enjoyed a new lease of life. Radicals in the "people-oriented" professions—social work, medicine, teaching and law—called upon professionals to become more accountable to those they served. Professional authority and autonomy were questioned.

A number of factors promoted this culture. The first two or three postwar decades were a time of sustained economic prosperity and high levels of employment. By the early 1970s, however, the postwar international political and economic order was experiencing some serious crises—American and Australian involvement in the Vietnam War was highly unpopular in some sections of the electorate in both countries, and increases in the price of oil by members of the Organization of the Petroleum Exporting Countries (OPEC) were producing an energy crisis as well as strong inflationary pressure in Western economies. Elites appreciated that greater community participation might head off a more fundamental challenge to the prevailing order.

Powerful social movements, mobilizing social minorities politically, were questioning in a radical manner the ends of both personal and social life. Beginning with the black rights movement in the United States in the 1960s and the Aboriginal rights movement in Australia, these movements eventually included the women's movement, which focused on gender inequality; the lesbian and gay movement, concerned with heterosexual oppression of homosexuals; the peace movement, concerned with the threat of nuclear war and the militarism of nation-states; and the green movement, concerned with the subordination of the natural environment to the material demands of the human species. Sharing a concern with individual needs, the new social movements highlighted the significance of social divisions based on gender, sexuality and race. Disillusioned with the hierarchic and bureaucratic nature of traditional political parties and trade unions, the new social movements sought to reconstruct civil society and create alternative forms of democracy.[1] Egalitarian interpersonal relationships and truly democratic decision making were valued as ends in themselves. They prefigured in current practice the societal-level change that the movements desired. Unlike traditional political parties, the movements did not seek state power but made specific demands on the state—whether for land rights, equal pay and affirmative action legislation, homosexual law reform, demilitarization or government measures to protect the natural environment. Some analysts of the new social movements argued that social conflict in postindustrial society was no longer primarily between capital and labor but between the loci of economic and political decision making and those who were reduced to dependent participation.[2]

The new social movements employed a rights-based language and held a worldview in which egalitarianism, democratic decision making and the sovereignty of the community were key elements. They demanded recognition of their rights to equality from the state and called for cooperative relations within their own communities and with the state. To the extent that these movements have been successful, the advance of their values has helped push cultural and social change in such a direction that the state must seek more to educate and persuade citizens than to coerce them into conforming to certain behaviors.[3]

From the late 1970s, two developments threatened the political idea of greater participation. First, the economies of the West experienced greater interdependence, due to greater trade volumes and greater movement of capital. National economies were now more vulnerable to external forces; the Australian economy, with prices for its commodities declining and its manufacturers inefficient, needed restructuring. Economic neoconservatives on both sides of Australian politics quickly assumed dominance, and deregulation, return to the market as distributor of resources and reduction of government activity became the watchwords. Economic criteria were applied to all human activities, and the public sector was reduced by privatization. Even where government continued to be involved—because the public interest required it, or an industry was too politically difficult to privatize—public quasi-markets were set up. Critics of the effect of neoconservatism on participation have since raised a number of important questions: whether citizens are motivated by more than material self-interest; whether contract administration is feasible when complex activities and a range of values are involved; whether there is evidence of increasing inequity; whether central accountability may become greater and accountability to citizens may diminish; and whether growth in contract administration may not reduce the public sector so much as to change its role.

Australian citizens in the 1990s were already participating extensively in civil society. Perhaps two in three Australians took part in at least one of a dozen "citizenship activities." These ranged across community service, education and other organizations. Four in ten citizens were committed to two or more activities. They were also active in specifically political matters—collecting signatures for a petition, going on legal protest marches or working on community problems. But citizens did not relate participation to the condition of the overall body politic. They felt that their actions did not influence government and bureaucracy. As few as one in ten believed that the federal government functioned for the benefit of all the people. The state (and the elected representatives of the people) were not trusted. If participatory mechanisms like community bodies and social movements, however, are to have an ongoing and effective role, they must appreciate the need to work with the many larger policy networks and communities that carry out detailed policy development in contemporary Australia.[4]

In the prewar era, doctors in Australia enjoyed considerable authority as members of a highly educated elite (in 1920, for example, while almost all Australians were literate, as many as 90 percent lacked secondary education). Moreover, biomedicine was being increasingly associated with the prestige of science. One surgeon, Sir Keith Jones, described the doctor-patient situation in the 1930s: "Doctors were paternalistic and patients very trusting. . . . Medical negligence claims were rare, although missed diagnoses were frequent and treatment mishaps a fact of life."[5] By the 1960s and 1970s, powerful critiques of medicine and health care, some from within medical ranks, were influencing public perceptions. A radical thinker, Ivan Illich, argued in *Medical Nemesis* (1975) that the more high-cost, high-technology medicine there was, the less healthy people were becoming. The health care system made people incapable of looking after themselves and deprived them of self-reliance. The first step, Illich believed, to reform was to "deprofessionalize" and "debureaucratize" health. A truly open market in health care was needed. This was the call, also, of those on the neoconservative side of politics influenced by free market economists like Milton Friedman. On the far left, a Marxist, Vicente Navarro, saw patient dependence on high-technology medicine as arising from capitalism's need to create new consumer needs and new markets. On this view, companies wishing to expand markets for health care products and technology were the drivers of growth in technological medicine.[6]

The self-help movement that swept Western countries at this time advanced arguments similar to those of critics of medicine like Illich. In the health area in Australia, self-help bodies like the Association for the Welfare of Children in Hospital and the Association for Relatives and Friends of the Mentally Ill became active in these years. Such groups (of which perhaps half a million existed in the United States by the late 1970s) were concerned with personal relations, social advocacy and "alternative" lifestyles as well as health. They emphasized peer leadership and guidance from lay, not professional, helpers—who themselves had been helped. They challenged the dependence on expertise that characterizes modern society, driven as it is by science and technology. Some groups, like the long-established Alcoholics Anonymous, accepted the prevailing social order. Others, especially those pursuing gender and sexual liberation, challenged the social and cultural order, including the organization of health care.

Consumerism was another international movement challenging medical authority. Following Ralph Nader's famous victory in automobile safety over the General Motors Corporation in the United States in the 1960s, the consumer movement quickly spread throughout the Western world. Governments enacted consumer protection legislation and appointed ombudsmen to investigate consumer complaints. Enhanced consumer rights consciousness pushed the growth of patient-initiated litigation against doctors and hospitals over the next couple of decades. A Medical Consumers Association was established in Victoria in 1974, and another two years later in New South Wales.[7]

Patients' rights and medical consumerism were particularly prominent in psychiatry, where control of patients' behavior and involuntary-restraint issues were fundamental to practice. Psychiatry was subjected to critiques that focused on issues of power and professional authority. The publication of Thomas Szasz's *Law, Liberty and Psychiatry* in 1963 had a dramatic impact. For Szasz, "mental illness" was an ideological construct that served the interests of social control. Indeed, an antipsychiatry model that drew on the critiques of Szasz, Ronald Laing and David Cooper—all psychiatrists—saw professional intervention as a form of deviance control, the political oppression of weaker citizens. That view was supported by sociological critiques of psychiatric hospitals as "total institutions" and also by revelations about the state misuse of psychiatry in the Soviet Union to contain political dissent. Whereas in the nineteenth century, psychiatrists had been influential in restraining the harshness of the law in relation to the death penalty, in the later twentieth century, the law was used to protect against abuse of patients' rights by psychiatry. In California the Lanterman-Petris-Short Act of 1972, and in Britain the Mental Health Act of 1983 strengthened legal and institutional protection of patients' rights.[8]

From the 1970s, mental health legislation in Australia gave more recognition to patients' rights. The 1974 Queensland Act limited detention of involuntary patients to twenty-one days; beyond that point, an appeal on behalf of the patient could be made to the Mental Health Review Tribunal. The 1977 South Australian Act had similar provisions, while it also restricted the use of controversial treatments like electroconvulsive therapy and psychosurgery. The 1983 New South Wales Act established a mental health advocacy service, offering legal assistance to patients pursuing their rights. The 1990 act and its associated policy embodied the principle of "least restrictive care."[9]

A language of rights is very compatible with the values of the new public health movement. One of the movement's key documents, the Declaration of Alma Ata, 1978, states that health is "a fundamental human right," that people have "the right and duty to participate individually and collectively in the planning and implementation of their health care."[10] The Ottawa Charter on health promotion, 1986, emphasized the sphere of the personal and interpersonal, and the role of the community, just as the manifestos of the new social movements did.[11]

Indeed, the new public health values are quite consistent with those of article 25 of the Universal Declaration of Human Rights, 1948, which states "Everyone has the right to a standard of living adequate for the health and well-being of himself and of his family, including food, clothing, housing and medical care and necessary social services."[12] The language of rights has in recent decades begun to permeate Australian political discourse. In 1966, Australia signed the International Covenant on Civil and Political Rights, an instrument intended to give more precise legal form to rights enunciated by the United Nations in the Universal Declaration of Human Rights, 1948. Australian enthusiasts for civil liberties were keen to see the covenant ratified; and the Fraser coalition federal government in 1979 created a Human Rights Commission. Conservative state premiers—Johannes Bjelke-Petersen of Queensland and Charles Court of Western Australia—strongly opposed creation of the commission, and as a result state laws did not come under its purview. Under federal Labor governments from 1983, the commission became more adventurous, concerning itself with human rights breaches under state jurisdiction even if it could not easily bring states to account. In 1993, for example, an outspoken human rights commissioner, Brian Burdekin, criticized Victorian legislation increasing police powers, including forcible fingerprinting of anyone over the age of fourteen years suspected of a crime. He argued that such legislation was at odds with both the international covenant on civil and political rights and the convention on the rights of the child (adopted by the UN General Assembly in 1989, it entered into force in 1990). But he could go no further than calling for commonwealth action to secure state compliance with international covenants.[13]

Unlike the United States and Canada, Australia does not have a bill of rights to protect individuals from arbitrary actions of government, because, as Mr. Justice Mason pointed out, "the founders [of the Australian constitution] accepted, in conformity with prevailing English legal thinking, that the citizen's rights are best left to the protection of the common law and because they were not concerned to protect the individual from oppression by majority will."[14] The Constitution guarantees few definite freedoms, but the High Court has identified some implied ones, especially freedom of political communication—the right of citizen and parliamentary representative to communicate. The court has held that the freedom has a wider ambit than direct communication between elector and elected. The limits of the ambit are unclear; however, public health legislation restricting speech, as in the case of advertising (of health-threatening products), runs in principle a risk of invalidation, because the public interest in free communication may be held to outweigh the public health interest in restriction. In 1994, Philip Morris, the cigarette company, asked the court to invalidate the commonwealth's Tobacco Advertising Prohibition Act of 1992 on the ground that it was contrary to an implied freedom of communication. Showing concern about the reach of the freedom-of-communication doctrine, the federal Labor government in 1995 had the act amended so that it might not contravene rights flowing from the constitutional freedom of political communication.

In Canada, the Quebec court of appeal had found in 1993 that similar prohibition of tobacco advertising did not infringe what is in that country the explicit constitutional right to free speech. However, in 1995 the supreme court of Canada overturned the decision, finding that freedom of commercial expression was a fundamental tenet of a free and democratic society. It might be prudent for those in Australia advocating restrictive public health legislation first to show that there is a need (for example, a causal connection between tobacco advertising and consumption) and second, that the burden produced by the restriction of freedom is not unduly greater than the benefit.[15]

Some state governments and the commonwealth promoted community participation in health services administration as early as the 1970s. We have looked in some detail at the Community Health Program initiated in 1973. Subsequently, district health councils were set up in Victoria, health and welfare councils in South Australia, the Consumer Advisory Network in Western Australia, the district health forums in Tasmania, the Health Issues Centre in Melbourne, the Public Interest Advocacy Centre in Sydney and the national Consumers' Health Forum in Canberra. In 1985–90, sixteen (of forty-three planned) district health councils were set up in Victoria, with the aim of promoting community participation and educating people about the factors that influence their health. Financial constraints hobbled the initiative, but the Victorian Consumer Health Voice from 1993 kept consumer advocacy alive. In the mid-1980s, consumer and community groups urged the federal health minister to strengthen consumer representation. When in 1987 a Health Department review supported the proposal, the Consumers' Health Forum (CHF) was created to allow consumer input into national policy making. By the mid-1990s, the CHF was responsible for selection and support of consumer representatives on more than eighty national health committees, which included those of the NHMRC and the commonwealth Health Department itself.

The community health movement was responsible for a major national initiative in support of community participation in the 1980s—the Community Health Accreditation and Standards Program (CHASP), which was developed to provide standards of quality and measures of effectiveness for community health services, including accountability to local communities. Initially developed as a review process in New South Wales in 1982–83, CHASP, with federal funding, reviewed fourteen community health centers in Victoria and South Australia. This resulted in publication of a manual of standards in 1985. After more work in these states and in Queensland, Tasmania and the ACT, a revised edition of the manual was brought out in 1991. This edition listed fifty-two standards (each with a list of indicators for assessing the service's level of achievement) covering the following areas: assessment/management of health problems; early detection; health promotion; community liaison, participation and advocacy; rights of consumers; client and program records; education, training and development; planning, quality assurance and evaluation; management; and work and its environment. From 1987, the commonwealth Health Department funded the Australian Community Health Association to promote the use of CHASP standards nationally.[16]

New South Wales pioneered mechanisms to deal with consumer health care complaints, establishing an independent Complaints Unit as early as 1984. It could investigate the work of, and prosecute, health care providers. The Victorian and Queensland complaints commissions, in contrast, pursued conciliation, while professional registration boards investigated and carried out prosecutions of health care professionals. In 1993, a National Health Strategy background paper recommended that the commonwealth draw up, with the assistance of consumer and community groups, a national charter of health rights akin to the Patients' Charter developed in Britain. The states and territories became obliged under the Medicare Agreements of 1993–98 to provide public hospital-services consumers with a Public Patients' Hospital Charter. This included the right to obtain free services as a public patient, to obtain them according to the criterion of clinical need, and to receive information on the services available to a public patient.[17]

HIV/AIDS, COMMUNITY PARTICIPATION AND HUMAN RIGHTS

The appearance in Australia of HIV/AIDS in the early 1980s raised in a very forthright way issues of both community participation and human rights. HIV/AIDS reinforced tendencies toward community involvement endorsed by the new public health perspective, because in the absence of a cure or vaccine, preventive education was central to control, and because the gay community played a leading part in preventive and educational work. Government encouraged community participation. Doctors and researchers worked with gay communities to promote condom use and availability; later, they worked to have needle exchanges established. High-risk groups—men having sex with men, hemophiliacs, injecting drug users, and prostitutes—were consulted by scientific and medical organizations, and were involved centrally in the task of prevention.

The pandemic has seen more than sixty million people infected and in the forty-five worst affected countries, it is projected that, between 2000 and 2020, sixty-eight million people will die prematurely from AIDS. In the early years much publicity was given to the threat to the populations of affluent countries like Australia, but over 95 percent of HIV-infected persons are residents of economically developing countries, a very great number of them in Africa and Asia. Not only has the virus spread very widely through African populations, but the high price of antiretroviral drugs combined with the poverty of African nations has largely prevented effective treatment. In countries like Zimbabwe, "therapeutic anarchy" in the absence of development of treatment guidelines has blighted treatment, even when drugs are available.[18]

In terms of mortality, morbidity and financial cost, the HIV/AIDS epidemic was potentially one of the most significant public health crises Australia has ever had to confront. The national policy response involved what a 1995 official evaluation called a "partnership between the affected communities, governments at all levels, and medical, scientific and health care professionals."[19] Australia was also fortunate to have the wealth, as well as enough state commitment to collective public provision, to offer high-quality health care and to support an extensive, and vitally important, educational program for high-risk groups. Under the able leadership of the federal health minister, Dr. Neal Blewett, a former professor of political science, a bipartisan approach to national policy formation was early established. Indeed, Australia was at the forefront internationally of initiatives in education and prevention, being the first country to test the blood supply for HIV and among the earliest to create an effective national strategy. The second official evaluation of the national HIV/AIDS strategy, concluded in 1995, that the epidemic among injecting drug users, sex workers, and heterosexuals had been contained. New HIV diagnoses among homosexually active men—among high-risk groups, male homosexual contact has been responsible for the greatest number of cases—had fallen from 2,284 in 1987 to 772 in 1994. In the Australian population as a whole, the transmission rate had stabilized at 2.7 new infections per hundred thousand people per year. But at mid-1995, the danger of an epidemic of HIV among Aboriginal and Torres Strait Island people seemed considerable. At June 1999, the cumulative figures for the epidemic in Australia were: HIV infections, 19,738; AIDS cases, 8,140; and deaths, 5,775.

It took the tragic, much-publicized deaths in late 1984 of three Queensland babies infected by blood from a gay donor to jolt the federal Labor government into providing national leadership, though the first Australian HIV/AIDS cases had been diagnosed as early as 1982–83. State and federal health ministers agreed that the states would ensure that high-risk people did not donate blood. From 1985, with an American blood test available, universal blood-donor screening was introduced. Free, accessible testing sites encouraged voluntary testing for HIV. Later, needle-exchange programs would be introduced. In May 1985, Dr. Blewett stated that in the absence of a vaccine or cure, the focus would be on education and prevention. In an innovative move, the federal government began direct funding of community-based organizations for educational and preventive work, as well as making funds available in the usual way via state and territory administrations. Until 1985, the commonwealth provided all funds, but thenceforth costs were shared between the central and state governments. In a particularly bold initiative, the commonwealth provided funds for the Australian Prostitutes Collective to develop health promotion and counseling services concerning HIV/AIDS and longer-established sexually transmitted diseases.

A National AIDS Task Force, reporting to the Australian Health Ministers' Advisory Committee, had been set up in 1984 to guide the work of the medical and scientific communities. The National Advisory Committee on AIDS (NACAIDS) was then created to guide efforts in the educational, social and legal areas. NACAIDS, headed by a well-known magazine editor, Ms. Ita Buttrose, came increasingly into conflict with the task force, headed by an eminent hematologist, Professor David Penington. NACAIDS put priority on promotion of safer sexual practices through community education, and it advocated partnerships between high-risk people and the health authorities. The task force put priority on testing of high-risk people and wanted medical leadership, not partnership. The gay community opposed compulsory testing, fearing discrimination against HIV-positive people. By mid-1986 Blewett had secured the agreement of Penington, Buttrose and the community-based AIDS councils to voluntary testing. However, conflict erupted again in 1987 over the controversial "Grim Reaper" mass education campaign. Devised by NACAIDS because it feared HIV was spreading into the heterosexual community, the campaign was aimed at the general public, not high-risk groups. The spread into the heterosexual community did not happen, but the campaign had the effect of raising general awareness of the epidemic and justifying greater public funding of services.

By 1988, the Penington-Buttrose conflict had evaporated, as both had left their advisory posts. Blewett could thus merge the task force and NACAIDS and form a new body, the National Council on AIDS. But the debate between advocates of the more traditional, medical approach and the new partnership approach continued. In 1989 Blewett had to defend his policy against claims by Dr. Bryce Phillips of the Australian Medical Association and Dr. Bruce Shepherd, orthopaedic surgeon, that AIDS had been "demedicalized." Shepherd convened a conference on the vexed question of compulsory testing of patients. Within medical circles, compulsory testing and contact tracing of sexual partners of infected people continued to be strongly supported. The states also varied in the degree to which they accepted Blewett's cooperation-based policy. Victoria, Western Australia and South Australia established cooperative relations with their respective AIDS councils. NSW was rather slow to develop community-based education programs. Conservative governments in Tasmania and Queensland refused to work with their councils in educational work directed at gay persons. With the advent of Labor governments in both states at the close of the 1980s, policy shifted toward more cooperation with gay groups and greater effort to educate schoolchildren about HIV/AIDS.

In 1988 Blewett had drawn up a policy discussion paper that was introduced in all parliaments and further developed through a process of consultation with interested groups throughout the country. The first national HIV/AIDS strategy for 1989–93 emerged from this policy process. The national strategy laid down six areas of action—education; prevention; treatment, care and counseling; community participation; research; and international cooperation. Although it had reservations about voluntary testing and about provision of condoms and needle-sterilizing equipment in prisons, the federal Liberal-National Party opposition expressed support for the strategy. There were few public attacks on the new strategy. In 1990 Blewett ceased to be health minister, but he left as his legacy a national policy consensus.

The second national strategy, 1993–94 to 1995–96, continued to focus on partnerships between governments, affected groups and health and scientific professionals. Education and prevention remained the centerpieces of national HIV/AIDS policy. Male homosexual sex and injecting drug use continued to be the primary routes of spread among adults at the close of the 1990s. Both the second and third national strategies were judged to have enjoyed great success in containing the spread of the virus. The fourth national strategy was implemented in mid-1999.[20]

The HIV/AIDS pandemic not only brought to the fore "new public health" issues of community participation and citizen partnership with government and health professionals but raised to first rank with respect to public health the issue of human rights. Where articulation of values has been common in medicine, it has been largely neglected in public health. From the time of Hippocrates to the 1960s, medical ethics essentially involved the doctor's duties to patients: nonmaleficence (not harming the patient) and beneficence (helping the patient). From the 1960s, under pressure from the patients' rights movement, respect for the autonomous decisions of the patient began to be added to the two traditional principles. At the same time, the principle of equity—fair, or even equal, shares of health care—began to be included as well. As we saw in the previous chapter, the concept of justice, or equity, has also powerfully influenced public health thinking about inequalities in health status in the last two to three decades, whether this thinking has been in terms of the impact on health of inequalities in material resources or of the impact of dignity-denying status inequalities.

Medicine in countries like the United Kingdom, the United States and Australia has since the 1970s very largely accepted the four ethical principles of nonmaleficence, beneficence, respect for autonomy, and justice. But public health has had difficulty in articulating its core values. Unlike medicine, public health is focused on the population, not the individual, and the primary determinants of health at the population level are social. Human rights, then—rather than medical ethics, with their focus on individual patient and doctor—would seem to offer an appropriate framework for values articulation in public health. After all, human rights set out to establish the social bases for human well-being, as Jonathan Mann so clearly recognized in his international work to contain the AIDS pandemic.[21]

In the later 1980s, the Global Programme on AIDS at the World Health Organization, under the leadership of Mann, made respect for human rights fundamental to its containment strategy. Mann recognized that human rights are not only worthy of respect in themselves but critical to winning the cooperation of infected people, itself vital to the success of preventive programs. In January 1988, a world summit of health ministers—148 countries were represented—was convened jointly by the British government and WHO. The summit issued the London Declaration on AIDS prevention, stating that human rights had to be protected and that discrimination (the potential for which was great in a killing disease commonly spread by illicit sex and illegal drug use) would work against successful containment. In May 1988, the World Health Assembly (that governs the WHO and is composed of representatives of the 191 member states) resolved unanimously that respect for the human rights and dignity of HIV-infected people and people with AIDS was vital to the success of national control programs and of the global containment strategy.[22]

Historically, human rights have developed in three "generations." First-generation rights were the civil and political rights—freedoms from state interference—that grew out of the experience of revolutionary constitutionalism in England, America and France in the seventeenth and eighteenth centuries. The second-generation rights—economic, social and cultural—grew out of the twentieth-century experience of wars of aggression and international economic depression. They were recognized in the Universal Declaration of Human Rights of the late 1940s. Some commentators have argued that the civil and political rights are more fundamental than the second-generation rights, that the latter are mere claims that the state is not compelled to meet. But the United Nations General Assembly has clearly stated that human rights are indivisible and interdependent and that promotion and protection must be accorded to both first and second-generation rights. Indeed, in recent years, a third generation—"solidarity" rights—has grown out of Third World dissatisfaction with the inequities of the prevailing, international economic and political order. At least six categories of solidarity rights have been identified, including: the right to economic, political, social and cultural self-determination; the right to economic and social development; the right to benefit from the "common heritage of mankind" and other information and progress; the right to peace; the right of humanitarian relief; and the right to a healthy environment. Not only are these collective rather than individual rights, but they require international cooperation to be attained. Further, they build upon the preceding categories of rights; they are historically cumulative.[23]

Public health emerged and developed within the nation-state and as part of the modern discourse on citizenship during the last two hundred years or so. The association of public health with human rights is particularly appropriate at this transitional stage of progression from the nation-state to a world political system. It has the advantage over citizenship that human rights seem more universal, being recognized by many nations; more contemporary, being able to transcend the nation-state; and more progressive, being unrelated to state management of people. Even so, in the shorter term a combination of human rights and citizenship institutions will be required for public health problems like HIV/AIDS; human rights can be employed against state repression of AIDS sufferers, when this occurs, while citizenship can be used to marshal support and resources, where these are available.[24]

That public health and human rights are complementary has begun to be recognized. Discrimination against HIV-infected persons or those living with AIDS—whether loss of employment, access to education or capacity to travel—encouraged dissimulation and unwillingness to participate in prevention. But denial of other human rights affects physical, psychological and social well-being. The right to association—people's capacity to talk and seek solutions to problems—can have such impact. Thus, it was a union of

Amsterdam drug users that came up with the idea of needle exchanges as a way to stop transmission of the AIDS virus through the use of contaminated syringes. Recognition of human rights is to be desired not simply for their instrumental value for public health objectives like containment of infection. They are also social goods in themselves. But since the greatest burden of HIV/AIDS has been carried by the poor and the stigmatized, it has become clear that absence of rights is a social-level risk factor for HIV/AIDS. Thus, preventive work with women in Africa and Asia is moving beyond education and individual behavior change to the more fundamental matter of their inferior status and lack of rights in strongly patriarchal societies. Because the future of public health lies in dealing with the structure and function of society, human rights offer a framework for both social analysis and action. Human rights have the added advantage of being already well developed within international law and international relations, as we have noted previously.

While the content of modern medical ethics is well developed and finds expression in international declarations like the International Code of Medical Ethics of the World Medical Association, public health lacks an explicit code. Part of the problem is preoccupation with methodology and technical expertise at the expense of conceptual substance and clarity about public health's identity. Jonathan Mann suggested that public health must act decisively in two areas to attain this clarity—that it must abandon its biomedical conceptual and linguistic heritage and adopt a human rights framework for the analysis of, and response to, the social determinants of health. Biomedical language and concepts do not take us far in understanding the effects of dignity-denying situations, especially the repetitive effects, on physical, psychological and social well-being. Yet we need to understand, and be able to express our understanding of, the "universe of human suffering." The contents of this universe must be named and described before they can be measured. Child abuse and domestic violence had no social reality until they were described and measured. A human rights framework is able to offer the clarity necessary if public health is to address properly its responsibilities. Since the conditions sustaining good health are social, public health must be involved in social change. Since the promotion of human rights has ethical dimensions, public health necessarily involves ethical issues. Just as the physician stands by the patient in his or her suffering even when the resources for cure and pain relief have been exhausted, so the public health practitioner must remain with vulnerable groups even when no effective measures are at hand. Public health is about development of new technologies, emerging diseases, and international changes in morbidity and mortality patterns. But it is also about greater understanding of the universe of suffering, which itself promises a fundamental shift in the conceptualizing of health. As Jonathan Mann observed, "Awareness of the limits of medicine and medical care, growing recognition of the health impacts of societal structure and function, globalization and consequent interdependence, and the sometimes active, sometimes ineffectual actions of nation-states, all intersect to lead toward a new vision of health."[25]

EMERGING AND REEMERGING INFECTIONS

From the beginning of recorded history, communication between different areas of the globe has been growing. Three periods may be identified—the period of geographical isolation; the period of intercontinental communication; and the current period of global interdependence. Taking cholera as an example, we may observe that it probably originated in Asia in ancient times, but only in the nineteenth century, with the advent of rail and steamship travel, did it spread quickly to other regions, especially Europe and the Americas. Generally, emerging infections have the same biological cause, which has operated over the millennia of recorded history—the dissemination of existing pathogens to new host populations. Since changes in the relationship between humans and the environment (changes in many cases instigated by humans) encourage this microbial spread, the control of microbial emergence is, in principle, feasible. A first step has to be establishment of a global network of disease surveillance centers. The monitoring of disease in urban areas of the tropical world, where many of the world's human microbe populations are concentrated, is particularly important.[26]

Perhaps the most damaging global emerging infection has been HIV/AIDS. But both tuberculosis and malaria have reemerged as serious, international threats. Moreover, both have developed strains resistant to antimicrobial drugs, as have other reemerging infections. By international standards, Australian TB and HIV/AIDS rates remain very low, and malaria has never been a major problem in this country. In very recent years, however, new infections have emerged in Australia: pig paramyxovirus, equine morbillivirus, and the Australian bat lyssavirus. Although these have been minor public health problems, they have generated a good deal of community concern. Japanese encephalitis, long endemic in Asia, is another recent emerging infection; so far, cases have been confined to North Queensland and the Torres Strait.[27]

TB remains a very significant health problem in economically developing countries; even in developed ones, if social conditions degenerate, TB cases proliferate. On WHO estimates, unless control measures increase over the next two decades, almost a billion new cases worldwide will be added to the 1.9 billion already suffering from active TB; 80 percent of active cases are located in twenty-two countries, most of which are in Africa and Asia. An estimated 10.7 million people have both HIV/AIDS and TB; the former causes the latter to progress much more quickly. Multidrug-resistant TB—resistant to isoniazid and refampin—looms as a serious international problem. It is a hundred times more costly to treat than nonresistant TB. It is especially rife in the former Soviet Union, because of breakdown of services, shortages of drugs and inadequate compliance with treatment. There are few drugs effective against multidrug-resistant strains. Even in affluent Britain, TB has in recent times been resurgent. In 2000–2001 there was a minor epidemic among students at a community college in Leicester, causing a certain amount of panic.[28]

Emerging infections other than HIV/AIDS include cryptosporidiosis, hepatitis C, Legionnaires's disease, and verocytotoxin-producing *Escherichia coli* 0157; reemerging infections other than tuberculosis include *Staphylococcus aureus, Neisseria gonorrhoeae,* and *Streptococcus pneumoniae.* The latter are reemerging because of antimicrobial resistance. Various environmental facts in contemporary life promote the spread of emerging and reemerging infections. The high number of aged persons in the populations of developed countries means that more people are in institutional care. Because of hospital early-discharge policies, many are vulnerable to infection. Further, there are many more people who are immune suppressed because of cancer chemotherapy, organ and tissue transplants or HIV/AIDS. At the other end of the life cycle, many more very young children are placed in creches and preschools because both parents work and the number of single-parent families has grown. There they are more susceptible to infections than within the family. The increasing speed and volume of international travel have provided vastly increased opportunities for diffusion of infections, and viruses, especially influenza, measles and rabies, have increased their global reach. The rapid, unregulated growth of cities in the developing countries has far outstripped the growth of water supply and sewerage infrastructures.

But the availability of suitable water cannot be assumed even in wealthy countries. In 1993 the intestinal parasite *Cryptosporidium parvum* contaminated the water supply in Milwaukee, Wisconsin, causing prolonged diarrhea in over four hundred thousand people, of whom about 4,400 were hospitalized and one hundred AIDS-affected persons died. Waterborne cryptosporidiosis occurred in England in 1989, and another outbreak (of five hundred confirmed cases) occurred in the Torbay area in 1995.

Although cryptosporidiosis associated with swimming pools had been noted in Australia, outbreaks connected with drinking water were considered most unlikely. Then, in July 1998, Sydney Water informed the NSW Health Department that *Giardia lamblia* cysts and Cryptosporidium oocysts had been found in unusually large numbers in Sydney's water supply. The public was told to boil water. After very heavy rainfall in the water catchment area in August, a second and then a third episode of contamination occurred. While chlorination had probably killed the Giardia, it would probably not have affected the Cryptosporidium, and although no increase in diarrheal illness was reported, there was concern about the possibly life-threatening effect of cryptosporidiosis on immuno-compromised persons. The repeated high counts of oocysts, however, were not easily explained, especially as water treatment systems had not failed, bacterial counts remained low, and diarrheal disease did not increase. Why, with Cryptosporidium levels high, had no disease resulted? Immunity of Sydneysiders from long exposure may be dismissed as an explanation, because no illness was reported among visitors to Sydney. Boiling of water probably helped, but not all people used boiled or bottled water. Probably the oocysts were dead or noninfective to humans, but at least some were viable, according to fluorescent in-situ hybridization in a few samples. While counts in some specimens were not confirmed in other laboratories, the existence of very high counts in others is definite; the sensitivity of surveillance methods may be questioned, yet similar methods had identified other waterborne outbreaks. It may, however, be concluded from the Sydney experience that open and coordinated management of catchment areas, storage, treatment plants and testing and distribution systems is essential for a clean and reliable water supply in a large, modern city like Sydney.[29]

Food-borne infections are also part of the emerging and reemerging infections picture. Contemporary eating habits and the organization of food production and distribution encourage their spread. In developed countries, purchase of food in bulk, eating of more meals outside the home and consumption of "fast foods," combined with mass production and international distribution of "ready to eat" foods, not only present opportunities for infection but increase the size of populations at risk. Intensive farming likewise encourages the spread of zoonotic infections pathogenic to humans. *Campylobacter jejuni* and *Campylobacter coli* (and Salmonellae) lie behind most notifications of food poisoning. Most cases of Campylobacter are connected with eating of poultry. Selection of poultry for volume of egg production and efficiency in food conversion rather than for resistance to disease has encouraged the spread of *Salmonella enteritidis* PT4. Growing consumption of poultry has made this pathogen the main cause of salmonellosis in human populations. In the United Kingdom in the 1990s, multidrug-resistant *Salmonella typhimurium* DT104 became the most common cause of food poisoning after PT4. Because it causes disease in sheep, pigs, and cattle as well as poultry, it can contaminate a large number of foods. Verocytotoxin-producing, entero-hemorrhagic *Escherichia coli* 0157 has produced comparatively few cases, but because of its high mortality and complications, it is an emerging infection of public health significance; an outbreak in Scotland in 1996 involved four hundred persons and produced twenty deaths.

A virulent strain of bovine spongiform encephalopathy (BSE), or "mad cow disease," in a cattle-to-cattle epidemic (which began with the chance appearance of BSE in an animal in the 1970s) developed in Britain through the practice of providing supplementary feeds of protein from bovine meat and bovine meal—a form of cannibalism. An epidemic in humans began in 1995; BSE leapt the species barrier as a result of human consumption of contaminated beef and produced a variant form of Creutzfeldt-Jakob disease (vCJD). By the end of 2000, 177,530 cases of BSE had occurred in Britain, as well as ninety cases of vCJD in the human population and approximately twenty deaths. The official bovine spongiform encephalopathy inquiry, chaired by Lord Phillips, a senior judge, reported in 2000. It saw misuse and misinterpretation of science as contributing to the human epidemic. It said that the government had not lied to the public but had offered misleading reassurance concerning the safety of beef.[30] The BSE epidemic in Britain appears to be coming under control. New British cases fell from 1112 in 2001 to 633 in 2002. New cases declined in other European countries between 2001 and 2002: Ireland (from 246 to 236), Portugal (110 to 32), Switzerland (42 to 14), France (274 to 184), Italy (50 to 21); Belgium (46 to 22), Germany (125 to 75), the Netherlands (20 to 14), and Denmark (6 to 1), but they increased in Spain (from 82 to 86).

In 1998, a Health Department study found that ten million people a year in Britain fell sick from food poisoning or contaminated water. The cost—health care and lost productivity—totalled 743 million pounds. In her submission to the official inquiry into BSE, Edwina Currie, a junior health minister in the Thatcher government who had been forced to resign because of egg-producer outrage at her claim that 60 percent of egg farms were infected with Salmonella, said of the Agriculture Ministry's approach to food safety: "They seemed to want to protect the industry . . . instead of putting public health as a primary concern."[31]

Australia to date has not had a case of BSE or vCJD reported. But risk-minimizing measures have been introduced: creation of an NHMRC Expert Committee to advise on measures against infectious spongiform encephalopathies; establishment of a National CJD Case Registry to pick up quickly cases of variant CJD; prohibition of feeding of ruminant protein to ruminants and a program to examine diseased cattle; refusal of blood donations by persons resident for six months or more in the United Kingdom in 1980–96, because CJD has been experimentally spread in animals by contaminated blood; and extension to imports from other European countries of a ban on importing of goods containing beef or beef products from Britain. Australia may soon take further measures to reduce risk of human-to-human transfer, including such measures adopted by Britain as greater use of disposable surgical instruments, more rigorous decontamination of nondisposable instruments, and more careful monitoring of vaccines prepared for human and bovine purposes. Scientific arrogance and commercial greed are interwoven in the emergence of BSE, and the lesson for public health concerns the dangers of market-driven deregulation. Greater state monitoring and regulation, not less, as the neoconservative marketeers want, are needed in an era when infectious disease so easily leaps species as well as geographic boundaries.[32]

Another aspect of the emerging and reemerging infections picture is antibiotic-resistant bacterial infections and nosocomial infections. Resistant strains of tuberculosis have already been mentioned. Resistant *Shigella dysenteriae* has killed thousands in refugee camps in Africa, and less lethal dysentery has become a formidable public health problem in the economically advanced world. With *Salmonella typhi* resistant to the cheaper antibiotics, Third World countries face very serious problems of control. Just as the emergence of vCJD is in part the result of commercial opportunism, so the widespread use of antibiotics in animals for commercial advantage has led to the emergence of resistant, nontyphoid Salmonellas that threaten the health of the human population. The excessive use of antibiotics in the First World has seen the establishment of methicillin-resistant *Staphylococcus aureus*. Penicillin-resistant *Streptococcus pneumoniae* has been shown to exist in as many as 25 percent of very young children. Enterococci and *Clostridium difficile* are nosocomial infections presenting major problems in hospitals, while resistant strains of gram-negative bacilli (*Escherichia coli, Citrobacter*, *Pseudomonas*, *Proteus*, *Klebsiella*, and *Serratia*) have become well established in hospital environments. Moreover, the health care organizational movement from hospital-based to community-based care may not so much be solving the problem as promoting the spread of antibiotic-resistant strains in the community.[33]

From a biological perspective, human populations are in competition with evolutionary changes in predatory infectious agents. In this race with microbial genes, the cost of relying on Darwinian selection alone in humans would be too great; huge fluctuations in human populations would result. We certainly possess protective technologies, like vaccines, antibiotics and medical-diagnostic tools. But we labor under great disadvantages: worldwide population crowding; widespread geographical mobility and great speed of travel; and considerable social, political, economic and hygienic inequalities. Short-term changes in equilibrium between human host and infectious agent may produce an overwhelming advantage for the latter, as in the 1918 influenza pandemic or the contemporary HIV/AIDS pandemic. Mutual accommodation can bring greater stability, although the appearance of infectious deviants can upset that equilibrium. Thus, with HIV, the disease may become more chronic as strains with longer latency predominate. But deviant strains may then arise to produce earlier lethality. As the eminent bioscientist Joshua Lederberg has stressed, this is a very complex, coevolutionary process of merger, union, bifurcation, and reemergence of new species. In such a binary association, unpredictable divergence may take place.

Genetic intervention may allow the human species to bypass the process of natural selection and random variation. But public health weapons, including education, already exist. However, these require the political will and investment of adequate resources. The Committee on International Science, Engineering and Technology of the U.S. National Science and Technology Council recently made a number of recommendations for dealing with global infectious disease threats: global and domestic surveillance of disease outbreaks, including establishment of laboratory capacity wherever needed; vector management and provision of safe water and food supplies; provision of community and professional education; support of research on causes of disease, pathogenic mechanisms, body defenses, vaccines and antibiotics; and development of the results of research in cooperation with pharmaceutical companies and construction of regulatory and incentive structures to promote this development.[34]

Emerging infectious diseases are a complex biological issue, but they are also a complex, social one. Human actions may enhance the pathogenicity or resistance to antimicrobials of mutations of infectious agents. Thus, the decline of malaria in the United States—an estimated one million cases a year still occurred in southern states (with a total population of twenty-five million) in the second decade of the twentieth century—resulted from agricultural development and socioeconomic factors more than from direct control measures. Social inequalities meant the poor could not afford better housing, drainage, or mosquito nets and repellents, so differential morbidity resulted. In the contemporary world, large social and economic forces arguably shape emergence of disease—as with international shipping practices and the movement of cholera from Asia to South America, or genocide and war in Rwanda and cholera outbreaks in Zaire. Yet the impact of social inequality on risk of infection is not acknowledged by some recent influential discussions of emerging infections, discussions that otherwise recognize the role of social factors.

The U.S. Institute of Medicine's report on emerging infections, for instance, does not recognize poverty or social inequality as causes of emergence. The Institute of Medicine identified as facilitators of the emergence of HIV urbanization, lifestyle mores, growing injecting drug abuse, international travel, and medical technology. Yet it is clear that HIV has spread globally along the fault lines of poverty and disempowerment—commercial sex and male migrant labor—as syphilis and gonorrhea did in colonial Asia and Africa in earlier times. Globally, the great majority of HIV-infected women are poor and disempowered by gender inequality. Gender inequality and poverty come together as a major risk factor for most women. Further, even social science studies of HIV/AIDS tend to neglect the impact of socioeconomic and gender status on mortality in HIV-infected people. Social inequalities have been convincingly shown to influence powerfully the contours of spread of the pandemic, as well as the course of infection in infected people. International and intranational economic disparities are influential, again, in the face of the high cost of antiviral drugs, currently twelve thousand to sixteen thousand dollars a year for the three-drug therapy. The upsurge of diphtheria in Russia in the early 1990s may be, and often is, explained by the falling away of vaccination practices. But this in turn is understandable only in terms of the chaotic socioeconomic change from state communism, with universal health services, to a free market economy, with resulting collapse of universal access to health services. The concern of standard epidemiology is with individual risk, and it gives no role to such socioeconomic phenomena. As epidemiologist Tony McMichael has observed, it is "oriented to explaining and quantifying the bobbing of corks on the surface waters, while largely disregarding the stronger undercurrents that determine where, on average, the cluster of corks ends up along the shoreline of risk."[35]

Emerging diseases do not halt at social or geographical borders. Unhappily for the poor, especially of the Third World, the considerable therapeutic benefits of medico-scientific knowledge too often fail to cross such borders. No major pharmaceutical company is researching a new tuberculosis drug, because, the great majority of sufferers being citizens of poor countries, there is not enough profit in it. If the eight million sufferers in poor countries all used such a drug for six months at an average total cost of eleven dollars per person, there would still not be enough profit in it to attract the companies. As Paul Farmer has noted, the study of borders more and more involves the study of social inequalities; thus, the U.S.-Mexican border, as much as any other border in the world, separates two populations with great differences in health status, health service entitlements and health service utilization. A more critical approach to the study of emerging and reemerging infections would have to include complexity, rather than (as now) dismantle it in the reductionist manner: "Effective analysis of emerging diseases must recognize the study of complexity as perhaps the central general scientific problem of our time."[36] Concepts and methods from the human and social sciences will be needed as much as will be those from molecular biology and other biomedical sciences.[37]

The need to understand and contain the pandemic of HIV/AIDS has led some epidemiologists to argue that a new paradigm for epidemiology is required. Mervyn and Ezra Susser have proposed that the pandemic needs to be understood at several levels of analysis: the molecular level, the intermediate level of specific social behavior of individuals, and at the population level. They suggest that it entails a new epidemiological paradigm, which they call "eco-epidemiology." They see the paradigm in terms of Chinese boxes, a nest of systems, each box containing a smaller one in successive levels of organization. The outer box would be the all-embracing physical environment. This in turn contains societies and populations, single individuals, individual physiological systems and ultimately molecules. Determinants and outcomes would be analyzed at the different levels of organization—within and across contexts, and in depth. The preventive approach would be to apply both information and biomedical technology in order to find effective leverage at different levels, from the contextual to the molecular.[38]

"PUBLIC HEALTH IN REVERSE": BIOLOGICAL WARFARE AND BIOTERRORISM

Biological warfare (and the more recent phenomenon, bioterrorism) may be defined as the deliberate use of microorganisms and toxins to produce disease or death in humans, livestock and crops. Biological weapons are particularly attractive to nonstate terrorists, because they involve raw materials that are comparatively easy to access, they are easy to transport, and they can pass through routine security systems without being detected.

The use of biological weapons has a long history. In the fourteenth century, Tatars besieging the Genoese-held city of Caffa in the Ukraine catapulted corpses of persons who had died of plague into the city to infect the defenders. Europeans in North America in the eighteenth century deliberately infected indigenes with smallpox. They may also have done so in Australia; British colonial authorities (or transported convicts) are alleged (evidence is virtually nonexistent) to have maliciously infected Aborigines in 1789, causing an epidemic in tribes of the Sydney region. In 1763 Sir Jeffrey Amherst, commander in chief of British forces in North America, urged Col. Henry Bouquet during the Pontiac uprising to "send" smallpox among the "disaffected" Indian tribes.[39]

In the last hundred years, biological and chemical weapons have evolved in four phases. The first phase saw the use of gaseous chemicals like chlorine and phosgene in World War I. The second saw the use of nerve agents like tabun (a cholinesterase inhibitor) and the development of anthrax and plague bombs in World War II. The third began during the Vietnam War, with the use of chemicals like Agent Orange to defoliate jungle and destroy crops, and with the use of "midspectrum" agents having chemical and biological features, such as auxins, bioregulators and physiologically active compounds. The fourth, now in progress, results from the genetic "revolution" and promises a variety of threats to living systems—organisms resistant to antibiotics and vaccines, organisms with greater aerosol and environmental stability, organisms with immunologic profiles not matching known diagnostic indicators, organisms undetectable by antibody-based sensor systems, and organisms operating as microfactories producing a toxin, venom or bioregulator.

Having expanded its bioweapons program during the Korean War, the United States had by the mid-1960s "weaponized" anthrax, *Pasteurella tularensis,* and *Bacillus globigii* as well as crop pathogens like stem rust. Public opinion forced the Richard M. Nixon administration into renouncing the use of biological weapons, and stockpiles were destroyed. Britain and France likewise declined to continue research, on practical as much as moral grounds—effective systems of delivery had proven difficult to develop.

From the 1970s the Soviet Union built under the *Biopreparat* program a considerable research and development capacity in biological weapons. Prior to its virtual closure by Boris Yeltsin in 1992, the program is estimated to have employed seventy thousand scientists and technicians. With unemployment widespread in the post-Soviet era, some are likely to have found work in Middle Eastern countries eager to develop their own bioweapons. It is believed that countries that now have the ability to deploy bioweapons include Iraq, Iran, Syria, Libya, China, North Korea, Russia, Taiwan and Israel. Sudan, India, Pakistan and Kazakhstan may also have such capacity.

In 1972 the Convention on the Prohibition of the Development, Production and Stockpiling of Bacteriological and Toxin Weapons and on Their Destruction came into being. But it has proven flawed in the vital areas of transparency, inspection, verification and enforcement, as attempts by United Nations inspectors to apply the provisions of the convention to Iraq after the Persian Gulf War showed. In 1998 President Bill Clinton authorized military attacks on sites in Sudan and Iraq, where biological weapons were allegedly being made. In 1999 a report of Congress stated that Iraq and North Korea had secretly stockpiled smallpox. Used against populations with large numbers unvaccinated—WHO had declared the world free of wild smallpox two decades earlier—the virus would be a formidable weapon.

At the same time the United States moved to strengthen its defenses against bioterrorism and biowarfare by stockpiling vaccines, training National Guard troops in biodefense, and generally pursuing a military-response model. Biodefense experts from within the ranks of public health quickly decried the emphasis on military preparedness, pointing out that state and local public health authorities, hospitals and medical practitioners were the real key to success in defense. The public health and the medical care systems would identify the pathogen, determine its mode of spread and treat its victims. These objectives are different from those of law enforcement, which seeks to apprehend the perpetrators of bioterrorism and obtain evidence with which to have them convicted.

Unlike the military's command mode of operation, modern public health tries to educate and engage the cooperation of citizens, respecting confidentiality as much as possible. A junior partner to law enforcement and the military in the response to what the U.S. Public Health Service has called "public health in reverse," public health faces the risk of losing the public confidence essential to its main task of promoting and preserving the citizens' health. Moreover, the new funds coming to public health for biodefense would not be available for most of its central concerns, like chronic disease control or child health promotion. Public health critics of this "dual use" notion of using funds from antibioterrorism to build much-needed public health infrastructure have asked if those advocating it now believe that the only answer to gross underfunding of public health is to make real public health needs a "caboose" attached to the military gravy train.[40]

The staging of the 2000 Olympic Games in Sydney caused Australian planning of responses to bioterrorist threats to be much upgraded. Health and

Emergency Management Australia developed management protocols and training manuals, while the NSW Health Department trained health workers. The commonwealth government provided twenty-three million dollars to cover the cost of improving the detective, protective and medical capacities of the Australian Defence Force.

At the same time Australia' s capacity to respond to malicious introduction of animal disease was tested in a joint exercise (Northern Shield) involving cooperation between state and federal agencies combatting exotic animal diseases on the one hand and the Australian Defence Force on the other. Animal-disease emergencies are normally dealt with under the Australian Veterinary Emergency Plan, considered to be the most advanced measure of its type in the world. It provides for nationally uniform strategies and operational approaches. Northern Shield was judged a success, although it must be said that had the exercise been held in the notorious wet season, when roads in Northern Australia become almost impassable, procedures would have been much more stringently tested. Nevertheless the exercise required military commanders to consider the complexities of dealing with animal disease emergencies, and animal health professionals to understand better the operational style of the Australian Defence Force.

In the aftermath of the 11 September 2001 terrorist attacks in New York and Washington and the subsequent malicious spread of anthrax by mail, Australia's acting chief medical officer, Professor John Mathews, reassured the country that protective measures against biological and chemical attacks were in place. These included training within health departments and with other agencies, medical treatment protocols applicable to civilian populations, supplies of pharmaceuticals, greater diagnostic and health surveillance capability, advisory and coordination arrangements, and access to information on international developments. He pointed out that the Australian Disaster Medicine Group (a subcommittee of the Australian Health Ministers's Advisory Council), the Communicable Diseases Network Australia and the Public Health Laboratory Network regularly shared information in preparation for any untoward event.

Soon after, the chief medical officer of the commonwealth, Professor Richard Smallwood, told citizens panicked into seeking vaccination against smallpox that the Federal Health Department had assured access to adequate quantities of vaccine in the very unlikely event of bioterrorists introducing smallpox into Australia. Even if the infection were introduced, he continued, a combination of measures—surveillance, quarantine, vaccination and treatment—would quickly contain its spread.[41]

ENVIRONMENTAL DEGRADATION AND HEALTH

The health problem presented by emerging and resurgent infections may be approached in terms of the evolutionary struggle between infectious agents and the human species. It may also be approached in terms of social and economic inequalities within and between national populations. We have already done both. But the problem is also usefully conceptualized in terms of the adverse effect on the natural environment of the economic development and population growth (the world's population increased by 1.244 billion in 1980–98) of the last 150 to two hundred years.

Since 1880 global average temperatures have increased by 0.3 to 0.6 degrees Celsius. The climate change will expand habitats favorable to vector-borne diseases by promoting changes from seasonal to perennial transmission and the entry of vectors into hitherto disease-free areas. Some analysts have suggested that 620 million more people in economically developing countries might be at risk of malaria by 2050. In 1985–95, higher temperatures or rainfall, sometimes in tandem with greater drug resistance, have produced epidemic malaria at high altitudes in Rwanda, Zambia, Swaziland, Ethiopia and Madagascar. A 1988 epidemic in the last-named country produced a hundred thousand deaths. The effects of climate change in Australia are likely to be much greater arbovirus and Murray Valley encephalitis virus activity. With vectors for malaria, dengue and yellow fever present, the establishment or reestablishment of these diseases is quite possible, and the most populated, hitherto temperate, southeastern parts of the country may then be at risk.[42]

Environmental degradation has proceeded well beyond pollution at the local level (itself a historical concern of public health) to the absolutely fundamental issue of whether the biosphere is able to sustain its life-maintaining capacity. Human societies, especially industrialized ones, are both running down resources—reducing biodiversity, depleting freshwater aquifers and fishing out the oceans—and dangerously overloading earth's "sinks" (like forests—carbon "sinks"—that remove carbon dioxide from the atmosphere for photosynthesis) with liquid and gaseous wastes, as depletion of stratospheric ozone and greater exposure to ultraviolet radiation, the buildup of atmospheric, greenhouse gases, and resulting world climate change and the global spread of organic pollutants all indicate. The emerging consequences of environmental degradation impinge adversely on the health of populations, whether these be more intense ultraviolet radiation, more extreme weather events, the effects of climate change on the reach of infectious diseases, lower-yield agriculture and fisheries, or the refugee problems resulting from major changes in the environment, like rising sea levels.

Some of the other First World countries seem to be doing rather better than Australia in addressing the issue of environment and health. In 1999–2000, the governments of the United Kingdom, the United States and Canada embarked upon investigation of the likely health effects of climate change. In 1998–99, the WHO Office on Environment and Health in Rome established a scientific panel to identify the early effects on health in Europe of climate change; the European Ministerial Conference on Environment and

Health, held in London in mid-1999, stressed climate change as an environmental health matter worthy of urgent effort by researchers and policy analysts alike. Efforts have been made recently in Australia to construct a national environmental health strategy. However, progress has been limited by uncertainty about the acceptance of ecologically sustainable development as a serious goal, by tight boundaries between sectors within government and between levels of government, and by staff reductions ("downsizing") with consequent loss of expertise.[43]

Since the late 1980s in Australia, a number of national reports have highlighted the great need for coordination of government action in environmental health. In the 1990s, public health people, both internationally and in Australia, began to discuss the health implications of environmental crises. Thus, in 1991 the third International Health Promotion conference in Sweden was concerned with supportive environments for health. In 1997, WHO published *Health and Environment in Sustainable Development*. This suggested that about 23 percent of preventable global ill health (at the head of which are diarrheal diseases, acute respiratory infections, malaria and injury) resulted from poor quality of the environment. In Australia, the Public Health Association in the 1990s finally addressed in policy the issue of ecological sustainability.

Various expert reports have also looked at environmental health. The 1988 *Health for All Australians* report (discussed in an earlier chapter) called for an adequate supply of quality drinking water for the whole country by 2000 and safe disposal of stored chemical wastes by the same year. Neither of these goals had been achieved by 2000. In the early 1990s, the NHMRC endorsed *Ecologically Sustainable Development: The Health Perspective*. This report proposed that planning for ecologically sustainable development include recognition of the fact that health and environment are interdependent; that the commonwealth develop a set of principles on ecology and health to be used in such planning; that environment and health guidelines, standards and indicators be employed; that the effectiveness of ecologically sustainable development be assessed; that mechanisms for public health and such development be part of accounting processes of relevant sectors; that a global program of research on the effects of environmental change be mounted to include information systems for disease surveillance, occupational health and safety and methods for dealing with negative effects on social health; and that priority in research be given to the interactions of economic development, the environment and physical and social health. Unfortunately, by the end of the 1990s not one of these proposals had been properly implemented. The NHMRC published in the mid-1990s a *National Framework for Environmental and Health Impact Assessment*. This report urged that health impact assessment routinely be part of any exercise in environmental impact assessment. At the same time, a report on national health goals and targets for 2000 pointed out the need for a national mechanism able to deal with environmental health. The National Public Health Partnership, established in 1996 (as we have noted) to improve collaboration between levels of government in public health, published in 1998 *Environmental Health in Australia—Towards a National Strategy.* Recognizing how management is split between levels of government, this discussion document called for more unified management. It introduced the idea of "charters of entitlement" and responsibilities for individuals, communities, governments, and businesses. It also proposed creation of a National Environmental Health Committee to advise the NPHP.

The failure to develop in Australia a national environmental health policy may be explained, at least in part, by the complexity of building meaningful bridges between the many departments and government agencies that would have to be involved, and the difficulty of covering the many particular areas of concern within the fields of health and the environment that would need to be included, as Charles Guest and others have pointed out.[44]

The failure also stems from the larger issue of the slowness of governments to take action about degradation of the natural environment itself. According to Stephen Boyden and others, besides the obstacles presented by the material interests of powerful companies in the private sector (and some governments), there are deep cultural reasons for the failure to take speedy action to rectify environmental problems, which many experts see as approaching the crisis point. Although a sympathetic worldwide environmental consciousness has grown prodigiously, especially among younger people, in the last three decades, too many people have still failed to appreciate that the well-being of human life is inextricably interwoven with that of the life forms of the rest of the biosphere. Falsely secure in their faith in science and technology, they ultimately rely on a "technical fix" to solve the problems of environmental degradation. Reinforcing this cultural issue is the fact that the time scales of such problems require a capacity to identify with, and be concerned about, the welfare of future generations, an altruism demanding a projection of empathy beyond the capacity of many people. Perhaps more importantly, the globally dominant system of free market economics can assign value to the natural environment only as a resource to be exploited. Moreover, the goal of ongoing economic growth is pragmatically and morally justified by mainstream economists and politicians alike as the only way to advance the material well-being of the disadvantaged within nations, as well as that of the disadvantaged nations themselves.

Just as the connection between wealth and health (beyond a minimum level) is being questioned, as we have seen earlier, on social grounds by researchers like Richard Wilkinson, that connection has been brought into serious doubt on environmental grounds as well. The creation of wealth through economic growth has been based on use of nonrenewable resources like fossil fuels. In conventional economic thinking, the environmental and social costs of economic growth are dismissed as externalities, without impact on the value of economic expansion. Thirty years ago, the economist E.F. Schumacher put the case for technologies not dependent on nonrenewable resources. More recently another economist, H.E. Daly, proposed a "steady-state" economy in which the rate of use of nonrenewable resources is not greater than the rate of development of renewable substitutes; the rate of use of renewable resources is not greater than the rate of their regeneration; and the rate of pollution is not greater than the rate of the natural environment to render it innocuous. While there are many signs of growing challenge, at least in economically developed countries, in the last three decades or so, to advertising-driven consumerism, the ideas of "alternative" economics remain outside the mainstream, where it is largely business as usual. Even the recently emerged discipline of health economics has become accepted by governments and health professionals because it is mainly concerned with efficiency of resource allocation within health care services and with microeconomic issues relating to treatment of illnesses, rather than larger problems of developing indices of sustainable health alternative to gross national product as measures of national accounting. (We will note below that in their work on determinants of health, Canadian economists Robert Evans, Greg Stoddart and colleagues have certainly addressed "big picture" issues.)[45]

FOOD SAFETY

The People's Health, volume 1 records how in the early twentieth century the Australian states individually introduced legislation specifically to control the quality and purity of food. In 1910, NSW convened a meeting of state representatives and representatives of business to get agreement on a common national code of standards. Further meetings were held in the interwar period. While a considerable degree of agreement was attained, a uniform approach to food policy could not be reached in the face of the insistence of the states on their individual sovereignty. The commonwealth lacked the constitutional power to impose a national food safety policy, as the Royal Commission on the Constitution of 1929 confirmed.

In the postwar era, two developments did much to advance the cause of a uniform approach. In 1955, the NHMRC Food Standards Committee was created to recommend safety standards. But governments reserved the right to decide about adopting recommended standards, and local pressures could lead to modification of recommended standards. Moreover, over time administrative responsibility for food policy migrated from one commonwealth department to another. Second, in 1981 the commonwealth and states (and the Northern Territory) agreed to establish the National Food Standards Council, made up of ministers who supervised standards. To achieve uniform food standards, use of this extraconstitutional mechanism had been necessary. A review of food regulation by the Commonwealth Business

Regulation Review Unit in 1988 found that the existing administration was costly to business and reduced the competitiveness of Australian food exports. In 1990, the states agreed to creation of an independent statutory authority, the National Food Authority. Under the supervision of the federal health minister, the authority was to develop uniform national food standards.

In the area of food policy, governments are caught in the continuing battle between the interests of business to keep costs down in order to maximize profits for shareholders and the interests of public health. The food manufacturing sector in the early 1990s in Australia represented 18 percent of total manufacturing employment and 21 percent of total manufacturing turnover. Under the Agri-Food Strategy of 1992, the federal government aimed to increase the value of food exports from $2.3 billion in 1992 to seven billion dollars in 2000. The strategy involved removal of government "impediments" to food industry growth. The National Food Authority saw regulations concerning food hygiene as an impediment to expansion of exports. For both Labor and Coalition governments in the 1990s, the desire to promote the economic well-being of industry has been a powerful influence on public health policy.[46]

In the late 1990s, two significant new issues in food safety emerged to throw into question the rationality of stressing commercial advantage to the detriment of public regulation. Bovine spongiform encephalopathy, which we have discussed above, arose in Britain in part because a change in rendering practices following deregulation permitted scrapie-like agents to survive in animal feed to infect cattle. The political context was one of support for food industry self-regulation.

In Britain, public disquiet about the second recent issue in food safety, genetically modified (GM) foods, has understandably followed from the experience of BSE and from the conflict between experts about the safety of GM foods. Caution would seem to be warranted, given the history of agents like low-level air pollution, originally thought to be harmless but now seen to be connected with heightened mortality. Part of the problem with GM foods, as with BSE, is the likely extended period before any adverse health effects become apparent. Careful monitoring of the ecological effect and of the health of those consuming GM foods would seem to be prudent. The British Medical Association has suggested that a moratorium on sale of GM foods be applied. The chief scientific adviser to the British government, Sir Robert May, and the chief medical officer, Dr. Liam Donaldson, urged that official studies of the impact of GM foods on health be instituted.

There are further legitimate concerns about GM foods. The use of antibiotic resistance as a marker to measure the success of genetic modification raises the fear that the GM food so modified might transfer antibiotic resistance to bacterial pathogens. Beyond these human health concerns are environmental and economic issues. Resistance to chemical herbicides might be spread from GM crops to weeds. Even more importantly, large-scale production of GM crops may adversely affect biodiversity. Those proposing cultivation of GM crops argue that they offer a solution to the imminent disaster of global famine when the problem of feeding eight billion people looms about 2020. Yet what little is known about the causes of famine would seem to indicate that the production of more food through a technological fix is too simplistic an answer. Availability of food is determined by a complex of economic, social and political factors, including the individual's possession of an income and a stable economic and social environment in which money may be exchanged for food. Moreover, poor countries may well face greater indebtedness to multinational suppliers of GM seed, increasing the international economic inequality that underlies the health inequality between rich and poor nations. Aggravating this potential problem is the use of the "terminator gene" in GM crops, so that farmers are forced to purchase fertile stock seed at each planting. Jeffrey Sachs, professor of international trade at Harvard University, has commented, "Transnational corporations and rich-country institutions are patenting everything from the human genome to rainforest biodiversity. The poor will be ripped off unless some sense and equity are introduced into this runaway process."[47]

The safety of GM foods is, of course, an issue also in Australia. The concerns that have been expressed overseas about privileging the interests of multinational food companies over the public health also exist here. The federal health minister, Dr. Michael Wooldridge, had been considering whether to appoint to the Genetic Manipulation Advisory Committee and the Interim Office of the Gene Technology Regulator an experienced and appropriately qualified public health professional to balance the current laboratory and clinical expertise on the two bodies. But the Howard coalition government had been pushing for a lenient GM labeling code for foods. In mid-2000, Australian and New Zealand health ministers overwhelmingly supported a code that requires thousands of packaged retail foods to carry labels indicating whether the food is genetically modified. The coalition government had wanted to exempt a wider range of foods from labeling, on the ground of the extra cost of labeling to the food industry, by requiring a 1 percent GM content before labels became mandatory. The Australia New Zealand Food Authority had proposed a more lenient code a year and a half previously, but this had been rejected by the state health ministers, who were probably stiffened in their resistance to leniency by opinion poll evidence that a very great majority of people wanted GM labeling.[48]

GENETICS AND PUBLIC HEALTH

While the interaction between genetic endowment and environmental conditions determines the health of a population, improvement of environmental conditions is the most cost-effective way to advance health. Environmental factors certainly bulk larger in health status differences between populations, as the considerable range of mortality rates from cardiovascular disease as between countries, or the effect of migration on such rates, would indicate. Genetic factors explain some of the range of mortality within a population, but even here it is how genetic disposition interacts with environmental factors that is significant. Moreover, since within a national population mortality may change radically over a few generations, as in the case of the mortality decline in economically developed countries since the late nineteenth century, change in environmental conditions rather than genetic change must be invoked.[49] Pure genetic determinism simply will not hold up.

Even so, public health genetics has a place in the future development of preventive strategies. Genetic approaches to prevention may be divided into "genotypic" and "phenotypic" categories. Prevention includes clinical intervention for susceptible individuals and population subgroups, environmental manipulation for the same, and behavioral change in susceptible individuals. Prevention of genetic disease has hitherto been carried out by advising patients not to have children or, following prenatal diagnosis, by destruction of the fetus. The ethical issues accompanying such genotypic prevention have been somewhat relieved by phenotypic prevention: clinical interventions on individuals with genetic susceptibilities and advice concerning risk from environmental determinants, like diet, for populations with different genetic susceptibilities. The effectiveness of phenotypic prevention has been limited, but there is reason to believe that it will improve as knowledge advances.

Privacy, confidentiality and informed consent are core ethical issues. From the specialist literature, the following principles may be isolated: the need to protect individual privacy, to ensure information is not a means of discrimination; to allow individuals to make informed choices; for health professionals to educate the public and their patients about the degree of uncertainty involved in many decisions; to advance public understanding of the concepts of predisposition and risk in relation to genetic testing and screening; and to avoid application of pressure to individuals to share sensitive genetic information. Discovery of a familial problem clearly has implications for the patient's family as well as the patient. Both the patient and practitioner have to resolve the question of whether, and then how, to inform other members of the family about the risk they face. Ethical questions are also raised by the issue of termination of the affected fetus, and by the matter of informed consent in children and in individuals with mental disability. Human genetics must be integrated into public health practice in the early twenty-first century. But in the late nineteenth century, public health, abjuring the task of confronting the deep social causes of premature mortality and morbidity, was seduced by the explanatory power of the new bacteriological knowledge and the call to identify high-risk populations. The lure of genetic control of disease must not be allowed again to distract public health from pursuing a broad, social conception of health.[50]

WHITHER PUBLIC HEALTH IN THE AGE OF GLOBALIZATION?

The history of public health in the second half of the twentieth century, particularly since the 1980s, saw disease prevention and health promotion gain ground in health policy in relation to the claims of curative and rehabilitative medicine. The rise to greater prominence of prevention and promotion has had much to do with the considerable and ever-rising costs of technologically driven curative medicine, which offers diminishing returns in terms of health gain but, so far, no magic cures for the leading causes of death in modern societies. Indeed, some philosophers of health, like the American Daniel Callahan, argue that even the richest countries can no longer afford an open-ended commitment to a curative medicine that aims to cure all disease and, mightily, to forestall death. Instead, Callahan wants an economically sustainable and socially just health system, in which caring, not curing, would be the primary task of health services.

Good health may be seen simply as the avoidance of pain and suffering. But viewed more comprehensively, it is the means to pursue a range of human goals. Human adaptability permits the pursuit of life goals with a range of levels of health. A good life is possible without complete healthiness. Unless perfect health, or the eradication of disease and disability, is the aim of the health system, good health becomes a question of how much illness and suffering is to be tolerated. Health is both an individual and social good to be pursued, but it is not an absolute one. Callahan points out that to function properly, social institutions require a sufficiency of healthy citizens. A robust, democratic polity in which the rule of law prevails requires the extensive participation of healthy people. The national economy needs their physical and mental labor. Nurturant and socializing institutions like families, churches and philanthropic organizations need a sufficiency of healthy people. The transmission of culture needs healthy children, able to learn. The military forces must have a continuing supply of healthy young recruits. The modest goal of sufficiency of health is to be preferred over the self-destructive goal of health perfection for all.

A sufficiency of health exists when the vast majority of citizens enjoy good enough health to perform their social roles. For children, there is sufficiency when most are healthy enough to be educated and go through normal mental and physical development; for adults, when the great majority can earn a living, carry out domestic duties and participate in community affairs; and for the aged, when a large majority live to perhaps eighty years while still participating in interpersonal and community activities. In economically advanced nations, something like an accepted average level of health exists, with most people expecting to die at the age of seventy-five or later. But some social groups have a health status less than the average. Equity requires collective effort to improve their health. The self-interest of the advantaged also points in this direction if infections and "social pathologies" are to be contained.

A balance has to be established between the social and the individual good. For much of the contemporary world, the social good and the individual good would be much advanced even by a health system limited to a decent, physical environment, clean and adequate food supply, good sanitation, immunization, antibiotics and trauma care. Generally available primary health care in tandem with a sound public health system would provide a level of health such that most people could function adequately in their social roles. When, however, the health system tries to meet individual needs that are beyond those met by this combination of basic health facilities, the costs of curative medicine grow massively.

Callahan, thinking generally of economically advanced countries but particularly of the United States, wants an economically sustainable, as well as a humane and just, health system. Even the citizens of the richest of nations can no longer afford, he argues, curative medicine organized to pursue heroically the cure of all disease. But caring for the sick individual is affordable. For Callahan, then, caring would be the first goal of any health service. Caring binds the sick and disabled to the community in the face of the alienation that sickness brings. It works against the individual's basic fear of abandonment. No final victory can be achieved over disease, but caring represents constant reassurance in the face of the chronic imperfections and uncertainties of life. An endless quest for cure per se can degenerate into objectification of the patient; caring promotes his or her dignity and humanity.

With caring at the masthead, medicine might adopt more limited goals—like assisting all citizens to enjoy full lives to about eighty years of age, compressing end-of-life morbidity to as short a time as possible, treating effectively chronic psychiatric disorders, and offering functional rehabilitation, where possible, to sustain engagement in everyday life.

In order of priority, the health system's objectives would now become:

- Caring, particularly for people not able to be cured or too costly to cure
- Implementation of public health strategies, particularly disease prevention and health promotion
- Provision of universally accessible primary and emergency health care
- Provision of advanced technological medicine like chemotherapy
- Provision of very advanced technological procedures like organ transplantation.

Callahan points out that a basic conflict exists between the contemporary wish for ever-improving health (the virtual denial of death) and the finiteness of human life. We cannot have, he asserts, both an equitable common health and unlimited medical progress. A properly resourced public health system, a universal primary care system, and widespread individual commitment to healthy lifestyles, along with universal access to high-quality education and high levels of decent employment and of social security, will ensure a generally healthy population. In such circumstances, advanced technological health care becomes very much less important. Public health has the demanding brief of working to change social and economic conditions that constrain healthy behavior and calling, at the same time, for personal responsibility for health practices.[51]

What stands in the way of achieving a health system embodying Callahan's priorities? First, there is the powerful, positive image of acute-care medicine and biomedical research as a realm of heroic struggle and dramatic achievement; there are considerable rewards, even fame and fortune, for successful practitioners. Second, strongly supporting this image is a deep-seated cultural belief in unlimited scientific progress. Critics have increasingly questioned both the fruits of science and scientific rationalism itself, but the belief remains well embedded in Western culture. Closely allied is a strong belief in individualism, which is especially influential in the United States but is prominent also in Australia and the United Kingdom. In recent years, with the discrediting of socialism and the collapse of Soviet communism, individualism and its economic expression, private enterprise, have spread unchallenged. The cultural and economic triumph of the market (rather than government) as the mechanism for distributing economic and societal goods has reached global proportions. Government enterprise and programs face a hostile ideological climate, even in the historical heartland of the welfare state, Europe. In the United States that hostility is deeply rooted, and it contributed to the failure of the campaign in the 1990s to introduce a universal, state-mandated, health care insurance scheme, even though a majority of Americans wanted it. The retreat of government from that effort was not a good sign for disease prevention and health promotion. These are irreducibly collective enterprises that must be pursued for the public good and that only government is fitted to supervise. Private economic interest and the maximization of profit are ultimately incompatible with the proper conduct of such activities.

Transition to a health system embodying Callahan's priorities might well take years, but a plan to initiate change in this direction could be drawn up now. Such a plan would need to show: first, how action to remove social-structural constraints on healthy behavior can be combined with encouragement of enhanced personal responsibility for health; and second, how technological medicine can be employed to deal with the gaps in health provision left even by the most effective public/personal-responsibility strategy. It will no doubt be difficult to reconcile impersonal, population-level measures with the persuasion of individuals to take responsibility for their own health. The danger of blaming the victim is always present when the voluntary element in behavior change is acknowledged. Efforts to change economic and social conditions producing low health status will have to be combined imaginatively with effective education and measures (some of them coercive) to induce personal behavior change.[52]

The Global Context of Public Health

Worldwide, poverty is the most significant cause of preventable mortality. Poverty blights the lives of more people now than two decades ago; 1.3 billion people, or 20 percent of the total population of the world, have daily incomes below one U.S. dollar. Even where such absolute poverty is unknown, as in the Western world, relative deprivation, as Marmot and others have shown, is related to inequalities in health status. Women, children, and the aged face the largest risks of poverty.

Gender inequality exists to a greater or lesser extent throughout the world, and it undermines health. The social subordination of women has combined historically with poverty to promote prostitution and so the spread of classical sexually transmitted diseases and, latterly, HIV/AIDS. In addition, efforts to control the spread have been critically undermined by gender inequality. The nineteenth-century system of compulsory treatment of prostitutes, initiated by Western countries at home and in their colonial empires to protect the health of military forces, was fundamentally flawed by gender bias. It focused on the women, leaving their male clients outside the reach of treatment and control. More recently, even when condom use was publicly promoted by governments in Asia and Africa to prevent the spread of the HIV/AIDS pandemic, unequal interpersonal power could ensure that condoms would not be used in the brothel or the marital bed. While the powerlessness of women in the negotiation of sexual relationships—everyday behavior may, of course, contradict norms even where an ideology of male superiority is especially powerful—should not be overstated, there seems to be no doubt that gender inequality puts women at great risk of HIV/AIDS in Asia and Africa.[53]

Growth of world population is interacting with two other processes—environmental degradation and economic globalization—to threaten global public health. The world's population is growing by about ninety million per annum. The developing countries will experience about 90 percent of future population growth. We have discussed the health effects of environmental degradation; developed countries disproportionately consume natural resources, contributing to degradation of the environment. While this continues, it is hardly reasonable to ask developing countries to forego consumption. Globalization of trade and capital flows seems to produce greater economic inequality within and between nations. While the final effect of the creation of the World Trade Organization (WTO) and greater free trade on public health has yet to become clear, some signs are emerging. The neoconservative ideology accompanying the spread of globalization looks to individual responsibility in health and welfare, as well as to the reduction of the role of government in favor of the market—in the name of lower taxes on capital and cheaper labor costs. The resulting reduction in government spending has much pressured state-funded health and welfare services.

One radical proposal for dealing with the economic growth that has produced environmental damage, and therefore health threats, is economist Herman Daly's idea of the "steady-state economy." In its emphasis on redistribution of income, the concept would also work to reduce the socioeconomic inequalities that underlie health inequalities. No quantitative increase (growth) of goods and services would take place in the steady-state economy, but qualitative improvement (development) would. In a capitalist, market-based economy, there is conflict between efficiency (allocation of resources) and equity (distribution of income). The market deals well with efficiency, but government intervention via taxes and welfare benefits is needed to redistribute income in the interest of equity. Daly adds a third factor—the ecological sustainability of resource use—again requiring government intervention. He proposes a revenue-neutral change from taxing labor and income to taxing resource "throughput" (the flow that starts with inputs of raw materials which are then converted into goods and services, and ultimately into waste outputs), with rates being determined by the scale of resource use that is considered ecologically sustainable. Under this regime, material living standards would cease their continuous rise, but the general living standard afforded by per capita resource use would provide "a good life," though that may well be more modest than the one many consumers in economically advanced economies now seek. The problem of poverty would be solved by a combination of population control, redistribution of wealth and income, and technical improvements in resource productivity.[54]

According to commentators like Colin Butler, there is a pressing need to change thinking about human welfare; in particular, key indices should not be purely economic but should take account of "natural capital," such as clean water, air, soil and forests, as well as of "social welfare," such as income distribution and levels of literacy, education, employment and human rights. He proposes instead of gross national product (GNP) the term "real national wealth" (RNW). This would allow quantification of natural capital and indices of human welfare. Thus, the RNW of the old Soviet Union would have been the resultant of the fact that it scored well on income distribution and employment but poorly on human rights and the natural environment; the RNW of New Guinea will decline drastically unless population growth is contained and the wealth coming from exploitation of its extensive mineral deposits is used for sustainable development.[55]

There are some positive signs at the international level. WHO has been revivified with the appointment of Dr. Gro Brundtland, who has a background in public health, as director general. The new Health for All policy involves the goal of reducing poverty. The World Bank has recently acknowledged that a strong state is vital to economic and social development. If the debt burden of developing countries is reduced and the worst effects of cutbacks in health services consequent on structural readjustment programs are reversed, their health status outlook will have a chance to improve. Indeed, it might be argued that opportunities for public health to become an important part of the WTO agenda do exist. The internal sovereignty of nation-states is being challenged in the area of health, for a variety of reasons—the activities of transnational corporations, the conditions set by the International Monetary Fund, attempts at health care reform by the World Bank and the terms laid down in bilateral aid agreements and in WTO agreements. There is a need to develop an international governmental structure to oversee a "global public health" process able to compensate for the negative health effects of the growing globalization of trade and investment; a process that might also bring into closer contact the health concerns of the developed and developing countries. But it is as yet unclear how this might be best be done. Some commentators propose that nation-states voluntarily place their internal sovereignty into a common pool; others want to strengthen the existing United Nations structure; while yet others want an all-inclusive mechanism bringing together government and nongovernment actors.[56]

Globalism and Health

Along with dangers to health and welfare, economic globalization seems to offer some opportunities. Limited evidence exists that environmental and social matters are beginning to be addressed in trade and investment agreements. The WTO has urged establishment of a World Environment Organization having the capacity to enforce agreed rules. The Montreal Protocol on Ozone-Depleting Substances employed the threat of trade sanctions to enforce almost complete observance of its requirements. This and two other multilateral agreements on the environment are identified in the North American Free Trade Agreement (NAFTA) as superordinate to trade and investment considerations. The WTO has been moving toward requiring governments to end subsidies that encourage environmental vandalism, like destruction of oceanic fish stocks by government-subsidized fishing fleets. On the other hand, most multilateral agreements promoting social and environmental protection, such as the United Nations Declaration of Human Rights, have only moral force. Some are directly challenged by wholly enforceable trade and investment agreements. The TRIPS agreement, which allows patenting of intellectual property, stands in the way of poor countries that want to use better technology. It is it at odds with the spirit of the Rio Agenda 21 agreement (the plan of action adopted at the United Nations conference on the environment and development held in Rio de Janiero in June 1992), and it can be enforced where the latter cannot.

Globalization has promoted international and intranational income inequalities. Trade and investment liberalization has overwhelmingly favored wealthy nations. More than 90 percent of direct foreign investment goes to North America, Europe, Japan and China. The global income growth (about five hundred billion dollars in 1995–2001) that has resulted from freer trade and investment goes to the rich nations. The least liberalized areas of trade—agricultural products and textiles—are the very ones where the poorer nations have comparative advantage over the rich. Agreements have been reached on trade in services, intellectual property investment, and competition policy, areas of vital interest to the rich nations; areas vital to the poor nations, like technology transfer and debt relief, have not enjoyed anything like the same priority. In these ways globalization has strongly advantaged the already-developed countries. Income inequalities within countries have also been worsened by this type of globalization, as neoconservative fiscal policies have deregulated markets and squeezed social welfare provision. Thus Canada, which had resisted the growth of income inequality through government redistributive policies, has abandoned many programs in order to become internationally more competitive. The result is that the number of low-income people in Canada is growing at a rate six times that of the population as a whole. One contemporary health analyst has proposed that modern plagues like HIV/AIDS are "indissociably linked" to local and global inequalities. That the linkage is not more generally recognized is, he suggests, in part the result of the fact that epidemiology concerns itself excessively with "validated" methodologies, ignoring the larger social and political factors that determine why some people become sick and others do not.

There have been some worrying cases under WTO and NAFTA in which health policies have been overturned on free trade grounds. Thailand was forced under the General Agreement on Tariffs and Trade (GATT) and other WTO agreements to allow American tobacco companies into the Thai market just when national tobacco-control legislation was being put in place. A WTO ruling negated a Japanese differential health-promoting tax policy favoring domestic spirits having lower alcohol content over imported spirits because the policy was seen to discriminate in favor of domestic products. The WTO forced the European Union to permit import of hormone-treated beef even though it had been banned as a health risk.

Deregulation of foreign investment and the availability of microcomputers have facilitated the movement of vast sums of money in and out of countries. Yet most of this money pursues short-term returns unrelated to the production of goods and services, the activities that actually create employment. Further, the financial crises that result from this free movement can be socially disruptive—as in the recent case of Mexico, where the poverty produced led to an increase in crime unprecedented in time of peace. The future impact of the General Agreement on Trade in Services (GATS) on state health services is another matter for concern. With the service industry rather than manufacturing destined to be the future source of profits in developed economies, global corporations, many based in the United States and Europe, need new markets. They see the billions spent by governments on health and social services as producing a new market expansion. American health maintenance organizations face both saturation of existing markets and attempts by government and employers to contain health-care costs. They are now looking to new opportunities overseas.

In 1994, national health and social services were defined at the Uruguay Round of WTO meetings as neither commercial nor part of a competitive market. They were thus protected from the provisions of GATS aimed at increasing private enterprise involvement in the service sector of the economy. But the WTO working party on domestic regulatory reform wanted to require states to outlaw, in the interest of a least-trade-restrictive approach, nonmarket mechanisms like cross-subsidization, universal risk pooling, solidarity and public accountability in funding and delivery of public services. Market mechanisms would have to replace such nonmarket devices, commonly used by governments to deliver national, universal health-care services. Governments failing to comply would encounter trade sanctions. Freedom of trade and investment are clearly being put ahead of health and welfare considerations. Not only is democratic government within the nation-state at risk, but the social welfare rights of citizens are threatened in places like Europe and Australia, where such rights have been strongly entrenched. In principle, both Australia's universal health insurance system, Medicare, and the universal pharmaceutical benefits scheme are jeopardized. The current round of re-negotiation of GATS is expected to conclude at the end of December 2002 but it will be the first in a series of rounds intended to expand the ambit of the agreement. Expansion will take place through increasing specific commitments, re-classifying services to broaden coverage, and introducing "horizontal" provisions covering all members, services, sectors and modes of supply.[57]

PUBLIC HEALTH IN THE UNITED STATES, THE UNITED KINGDOM AND AUSTRALIA

In late 1988, after a two-year study, the Institute of Medicine (IOM) made public its report on public health in the United States, *The Future of Public Health*. The study found the system in disarray, with inadequate capacity to carry out essential public health functions, disjointed decision making (made worse by lack of necessary data bases), no effective leadership, and a poor public image that worked against the growth of community support. In the decade following the report, programs to make better connections between academics and public health practitioners were developed. Progress was made in the organization of state health agencies and in development of public health infrastructure. However, inadequate funding at the local level has retarded implementation of the recommendations of the IOM. Of $940 billion a year spent on health services, less than 1 percent has gone to prevention; experts believe that 6 percent is an appropriate level of investment. Public health agencies in the mid-1990s were still carrying the additional burden of providing last-resort, health care for the poor, restricting their capacity to address population health problems. The size of the burden can be appreciated by realizing that one in two children from minority populations was living in poverty and at least thirty-nine million Americans had no health-care insurance.[58]

As late as 1995, the U.S. surgeon general, Dr. M. Joycelyn Elders, could state, "Our public health system is underfunded, undersupported, and underappreciated. . . . We do not have the education and training to build the kind of health leadership that we need for the 21st Century." Yet public health has been responsible for the majority of extra years of life enjoyed by the American people; only five of the thirty extra years of average life expectancy are attributable to "sick care advancements."[59]

In the United Kingdom, the emphasis in public health development for a very long time has been on public health medicine. Other public health professionals were institutionally and ideologically less central, although recently there have been some hopeful signs of change. Not surprisingly, then, academic public health has been dominated by public health doctors. Moreover, academic public health has not been organizationally well related to the world of public health practice. Until very recently, public health was professionally fragmented, with three organizations representing the cause. The Public Health Alliance (PHA), formed in 1987, decided from the outset to remain nonparty political. In its commitment to multidisciplinarity, it took as its model the Canadian and the long-established American Association of Public Health. Doctors were not numerous as members. Committed to nonhierarchical organization, it wanted to attract members from voluntary bodies and from the field of community development. Throughout the 1990s, its great concern, as expressed in surveys of members, was poverty and health. In 1991 the Association for Public Health (APH) was established, with the assistance of the Health Education Authority. It sought to attract a health professional membership and to champion the cause of the concept of health gain. The organizational fragmentation of public health in Britain was made clear when the World Federation of Public Health Organisations, rejecting the membership applications of the PHA and two other public health bodies from the United Kingdom, observed that none of them was able to show that it was working toward integration. Finally, in 1999, the APH, the PHA and the Public Health Trust came together to form the UK

Public Health Association. Its core values were stated to be equity, social justice, sustainable development and the right of everyone to good health.[60]

We have seen that historically in Australia, as in the United Kingdom and the United States, public health has been subordinate to medical and hospital care in national health policy and that this has been the case despite good evidence that public health has played a larger role in bringing down death rates during the modern mortality decline of the last 120 years or so. Given the historical achievements of public health, it should have a direct role in monitoring all government policy initiatives influencing population-health status and in advising government in the light of its findings. For this, a status equal to that of health care is needed. In the Westminster system of cabinet government that operates in Britain and Australia, a minister of public health with an administration independent of the established Health Department might be one way to achieve this. The Blair Labor government, on assuming office in 1997 in Britain, appointed the first minister for public health, the Right Honorable Tessa Jowell. Unfortunately, she remained in the ranks of the more junior ministers and was not included in the cabinet.[61]

Another way to make a larger organizational "place" for public health would be to recast national health policy in more comprehensive terms, as Lewis and Leeder have recently proposed for Australia.[62] Recasting of policy might be accompanied by institutional innovation. A new advisory body on health, a Prime Minister's Health Council (with strong representation for public health), might be set up along the lines of the Council on Science and Technology. In addition a National Health Forum might be convened to discuss development of a more comprehensive health policy that takes account of the determinants of health inside and outside the health system and addresses the politically difficult issue of social inequalities in health. Like the National Constitutional Forum, this body would be composed of representatives elected by citizens and government appointees, briefed by health experts before its deliberations.

In Australia, the stated concern of the commonwealth Department of Health and Aged Care is with health services, not health. It views itself as "the leader in promoting, developing and funding world-class health and aged care services for all Australians" and as using a "targeted approach to disease management and to addressing the health risks of particular individuals and communities."[63] This may be contrasted with the overt recognition of Health Canada, the Canadian federal health department, of the relationship between health status, and social and environmental factors: "Health Canada recognises that health depends on more than a good health care system. Factors such as income, education, social support networks, the environment, and employment and working conditions determine health and well-being. The Department focuses on this wide range of personal and collective circumstances when developing strategies to promote health."[64] Health Canada's broad picture of the determinants of health reflects a conception of population health that owes much to the work of economists Robert Evans and Greg Stoddart over the last decade or so. In its desire to move the primary focus of health policy away from health care, this conception is in agreement with modern health promotion, although it is concerned with economic growth as the source of health gain rather than with income redistribution, which is the aim of health promotion. Whatever the case, health policy must integrate biological, social and economic considerations in a multisectoral strategy rather than focus simply, as now, on efficient, effective health care.[65]

The population health approach identifies health determinants at the collective as well as the individual level and outside the health system as well as within it: income and social status, social support networks, education, employment and working conditions, physical environments, personal health practices and coping skills, healthy child development, genetic endowment, health resources, gender and culture. It requires action across a range of modalities: health promotion, disease and injury prevention, risk assessment, policy coordination, medical treatment, rehabilitation and palliative care. Evans and Stoddart stress that "appropriate conceptualisation of the determinants of health is a necessary but not a sufficient condition for serious reform of health policy."[66]

Proponents of health promotion in Canada and elsewhere themselves have traditionally taken a broad approach to health, integrating social, economic and political factors with biological ones and wanting to move beyond even equitable health services to deal with determinants outside the health system. But population health began in the early 1990s to challenge health promotion in Canadian health circles as the alternative to biomedicine. As already noted, the two have much in common. Indeed, in 1996 Health Canada synthesized them in the "population health promotion" model (of which more later).[67]

While Evans and Stoddart present compelling evidence for the significance of the social and economic determinants of health, they do not offer an integrated explanation for the widely observed phenomenon of the social gradient in health status. An English health researcher, Richard Wilkinson, offers such an explanation. It involves the two dimensions of "materiality" and "meaning," or economic and cultural—material resources we possess and how we understand our being in the world, with both related to our place in the social hierarchy. Thus, the Evans and Stoddart population health model's concern with the biological and psychosocial pathways connecting low social status and poor health needs to be supplemented by concern with the economic, social and political forces keeping the structural inequities in place. This concern with structural inequities has been characteristic of health promotion.[68]

What, then, are the significant differences and similarities between population health and health promotion? One difference has been mentioned already—where population health looks to an increase in wealth to advance health status, health promotion says there must be a redistribution of wealth to poorer groups. Another difference is that while health promotion has not usually offered a convincing analysis of the determinants of health, population health has. Yet another is that health promotion places an ultra-democratic emphasis on community development and participation, where population health does not even seek to do so. (Indeed population health has been developed by an elite group of researchers at the Canadian Institute of Advanced Research, and their main aim has been interpreting scientific evidence concerning health determinants, not promoting community control of the social production of health.) However, both share the view that social structure and processes are critical to the production of health. They both want to see the focus of health policy shifted from the biology and the health behavior of the individual.[69] Australia needs a more comprehensive national health policy, one that reflects the growing evidence about the considerable importance of social and economic factors and that, like Canada's policy, marries the best of population health and health promotion strategies. We noted in an earlier chapter that from the mid-1980s the commonwealth demonstrated a greater willingness to take national initiatives in disease prevention and health advancement, although under neoconservative Coalition governments since 1996 the focus of public health has returned to more traditional medical or behavioral concerns.

Earlier, we listed the priorities identified by Daniel Callahan as appropriate to economically sustainable and socially equitable health services. A comprehensive Australian health policy drawing on Callahan's priorities for the health services and on a model integrating population health and health promotion would have the following features. First, it would embody Callahan's order of priorities in health services: emphasis on caring for patients; pursuit of public health measures; primary and emergency medical care; advanced technological medicine (like chemotherapy); and, finally, very advanced technological medicine (like organ transplantation). Second, at the population level, it would employ what Health Canada has termed "the population health promotion" model. The model requires action on a range of health determinants using health promotion strategies proposed in the Ottawa Charter for 1986 and intervention at various levels of social organization from the individual to society as a whole.

There are five health promotion strategies: reorientation of health services from sickness care to health advancement; development of personal, health-related skills in individuals; creation of socially supportive environments; construction of health-advancing public policy; and strengthening of community action in support of health. Nine health determinants are to be addressed: income and social status, social support networks, education, working conditions, physical environments, biology and genetics, individual health practices and coping skills, healthy child development and health services.

A number of assumptions that incorporate various values underlie the model. These are:

1. All health determinants need to be acted upon.
2. As well as acting on determinants for which they are directly responsible, health organizations try also to influence other government policies affecting health.
3. Interventions may be made at any level of social organization, but there will also be an effort to achieve overall coordination of such activities.
4. Change at the macrolevel of social values and structure is required to reduce inequalities in health status.
5. Individual health status results from personal health behavior and the effect of social and physical environments; environments impact psychologically as well as physically on the health of individuals.
6. Social environments in which a high degree of equity exists and relationships based on mutual respect and support rather than differential power and status promote health.
7. Disease prevention, health protection and health care complement health promotion.
8. Community participation in policy development and implementation is necessary if people are to influence the determinants of their health.

These assumptions reflect a social conception of health in which the full range of health determinants is addressed, high priority is given to reduction of health status inequalities and the values of caring, equity, and democratic participation figure prominently. A comprehensive national policy reflecting a social conception of health would see health sector bodies continuing to provide direct service but would see them also serving indirectly by influencing other sectors of government (and the private sector) to pursue policies promoting health. A comprehensive policy recognizes that the majority of health determinants lie outside the health care services; accordingly, economic, educational, environmental and social welfare policies become as important as health services policy itself. However, if the health care services are to respond equitably to the disproportionate burden of ill health carried by the socially disadvantaged in Australia, Medicare—the universal, state-financed, health insurance scheme—must continue. A social conception of health is central to a comprehensive health policy addressing all major health determinants and the causes of health inequalities. The proper pursuit of health policy now requires the federal government to attend seriously to the connections between health on the one hand and economics, social welfare and education on the other.[70]

CIVILIZING GLOBAL CAPITALISM IN THE INTERESTS OF HEALTH ADVANCEMENT

There is a clear parallel between the process of civilizing free market capitalism in nineteenth-century Britain—the pioneer of both industrial capitalism and modern public health—and the need to civilize global capitalism at the beginning of the twenty-first century. Just as environmental interventions were made in the form of publicly funded clean water supplies, sewerage and other public health infrastructure to promote the collective health of the British people seriously damaged by free market economic growth, so social and environmental agreements need to accompany international agreements to liberalize trade and investment today to protect global health against the effect of free market capitalism. The same struggles entered into nationally 150 years ago have to be pursued at the global level today.

For a large part of the eighteenth century, average mortality had been falling in Britain. But from the 1820s to the 1870s, a half-century of unprecedented free market economic expansion, life expectancy remained stagnant. Indeed, in the 1830s and 1840s, the fast-growing industrial cities like Manchester, Liverpool and Glasgow had life expectancies as low as those in the period of the Black Death in the fourteenth century. In a time of sharp growth in national income, the urban incidence of the diseases of crowding and insanitation (infant diarrheal disease, typhus, typhoid and cholera) was increasing. The environmental degradation that underlay this epidemiological pattern resulted from three social changes (which in turn resulted from the free market style of economic expansion). In the first place, capital accumulation, vigorous entrepreneurial activity and siphoning off of various types of rents were producing great inequality of income and wealth. Second, rural immigrants were flooding into urban areas, where they took the worst-paid employment. Finally, urban segregation saw the wealthy leave urban centers for the cleaner, more salubrious outer areas. Poorly paid workers occupied poor-quality rental housing in the city, thus contributing to the process of capital accumulation by employers and property owners, which itself powered the free market, economic expansion.

Local government reforms to rectify environmental deterioration in the cities were delayed until the late 1860s because of the new political power of small capitalists and property owners, who above all wished to avoid funding municipal improvements. In an age of absolute belief in nonintervention in the working of the market at the local or national level, low municipal rates were matched by low spending on welfare through the Poor Law. Indeed, the Poor Law of 1834 reduced welfare spending on the disabled and the poor from 2 to 1 percent of national product. The "economy" campaigns of nineteenth-century British liberalism are today paralleled by the "restructuring" and welfare minimization demanded by neoconservative advocates of unrestricted economic globalization, as Simon Szreter has recently pointed out.[71]

Industrial and commercial rather than health-promoting considerations lay behind expansion of municipal water supplies in the two decades or so from the late 1840s, after the 1848 Public Health Act allowed local government to obtain central government funds for water and sewerage infrastructure. Water was a vital industrial input, and this was the key reason for the laying of new water mains. The complementary development of commercially unimportant underground sewerage systems was small, despite the 1854 cholera epidemic. The Sanitary Commission of 1871 noted that most provincial cities had failed to construct arterial sewerage systems. Further, prior to the 1870s, mass connection of individual dwellings to the water supplies did not advance far.

Significant political changes ensured that from the close of the 1860s investment in the urban environment, especially domestic water supplies and sewerage systems, advanced at a greater pace. Able, new men from the urban elite, supported by an increasingly professionalized municipal officer corps, preached the gospel of civic pride and civic improvement in place of liberal "economy." At the same time, the urban electorate widened beyond the control of the entrenched petty bourgeoisie to include "respectable" working men, as the Reform Act of 1867 and the Municipal Franchise and Assessed Rates Acts of 1869 created broader national and local franchises. Long-term loans at low interest and profits from local gas, electricity and transport services were used to finance the building of new health-promoting infrastructure. Expectation of life at birth in England and Wales rose significantly in these decades of revivified urban government.

The paradigmatic case of Britain in the nineteenth century points up the central importance of community participation in the political process. Extension of the vote to the working class, combined with leadership drawn from imaginative members of the new, urban elite, ensured that collective health and environmental problems were addressed effectively. The development of new sources of public funding generally acceptable to taxpayers was another significant factor. The importance of the mediatory role of the "state" (embracing not only the central government and bureaucracy but local government and public-service professions as well) in managing an equitable relationship between the market-driven economy and the health of the population is clear.

The lesson from nineteenth-century Britain is that to balance the health and welfare costs produced by the contemporary market economy, driven by trade and investment globalization, the civic institutions of participation and trust—the "social capital"—of modern societies must be nurtured and encouraged at the national level. At the international or global level, various stratagems must be pursued. Nongovernment organizations are already pushing to give superordinate status to social and environmental goals in WTO matters, as against business support for the superordinancy of economic goals. The Public Health Associations of Canada, the United

Kingdom and Australia, the World Federation of Public Health Associations and the International Union of Health Promotion and Education have advocated enforceable social and environmental agreements to accompany multilateral trade and investment agreements.

New forms of international governance are required, forms that include nongovernment organizations as well as nation-states and established international organizations like the United Nations (UN). UN bodies (including the WHO) and the World Bank are already trying partnership approaches. But this more inclusive process must go beyond cooperation to joint decision making. Two ideological developments would facilitate this process: first, as in the debate about the environment, health should be reframed as a "commons" (defined as physical or biological systems outside the jurisdiction of one nation-state but valued resources of two or more); second, health should be identified as a "global public good," the benefits of which extend across national borders, generations and population groups. Health demands a public policy response that is global.

If we take a long-term view of the process of globalization of trade and finance since the nineteenth century, we may identify two types of "institutional defense mechanism" against the process. The first involved in the late nineteenth and early-twentieth-century establishment of economic and social compensations at the level of the nation-state, especially tariff protection, monetary policy regulation and immigration restriction. The second involved attempts to develop international rules that from the 1920s were pursued through international bodies like the League of Nations. After the radical, nationalist responses of fascism and Stalinism to this interwar internationalism and the resulting violence of the Second World War, there was a return to internationalism in the United Nations and the International Monetary Fund. In the 1990s, the defense against globalization (ethnic exclusivism and anachronistic religious fundamentalism apart) consists largely of diffuse anger about a variety of targets, from multinational corporations to global capital. This anger has given rise to a loose antiglobalist coalition mainly calling for capital and immigration controls. But it has not yet produced a coherent, intellectual and policy alternative. The reaction against globality has also been hampered by the lack of plausible alternative national models of success. Yet if the historical pattern (of swings for and against globalization) of the last two centuries still holds, we may anticipate a full pendulum swing against globality to develop soon.[72] The historical record shows that globalization is neither monolithic nor inevitable. Historically, it has been a discontinuous process, and it has been as much resisted as promoted by human agency. Indeed, one social scientist has suggested that globalization begs to be engaged and given form.[73]

Public health activists can contribute to the shaping of globalization and the civilizing of global capitalism in a number of ways: by participating in multi-actor meetings where the difficult issues of reconciliation of social and environmental with trade and investment goals can be explored; by showing the likely health effects of liberalization of trade and investment before it is implemented; and by lobbying national governments for some degree of regulation of international capital flows. One example of the last is the proposed Tobin, or financial transaction, tax, for which support has come from a number of countries. A small fee would be levied on all trade in stocks, bonds, currencies, options, futures and derivatives contracts. While not penalizing long-term investment, this tax would make the very short-term global movement of capital, which is so destabilizing to national economies, very expensive. Moreover, by bringing in $150 billion or more a year, it would fund the efforts of poor nations to implement social and environmental agreements.[74]

In this age of economic globalization, public health must, as it did in nineteenth-century Britain, become heavily involved in the political process in order to overcome the negative effects on the health of the people of unfettered market-driven economic growth. It must be an important contributor to the civilizing of global capitalism, just as it helped civilize industrial capitalism in the nation-state 150 years ago.

NOTES

1. V. Burgmann, *Power and Protest: Movements for Change in Australian Society* (Sydney: Allen and Unwin, 1993), 4.
2. Ibid., 10.
3. Ibid., 1–7; T. Dalton, "Participation. Influencing Policy in Troubled Times," in *Keeping It Together: State and Civil Society in Australia*, ed. A. Farrar and J. Inglis (Leichhardt: Pluto Press, 1996), 188–89.
4. Dalton, "Participation. Influencing Policy in Troubled Times," 190–205.
5. Sir Keith Jones, "Medicine and the Law: Thirties Style," *Medical Journal of Australia* 161 (1994): 21.
6. E. Bates, "The Consumer and the Health Care System," *Community Health Studies* 11(2) (1978): 73–75.
7. Ibid., 78.
8. C. Crawford, "Medicine and the Law," in *Companion Encyclopedia of the History of Medicine*, ed. W.F. Bynum and R. Porter (London: Routledge, 1993), 1632–33.
9. See M. Lewis, *Managing Madness: Psychiatry and Society in Australia 1788–1980* (Canberra: AGPS Press, 1988), 91–93; G.A. Edwards, "Psychiatric Treatment and Services in Australia, 1914–1994," *Medical Journal of Australia* 161 (1994): 44.
10. *Declaration of Alma Ata: Adopted at the International Conference on Primary Health Care Alma Ata, USSR, 6–12 September 1978* (Geneva: World Health Organization [hereafter WHO], 1978), Section I, VI.

11. G.R. Palmer and S.D. Short, *Health Care and Public Policy: An Australian Analysis* (South Melbourne: Macmillan Education Australia, 1994), 214.

12. Quoted in R.R. Winton, "Health, Medicine and Human Rights," in *The Health Problems of the Nation,* ed. J. Birman (Perth: Extension Service University of Western Australia, 1974), 14.

13. A. Hermann, *Alan Missen, Liberal Pilgrim: A Political Biography* (Woden, ACT: Poplar Press, 1993), 138–41; M. Daly, "Human Rights Record Poor: Burdekin," in *Human Rights,* ed. K. Healey (Wentworth Falls, NSW: Spinney Press, 1993), 14.

14. Quoted in C. Reynolds, "Public Health and the Australian Constitution," *Australian Journal of Public Health* 19(3) (1995): 246.

15. Ibid., 244–48.

16. Palmer and Short, *Health Care and Public Policy,* 316–18; D. Fry, "Quality Assurance and Community Health Services," in *Community Health: Policy and Practice in Australia,* ed. F. Baum, D. Fry and I. Lennie (Leichhardt, NSW: Pluto Press, 1992), 132–34.

17. Palmer and Short, *Health Care and Public Policy,* 321–22.

18. Ibid., 237; R. Horton, "African AIDS beyond Mbeki: Tripping into Anarchy," *Lancet* 356 (2000): 1542.

19. Quoted in M. Lewis, "Control of STDs and the History of Public Health in Twentieth Century Australia," unpublished paper, Microbiological Unit Centenary Conference, University of Melbourne, 1998, 8.

20. Ibid., 8–12; Palmer and Short, *Health Care and Public Policy,* 238–41.

21. K.C. Calman and R.S. Downie, "Ethical Principles and Ethical Issues in Public Health," *Oxford Textbook of Public Health,* ed. W.W. Holland, R. Detels and G.E. Knox (Oxford: Oxford University Press, 1997), vol. 1, 392–93; J.M. Mann, "Medicine and Public Health, Ethics and Human Rights," *Hastings Center Report* 27(3) (1997): 7–8.

22. J.M. Mann and K. Kay, "Confronting the Pandemic: The World Health Organization's Global Programme on AIDS, 1986–1989," *AIDS* 5 (Supplement 2): S221–28.

23. S. Davidson, *Human Rights* (Buckingham: Open University Press, 1993), 41–44.

24. B.S. Turner, "Outline of a Theory of Human Rights," in *Citizenship: Critical Concepts,* ed. B.S. Turner and P. Hamilton (London: Routledge, 1994), 469–70.

25. Mann, "Medicine and Public Health, Ethics and Human Rights," 9–13.

26. S.S. Morse, "Global Microbial Traffic and the Interchange of Disease," *American Journal of Public Health* 82(10) (1992): 1326–27.

27. "Emerging and Re-emerging Infections: How Are We Doing?" *National Public Health Partnership News* 5 (1998): 1–2.

28. D. Satcher, "Tuberculosis: Battling an Ancient Scourge," *JAMA* 282 (21) (1999): 1996; AM/ABC Radio, 5 April 2001.

29. P. Wall and R. Stanwell Smith, "Communicable Disease Challenges and Control," in *Progress in Public Health,* ed. G. Scally (London: F.T. Healthcare, 1997), 139–44; G.L. Gilbert, "From Broad St. to Prospect via Milwaukee: Water Contamination and Human Disease," *Inoculum* 8(1) (1999): 4–6.

30. Quoted in S. Leeder and A. Dominello, "Mad Cow Disease," *In Touch* 18(2) (2001): 1.

31. Quoted in *Sydney Morning Herald*, 21 November 1998.

32. Leeder and Dominello, "Mad Cow Disease," 1–2; C.L. Masters, "The Emerging European Epidemic of Variant Creutzfeldt-Jakob Disease and Bovine Spongiform Encephalopathy: Lessons for Australia," *Medical Journal of Australia* 174 (2001): 160–61.

33. Wall and Stanwell Smith, "Communicable Disease Challenges and Control," 147–48.

34. J. Lederberg, "Infectious Disease as an Evolutionary Paradigm," *Emerging Infectious Diseases* 3(4) (1997): 418–23.

35. Quoted in P. Farmer, "Social Inequalities and Emerging Infectious Diseases," *Emerging Infectious Diseases* 2(4) (1996): 265.

36. Quoted in ibid., 266.

37. Ibid., 259–67; M. Lewis and S. Bamber, "Introduction," in *Sex, Disease and Society: A Comparative History of Sexually Transmitted Diseases and HIV/AIDS in Asia and the Pacific,* ed. M. Lewis, S. Bamber and M. Waugh (Westport, Conn.: Greenwood Press, 1997), 2–15; L. Garrett, *Betrayal of Trust: The Collapse of Global Public Health* (New York: Hyperion, 2000), 576–77.

38. M. Susser and E. Susser, "Choosing a Future for Epidemiology: II. From Black Box to Chinese Boxes and Eco-Epidemiology," *American Journal of Public Health* 86(5) (1996): 674–77.

39. E.J. DaSilva, "Biological Warfare, Bioterrorism, Biodefence and the Biological and Toxin Weapons Convention," *Electronic Journal of Biotechnology* 2(3) (1999): 2; G.W. Christopher, T.J. Cieslak, J.A. Pavlin and E.M. Eitzen, "Biological Warfare: A Historical Perspective," *JAMA* 278(5) (1997): 412–13: N. Butlin, *Our Original Aggression: Aboriginal Populations of Southeastern Australia 1788–1850* (Sydney: George Allen and Unwin, 1983), 21–22: F. Fenner, D.A. Henderson, I. Arita, Z. Jezek and I.D. Ladnyi, *Smallpox and Its Eradication* (Geneva: WHO, 1988), 239.

40. DaSilva, "Biological Warfare, Bioterrorism, Biodefence and the Biological and Toxin Weapons Convention," 4; Garrett, *Betrayal of Trust,* 482–544; H.W. Cohen, R.M. Gould and V.W. Sidel, "Bioterrorism Preparedness: Dual Use or Poor Excuse?" *Public Health Reports* 115(5) (2000): 403.

41. W. Pyper, "Bioterrorism: Are We Ready?" www.publish.csiro.au/ecos/Ecos101/ecos101a.htm (accessed 16 November 2001); I. Douglas, "Defence against Emergency Diseases," *Australian Veterinary Journal* 79(1) (2000): 18–19; "Statement by Australia's Acting Chief Medical Officer, Professor John Mathews," www.health.gov.au/pubhlth/strate . . . munic/factsheets/anthrax_statement.htm (accessed 16 November 2001); "Statement by the Commonwealth Chief Medical Officer: Smallpox Is a Low Threat in Australia," www.health.gov.au/pubhlth/strate . . . munic/factsheets/smallpox_statement.htm (accessed 16 November 2001).

42. E.K. Jackson, "Climate Change and Global Infectious Disease Threats," *Medical Journal of Australia* 163 (1995): 570–72: F. Baum, *The New Public Health: An Australian Perspective* (Melbourne: Oxford University Press, 1998), 266–67.

43. A.J. McMichael and C.S. Guest, "Doctors and the 'Environment,'" *Medical Journal of Australia* 171 (1999): 576; C. Guest, R. Douglas, R. Woodruff and T. McMichael, "Health and the Environment," *Tela: Environment, Economy and Society* 1 (1999): 1.

44. Guest, Douglas, Woodruff and McMichael, "Health and the Environment," 3–26; *Health and Environment in Sustainable Development: Five Years after the Earth Summit* (Geneva: WHO, 1997), executive summary, chap. 5.

45. Baum, *The New Public Health,* 249–51, 436–39.

46. J. Smith, "The Journey towards a National Food Safety Policy," in *Health Policy in Australia,* ed. H. Gardner (Melbourne: Oxford University Press, 1997), 158–62.

47. Quoted in S. Leeder, "Genetically Modified Foods: Food for Thought," *Medical Journal of Australia* 172 (2000): 174.

48. M. Metherell and A. Stevenson, "Coming to Your Kitchen: Food with All the Facts," *Sydney Morning Herald,* 29 July 2000.

49. R. Beaglehole and R. Bonita, *Public Health at the Crossroads: Achievements and Prospects* (Cambridge: Cambridge University Press, 1999), 44–45.

50. Ibid., 211; R. Zimmern, "Genetics," in *Perspectives on Health,* ed. S. Griffiths and D.J. Hunter (Oxford: Radcliffe Memorial Press, 1999), 132–38.

51. D. Callahan, *What Kind of Life: The Limits of Medical Progress* (Washington, D.C.: Georgetown University Press, 1990): 103–37; D. Callahan, review of R.G. Evans, M.L. Barer and T.R. Marmor, eds., "Why Are Some People Health and Others Not? The Determinants of Health of Populations," *Journal of Health Politics, Policy and Law* 21(4) (1996): 885–86; D. Callahan, *False Hopes: Why America's Quest for Perfect Health Is a Recipe for Failure* (New York: Simon and Schuster, 1998), 23, 173–87, 270–74.

52. Callahan, *False Hopes,* 186–201.

53. See Lewis and Bamber, "Introduction," 6–7; P.W. Setel, "Comparative Histories of Sexually Transmitted Diseases and HIV/AIDS in Africa: An Introduction," in *Histories of Sexually Transmitted Diseases and HIV/AIDS in Sub-Saharan Africa,* eds. P.W. Setel, M. Lewis and M. Lyons (Westport, Conn.: Greenwood Press, 1999), 8–9.

54. R. Gittins, "Cutting to the Root of the Anti-Globalisation Debate," *Sydney Morning Herald,* 5–6 May 2001.

55. C. Butler, "Overpopulation, Overconsumption, and Economics," *Lancet* 343 (1994): 584.

56. R. Beaglehole and R. Bonita, "Public Health at the Crossroads: Which Way Forward?" *Lancet* 351 (1998): 592; I. Kickbusch and E. de Leeuw, "Global Public Health: Revisiting Healthy Public Policy at the Global Level," *Health Promotion International* 14(4) (1999): 286.

57. P. Farmer, *Infections and Inequalities: The Modern Plagues* (Berkeley: University of California Press, 2001), 281; R. Labonte, "Globalism and Health: Threats and Opportunities," *Health Promotion Journal of Australia* 9(2) (1999): 129; P. Laris, "Public Health Alert: Risk of GATS Infection," *In Touch* 18(3) (2001): 1; A.M. Pollock and D. Price "Rewriting the Regulations: How the World Trade Organisation Could Accelerate Privatisation in Health-Care Systems," *Lancet* 356 (2000): 1995; "Trading Public Health for Private Wealth," *Lancet* 356 (2000): 1941.

58. B. Walker, "The Future of Public Health: The Institute of Medicine's 1988 Report," *Journal of Public Health Policy* 10 (1989): 19–31; M.J. Elders, "The Role of Public Health in Improving the Health of America," *Journal of Public Health Policy* 16 (1995): 134–35; Beaglehole and Bonita, "Public Health at the Crossroads," 591.

59. Elders, "The Role of Public Health in Improving the Health of America," 134.

60. Beaglehole and Bonita, "Public Health at the Crossroads," 591; J. Upward, *Rethinking Public Health: The First 10 Years of the Public Health Alliance* (Birmingham: Public Health Alliance, 1998), 23–27; *UKPHA. UK Public Health Association* (Birmingham: UKPHA, [1999]), n.p.

61. S. Griffiths and D.J. Hunter, "Introduction," in *Perspectives in Public Health,* ed. S. Griffiths and D.J. Hunter (Abingdon: Radcliffe Medical Press, 1999), 1; Beaglehole and Bonita, "Public Health at the Crossroads," 592.

62. See M.J. Lewis and S.R. Leeder, *Where to from Here? The Need to Construct a Comprehensive National Health Policy* (Sydney: Australian Health Policy Institute at University of Sydney, 2001), 1–47.

63. Quoted in M. Frommer, A. Shiell and G. Rubin, "Perspectives on Population Health," unpublished paper, Australian Centre for Effective Healthcare, University of Sydney, 4 April 1999, 4.

64. Quoted in ibid., 3–4.

65. J.W. Frank, "The Determinants of Health: A New Synthesis," *Current Issues in Public Health* 1 (1995): 233–37; A. Robertson, "Shifting Discourses on Health in Canada: From Health Promotion to Population Health," *Health Promotion International* 13(2) (1998): 157.

66. R.G. Evans and G.L. Stoddart, "Producing Health, Consuming Health Care," in *Why Are Some People Healthy and Others Not? The Determinants of Health of Populations,* ed. R.G. Evans, M.L. Barer and T.R. Marmor (New York: Aldine de Gruyter, 1994), 60.

67. Frank, "The Determinants of Health," 237; Health Canada, "Health Promotion in Canada: A Case Study," *Health Promotion International* 13(1) (1998): 14.

68. B. Poland, D. Coburn, A. Robertson and J. Eakin, "Wealth, Equity and Health Care: A Critique of a 'Population Health' Perspective on the Determinants of Health," *Social Science and Medicine* 46(7): 790–91; M.V. Hayes and J.R. Dunn, *Population Health in Canada: A Systematic Review* (Ottawa: Canadian Policy Research Networks, 1998), 3.

69. M. O'Neill, A. Pederson and I. Rootman, "Health Promotion in Canada: Declining or Transforming?" *Health Promotion International* 15(2) (2000): 138; J.R. Dunn and M.V. Hayes, "Toward a Lexicon of Population Health," *Canadian Journal of Public Health* 90 (Supplement 1) (1999): S9.

70. Hayes and Dunn, *Population Health in Canada,* 54; Health Canada, "Developing a Population Health Model," www.hc–sc.gc.ca/hppb/phdd/php3.html (accessed 13 October 2000).

71. S. Szreter, "Rapid Economic Growth and 'the Four D's' of Disruption, Deprivation, Disease and Death: Public Health Lessons from Nineteenth-Century Britain for Twenty-first-Century China?" *Tropical Medicine and International Health* 4(2) (1999): 146–49.

72. H. James, *The End of Globalization: Lessons from the Great Depression* (Cambridge, Mass.: Harvard University Press, 2001), 217–24.

73. M.F. Guillen, "Is Globalization Civilizing, Destructive or Feeble? A Critique

of Five Key Debates in the Social–Science Literature," *Annual Review of Sociology* 27 (2001): 255.

74. Szreter, "Rapid Economic Growth and 'the Four Ds' of Disruption, Deprivation, Disease and Death," 146–52; Labonte, "Globalism and Health: Threats and Opportunities," 130–32; Kickbusch and de Leeuw, "Global Public Health," 286–87.

Selected Bibliography

Baum, F. *The New Public Health: An Australian Perspective*. Melbourne: Oxford University Press, 1998.

Baum, F., D. Fry, and I. Lennie, eds. *Community Health. Policy and Practice in Australia*. Leichhardt, NSW: Pluto Press Australia, 1993.

Beaglehole, R., and R. Bonita. *Public Health at the Crossroads: Achievements and Prospects*. Cambridge: Cambridge University Press, 1999.

Bunton, R., and G. Macdonald, eds. *Health Promotion: Disciplines and Diversity*. London: Routledge, 1992.

Bury, M. *Health and Illness in a Changing Society*. London: Routledge, 1997.

Callahan, D. *False Hopes: Why America's Quest for Perfect Health Is a Recipe for Failure*. New York: Simon and Schuster, 1998.

Duffy, J. *The Sanitarians: A History of American Public Health*. Urbana: University of Illinois Press, 1990.

Evans, R.G., M.L. Barer, and T.R. Marmor, eds. *Why Are Some People Healthy and Others Not? The Determinants of Health of Populations*. New York: Aldine de Gruyter, 1994.

Garrett, L. *Betrayal of Trust: The Collapse of Global Public Health*. New York: Hyperion, 2000.

Hayes, M.V., and J.R. Dunn. *Population Health in Canada: A Systematic Review*. Ottawa: Canadian Policy Research Networks, 1998.

Kunitz, S.J. *Disease and Social Diversity: The European Impact on the Health of Non-Europeans*. New York: Oxford University Press, 1994.

Lancaster, H.O. *Expectations of Life: A Study in the Demography, Statistics, and History of World Mortality*. New York: Springer-Verlag, 1990.

Lewis, M. *Managing Madness: Psychiatry and Society in Australia 1788–1980*. Canberra: AGPS Press, 1988.

———. *A Rum State: Alcohol and State Policy in Australia*. Canberra: AGPS Press, 1992.

———. *Thorns on the Rose: The History of Sexually Transmitted Diseases in Australia in International Perspective.* Canberra: Australian Government Publishing Service, 1998.

Lewis, M., and S. Leeder. "History of Public Health in Australia since 1945." In *Infectious Disease in Humans,* ed. B. Furnass. Canberra: Nature and Society Forum, 1998.

———. *Where to from Here? The Need to Construct a Comprehensive National Health Policy.* Sydney: Australian Health Policy Institute, University of Sydney, 2001.

Palmer, G.R., and S.D. Short. *Health Care and Public Policy: An Australian Analysis.* South Yarra: Macmillan Education Australia, 2000.

Reid, J., and P. Trompf, eds. *The Health of Immigrant Australia: A Social Perspective.* Sydney: Harcourt Brace Jovanovich, 1990.

———. *The Health of Aboriginal Australia.* Sydney: Harcourt Brace Jovanovich, 1991.

Sax, S. *A Strife of Interests: Politics and Policies in Australian Health Services.* Sydney: George Allen and Unwin, 1984.

Starr, P. *The Social Transformation of American Medicine: The Rise of a Sovereign Profession and the Making of a Vast Industry.* New York: Basic Books, 1982.

Stiglitz, J. *Globalization and Its Discontents.* Camberwell, Victoria: Penguin Books, 2002.

Szreter, S. "Rapid Economic Growth and 'the Four Ds' of Disruption, Deprivation, Disease and Death: Public Health Lessons from Nineteenth-Century Britain for Twenty-first-Century China?" *Tropical Medicine and International Health* 4(2) (1999): 146–52.

Tuohy, C.H. "Dynamics of a Changing Health Sphere: The United States, Britain and Canada." *Health Affairs* 18(3) (1999): 114–34.

Vagero, D. "Health Inequalities as Policy Issues: Reflections on Ethics, Policy and Public Health." *Sociology of Health and Illness* 17(1) (1995): 1–19.

Veenstra, G. "Different Worlds: Three Approaches to Health Research." *Canadian Journal of Public Health* 90 (Supplement 1) (1999): S18–21.

Wilkinson, R., and M. Marmot, eds. *Social Determinants of Health: The Solid Facts.* Copenhagen: WHO Regional Office for Europe, 1998.

Wills, C. *Yellow Fever Black Goddess: The Coevolution of People and Plagues.* Reading: Addison-Wesley, 1996.

Index

About the Author

MILTON J. LEWIS is Senior Research Fellow in the Department of Public Health and Community Medicine at the University of Sydney. With degrees from the University of New South Wales and the Australian National University, Lewis has worked in higher education institutions in Australia, the United Kingdom, and New Guinea. He has published widely on the history of medicine and public health. He is a member of several Australian and overseas associations concerned with the history of medicine and health, and he was chairperson of the organizing committee of the First National Conference of the Australian Society of the History of Medicine held in Sydney in 1989.